KV-731-253

ADVANCES IN MODELLING AND CLINICAL APPLICATION OF INTRAVENOUS ANAESTHESIA

ADVANCES IN EXPERIMENTAL MEDICINE AND BIOLOGY

Editorial Board:

NATHAN BACK, *State University of New York at Buffalo*

IRUN R. COHEN, *The Weizmann Institute of Science*

DAVID KRITCHEVSKY, *Wistar Institute*

ABEL LAJTHA, *N. S. Kline Institute for Psychiatric Research*

RODOLFO PAOLETTI, *University of Milan*

A Continuation Order Plan is available for this series. A continuation order will bring delivery of each new volume immediately upon publication. Volumes are billed only upon actual shipment. For further information please contact the publisher.

ADVANCES IN MODELLING AND CLINICAL APPLICATION OF INTRAVENOUS ANAESTHESIA

Edited by

Jaap Vuyk
Leiden University Medical Centre
Leiden, The Netherlands

and

Stefan Schraag
University of Ulm
Ulm, Germany

Kluwer Academic / Plenum Publishers
New York, Boston, Dordrecht, London, Moscow

Proceedings of the European Society for Intravenous Anaesthesia (EuroSIVA) held in Vienna, Austria in 2000, Gothenburg, Sweden in 2001, and Nice, France in 2002.

ISBN 0-306-47705-X

©2003 Kluwer Academic/Plenum Publishers, New York
233 Spring Street, New York, N.Y. 10013

http://www.wkap.com

10 9 8 7 6 5 4 3 2 1

A C.I.P. record for this book is available from the Library of Congress

All rights reserved

No part of this book may be reproduced, stored in a retrieval system, or transmitted in any form or by any means, electronic, mechanical, photocopying, microfilming, recording, or otherwise, without written permission from the Publisher, with the exception of any material supplied specifically for the purpose of being entered and executed on a computer system, for exclusive use by the purchaser of the work

Printed in the United States of America

LIST OF CONTRIBUTORS

Luc Barvais
Erasme University Hospital, Belgium

Valerie Billard
Institut Gustave Roussy, France

Tiziana Bisogno
Institutes di Biomolecular Chemistry and Cybernetics, Italy

Fred Boer
Leiden University Medical Center, The Netherlands

Alain Borgeat
Orthopedic University Clinic, Switzerland

Aurélie Bourgoin
Hopital Nord, France

Jim Bovill
Leiden University Medical Center, The Netherlands

Albert Dahan
Leiden University Medical Center, The Netherlands

George Ekatodramis
Orthopedic University Clinic, Switzerland

Frank Engbers
Leiden University Medical Center, The Netherlands

Pierre Fiset
Hopital Royal Victoria,Canada

Iain Glen
Glen Pharma Limited, UK

Armin Holas
University Hospital Graz, Austria

Thomas Henthorn
University of Colorado Health Sciences Center, USA

Gavin Kenny
Glasgow Royal Infirmary, UK

Jordi Mallol
Facultat de Medicina i Ciències de la Salut, Spain

Vinzenco Di Marzo
Institutes di Biomolecular Chemistry and Cybernetics, Italy

Diederik Nieuwenhuijs
Leiden University Medical Center, The Netherlands

Martijn Mertens
Leiden University Medical Center, The Netherlands

Claude Meistelman
University Hospital Nancy, France

Vincenzo di Marzo
Istituto per la Chimica di Molecole di Interesse Biologico, Italy

Charles Minto
University of Sydney, Australia

Eric Mortier
University Hospital of Gent, Belgium

Erik Olofsen
Leiden University Medical Center, The Netherlands

Luciano De Petrocellis
Institutes di Biomolecular Chemistry and Cybernetics, Italy

Marije Reekers
Leiden University Medical Center, The Netherlands

Johan Ræder
Ullevaal University Hospital, Norway

Raymonda Romberg
Leiden University Medical Center, The Netherlands

Rolf Sandin
Länssjukhuset, Sweden

Elise Sarton
Leiden University Medical Center, The Netherlands

Thomas Schnider
Kantonsspital, Switzerland

Stefan Schraag
University of Ulm, Germany

Frederique Servin
C.H.U. Bichat-Claude Bernard, France

Michel Struys
University Hospital of Gent, Belgium

Francesco Sureda
Facultat de Medicina i Ciències de la Salut, Spain

Nick Sutcliffe
Healthcare International, UK

Xavier Viviand
Hopital Nord, France

Jaap Vuyk
Leiden University Medical Center, The Netherlands

PREFACE

Since its launch in 1998 the European Society for Intravenous Anaesthesia (EuroSIVA) has come a long way in providing educational material and supporting the research and clinical application of intravenous anaesthesia. After the first two annual meetings held in Barcelona and Amsterdam in 1998 and 1999, three other successful meetings took place in Vienna, Gothenburg and Nice in 2000, 2001 and 2002. Next to these main meetings, starting in the year 2000, a smaller winter meeting has been organised every last week of January in Crans Montana, Switzerland. Both the main summer and the winter meetings breathe the same atmosphere of sharing the latest on intravenous anaesthesia research in the presence of a friendly environment and good company. Since the first meetings the educational tools of EuroSIVA have increased in quantity and technical quality allowing digital slide and video presentation along with the use of the computer simulation program TIVAtrainer during the speaker sessions and the workshops. Furthermore, EuroSIVA now exploits a website www.eurosiva.org that allows for continuous exchange of information on intravenous anaesthesia, the TIVAtrainer, the EuroSIVA meetings and online registration for these meetings. The EuroSIVA is currently engaged in friendly contacts with the Asian Oceanic Society for Intravenous Anaesthesia (AOSIVA), the United Kingdom Society for Intravenous Anaesthesia (UKSIVA), the Korean Society for Intravenous Anaesthesia (KSIVA), the European Society of Anaesthesiology (ESA) and the International Society for Applied Pharmacology (ISAP). This book now is the result of the joint efforts of participants of the EuroSIVA meetings in Vienna, Austria in 2000, Gothenburg, Sweden in 2001 and Nice, France in 2002. Consequently, the book provides an in-depth view on the current state of research and clinical application of intravenous anaesthesia. The book, that has been supported by AstraZeneca, is divided into 3 sections with subjects on pharmacokinetic and dynamic modelling of anaesthetic action, monitoring and clinical application of intravenous anaesthesia and lastly, on the determination and meaning of effect sites of anaesthetic action. The book will be of educational value to all those professionals that are involved in the science and clinical application of intravenous anaesthesia.

Jaap Vuyk, September 2002, Leiden, The Netherlands

CONTENTS

PHARMACOKINETIC AND DYNAMIC MODELLING

MONITORING AND CLINICAL APPLICATION OF INTRAVENOUS ANAESTHESIA

EFFECT SITES OF ANALGESIC AND ANAESTHETIC ACTION

SECTION 1

PHARMACOKINETIC AND DYNAMIC MODELLING

BASIC PHARMACOKINETIC PRINCIPLES FOR INTRAVENOUS ANAESTHESIA

Frank Engbers[*]

1. INTRODUCTION

The ultimate aim of pharmacological research is to describe the dose-effect relationship of drugs. This relationship is difficult to describe because it is time dependent. A phase difference exists between the moment of administration of the drug and the observed effect. Furthermore, continuous measurement of the effect of a drug is not always possible. If blood concentrations of the drug can be measured then the dose-effect relationship is divided into a dose-concentration relationship (pharmacokinetics) and a concentration-effect relationship (pharmacodynamics).

The usual assumption is that no time dependency exists in the concentration-effect relationship e.g. that the same concentration will give the same effect (in comparable circumstances). In other words: the time dependent processes are all enclosed in the dose-concentration relationship. If this assumption was factual then a scientifically defined dose-effect relationship could be clinically utilized by designing a dosage scheme with the help of pharmacokinetics that will obtain a required concentration. While this assumption may be true for most drugs e.g. for antibiotics, for intravenous anaesthetics this is not the case. In intravenous anaesthesia additional concepts and parameters are necessary to understand and take advantage of published concentration-effect relationships. In this chapter some basic pharmacokinetic principles, in relation to intravenous anaesthesia will be described.

[*] Frank H.M. Engbers, Department of Anaesthesiology P5-38, Leiden University Medical Center, 2300 RC Leiden, The Netherlands.

Advances in Modelling and Clinical Application of Intravenous Anaesthesia
Edited by Vuyk and Schraag, Kluwer Academic/Plenum Publishers, 2003

3

2. PHARMACOKINETIC MODELS

A pharmacokinetic experiment usually produces measured blood concentrations at discrete time intervals. To estimate the blood concentrations between the measurements a function is necessary to interpolate the data points. This function can be obtained on the basis of a model. To construct such a model several approaches are available. We can try to understand what is happening to the drug in the body by applying our knowledge of physiological processes and construct a physiological model. Because it is impossible to obtain information from a few blood samples on the pharmacokinetic properties of the individual tissues and organs, the physiological model has to be based on an extremely simplified circulatory system.

In contrast with the physiological approach the body may be looked at as a single or multiple compartment system in which the drug is absorbed, distributed and eliminated without making an assumption on the body composition or the drug transport. Although the physiological model in the end may be much better adaptable to the dynamically changing physiological state of the patients that receive intravenous anaesthesia, until now the compartmental models are more widely used because of their simplicity, reproducibility and mathematical robustness. Recently, models have been proposed that are hybrids between pure compartmental models and physiological models.[1]

Refinement of the pharmacokinetic models by adding complexity should always be balanced against the clinical usefulness. The aim of intravenous anaesthesia is to obtain and maintain a predictable effect that can be adjusted, rather than to maintain a constant blood concentration.

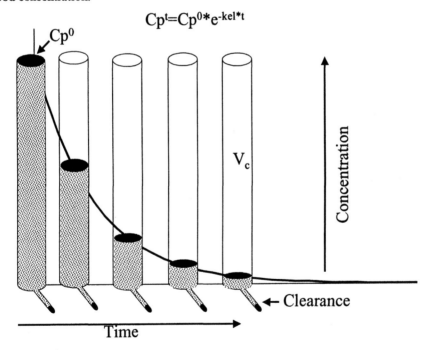

Figure 1. The 1-compartment model.

3. ABSORPTION, DISTRIBUTION AND ELIMINATION

The 3 basic processes that determine the dose-concentration profile are absorption, elimination and distribution. Because during intravenous anaesthesia the drug is injected the absorption process plays obviously no part. As an example we may take a 1-compartment model (Figure 1). This compartment has a volume (V) and drug will be removed from this compartment by excretion or metabolisation. Calculating the volume is straightforward. After a dose D (e.g. 1000 mg) is given, the concentration C (e.g. 0.2 mg/ml) is measured so the volume equals D/C (e.g. 5000 ml). In compartmental modelling the assumption is made that immediate mixing occurs. Influences of drug transport mechanisms and site and speed of sampling are not incorporated. Suppose that the drug in the above example was absorbed by another substance and the measured concentration consequently was 10 times less (0.02 mg/ml) then the calculated volume would have to be 10 times bigger (50000 ml). It is clear from this example that there is not a clear relationship between the volume(s) of a pharmacokinetic compartmental model and the physiological compartments of the body but also that the laboratory methods used for measuring the blood concentrations and the moment and site of sampling may highly influence the central compartment volume of the pharmacokinetic model.[2]

Now the initial volume is determined, the elimination has to be estimated. Just as the kidneys clear a fixed amount of blood in time we can for most drugs assume that a fixed part of volume V in time will be cleared of the drug (clearance; k_{el}). At a high concentration a larger absolute drug mass will be eliminated than with a low concentration (Figure 1) and thus the amount of drug removed will decrease with the decreasing concentration. So, the change in the drug concentration (dC/dt) is a fixed constant (k_{el}) times the blood concentration;

$$\frac{dC_p}{dt} = -k_{el} \bullet C_p .$$

After integration this can be written as

$$C_p^t = C_p^0 \bullet e^{-k_{el} \bullet t},$$

where C_p^t is the concentration at time t and C_p^0 is the concentration when the decay curve is started immediately after the bolus. The clearance is formulated as $V \bullet k_{el}$. The unit of k_{el} is time^{-1}. This rate constant can also be expressed as a half-life: $t\frac{1}{2}_{kel} = \frac{\ln(2)}{k_{el}} = \frac{0.693}{k_{el}}$. This is called the elimination half-life. It is the time required for the process represented by the rate constant to be half completed. Starting with drug concentration C after one half-life the concentration will be ½ C, after another half-life it will be ½ . ½ C = ¼ C and so on. Please remember that this is only true for a 1-compartment model. The change (dC/dt) of the concentration (tangent of the concentration curve) is linearly decreasing. If the decay curve of a 1-compartment model is drawn on a logarithmic scale then it will create a straight line (Figure 2). Because the amount of drug eliminated is only dependent on the concentration, the elimination process is said to be a first order process. The terminology is adapted from chemistry where a reaction that is only dependent on one reaction product is called a first order reaction.

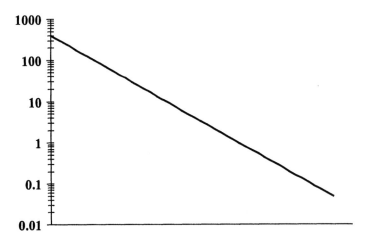

Figure 2. One compartment model on logarithmic scale.

With a zero order process the amount of drug eliminated is independent on the drug concentration and therefore constant in time. It is possible that a first order process like elimination, that is dependant on e.g. enzymatic metabolisation, may become a zero order process when the break down capacity gets saturated. Drugs that are less potent need a higher concentration to exhibit an effect. If the metabolisation system of these drugs (or their metabolites) can be saturated easily, inhibited by other drugs or deteriorates in old age or disease, then they are more likely to exhibit this effect. These are dangerous drugs for continuous IV application for the reason that if the infusion rate exceeds the maximum elimination capacity, the blood concentration will continue to rise due to real accumulation. The effect of the drug can be extremely prolonged in such a case.[2]

If the decay curve of all drugs could be described by a 1-compartment model then the shape of the decay curve would be similar. This is not the case. Drugs are different not only in the clearance and initial volume but also in the way they distribute and redistribute through the body. The first part of the decay curve is often steep because drug is distributed from the central compartment (where the samples are taken from) to other compartments and later on if the concentration gradient between the central compartment and other parts of the body is reversed the drug will redistribute to the central compartment, thus flattening out the decay curve. By adding more exponential functions the shape of this curve can be described more adequately. For most drugs 3 functions are adequate. In formula:

$$C_p^t = A \bullet e^{-\alpha \bullet t} + B \bullet e^{-\beta \bullet t} + C \bullet e^{-\gamma \bullet t}$$

The half-life represented by γ is called the terminal elimination half-life. Because the decay curve is not only dependent on γ it is not valid to say as for the 1-compartment model that after one elimination half-life the concentration will be halved after a bolus or even after a prolonged infusion. The individual exponential terms will produce a straight line when drawn on a logarithmic scale, the sum of the exponents will not.

$$Cp^t = A \cdot e^{-\alpha t} + B \cdot e^{-\beta t} + C \cdot e^{-\gamma t}$$

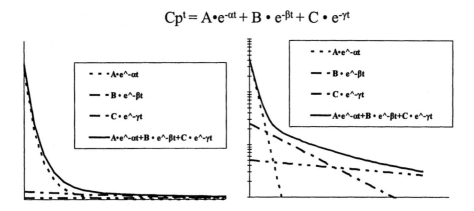

Figure 3. The 3-exponential curve leading to a 3-compartment model

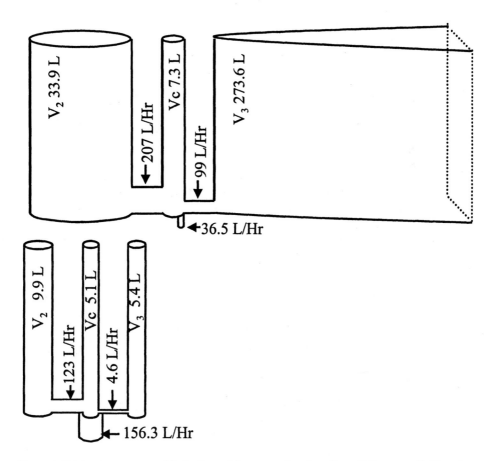

Figure 4. The 3-compartment models for fentanyl (upper panel) and remifentanil (lower panel). The volumes and clearances are drawn in scale.

Another mathematical approach to compartmental pharmacokinetic analysis is through construction of a 3-compartment model by defining the clearances and volumes of the various compartments. Both approaches are related but not mathematically the same. With the help of these compartments distribution and redistribution of the drug through the body can be modelled. It is clear from Figure 3 that the 3 exponential functions into which the drug concentration curve is decomposed each have their impact at different time frames. It is impossible to determine the half-life of the transport between the central compartment and the third compartment with blood samples only taken during the first 2 hours if this half-life is assumed to last 5 hours or more. This is the reason that in one study a 2-compartment model is sufficient while in another study with longer sampling times a 3-compartment model is required. The concentration-time curves of some drugs can be fitted well using a 2-compartment or even a 1-compartment model, even for a prolonged period. The drugs used in intravenous anaesthesia usually require a 3-compartment model. In figure 4 the 3-compartment models for remifentanil and fentanyl are drawn in scale with the compartmental volumes and inter-compartmental clearances.

Although in the 3-compartment model more exponential functions are involved it is still a first order kinetic system. The model is assumed to be linear meaning that doubling the dose will double the concentration and that therefore the concentration curve of one dosage may be superimposed on a curve that is the result of another dosage.

Table 1. The pharmacokinetic parameters of some anaesthetic agents.

	Vc (L)	V_2 (L)	V_3 (L)	Cl (L/h)	Cl_2 (L/h)	Cl_3 (L/h)	$T\frac{1}{2}k_{e0}$ (min)
Propfol[12]	15.9	32.4	202	113.6	106.9	40	2.6
Midazolam[13]	31.5	53	245	25.8	33.6	23.4	5.6
Thiopentone[14]	5.53	33.7	152.1	12.9	159.3	35.5	1.17
Fentanyl[15]	7.35	33.94	275.6	36.5	207.7	99.2	5.8
Alfentanil[16]	7.77	12.0	10.5	21.4	48.5	7.9	1.1
Sufentanil[17]	11.48	25.1	88.3	61.3	241.1	53.0	5.8
Remifentanil[9]	5.122	9.9	5.4	156.3	123	4.6	1.16

4. APPLICATION OF PK TO DEVELOP A DOSING SCHEME

4.1. Infusion

We may use the pharmacokinetic formulas to calculate a blood concentration at any time knowing the drug input and the kinetics. Reversing this process to calculate a required dose to obtain a blood concentration is more complicated and especially for the requirements in anaesthesia hardly sufficient. As an example fentanyl and remifentanil will be discussed in the development of an infusion scheme for these agents that provides a stable, clinical effective concentration.

In a first order system the mass of the eliminated drug is dependent on the concentration. When drug is infused continuously there will be a point in time where the amount of drug eliminated is in balance with the drug input. From that moment on the blood concentration will stop increasing and stay constant. This is called the steady-state and it is easy to see that in the case of a 3-compartment system the drug concentration has to be equal in all compartments. The only drug lost now is that by the clearance from the central compartment. So the infusion rate that will bring a steady state concentration in the end equals the amount of drug cleared from the central compartment:

Rate = (Css • Vc) • k_{el} or R = Css • Clearance. If a drug has a large volume of distribution like fentanyl then it will take quite a while before this steady-state situation will occur. With the patient and drug data from Table 1 the following calculations can be made. Remifentanil Css (concentration desired): 5 ng/ml, Cl = 2606 ml/min, the infusion rate is then 5 • 2606 = 13030 ng/min/1000 = 13.03 µg/min/70 = 0.186 µg/kg/min.

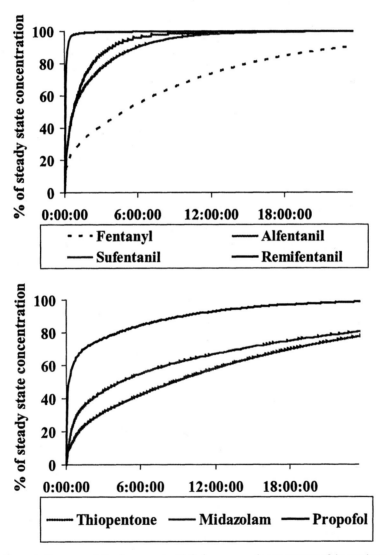

Figure 5. Concentration curves following a constant infusion expressed as percentage of the steady state concentration.

For fentanyl: Cl = 608 ml/min and Css : 2.5 ng/ml. The required infusion rate then is 2.5 ● 608 = 2.5 ● 608 = 1520 ng/min/1000 = 1.520 µg/min/70 = 0.0217 µg/kg/min = 1.302 µg/kg/h. With Fentanyl it will take about 20 h to reach 90% of the Css, with remifentanil it will only take 20 min. Although the principle of reaching a fixed concentration by infusion is true for all drugs (that follow first order elimination) the shape of the curve is different for each drug. Figure 5 shows these curves over 24 hour period for some anaesthetic drugs when the concentration is expressed as a percentage of the steady state concentration. Note that drugs like fentanyl, thiopentone and midazolam are still not at their steady state level after 24 hours. To decrease the time that the concentration is below the Css, a loading dose may be given.

4.2. The loading dose

The most obvious loading dose is the bolus that will bring the central volume to the required concentration immediately (Bvc).[3] The amount of drug required to achieve Css in the central compartment is: Bvc = Css · V. For remifentanil: Vc=5122 ml, Css=5 ng/ml and Bvc = 5 · 5122 = 25610 ng = 25.6 µg/70 kg = 0.366 µg/kg. For fentanyl: Vc=7350 ml, Css=2.5 ng/ml and Bvc=2.5 · 7350 = 18375 ng = 18.4 µg = 0.262 µg/kg. Because of the linearity of the pharmacokinetics the results of the bolus and the infusion calculation may be added or superimposed. It is clear that in the case of fentanyl this bolus dose does not add too much in the attempt to create a clinical effective concentration. In the case of remifentanil there still is a 'dip' in the blood concentration but clinically we will note an improvement of the effectiveness. Theoretically, the complete distribution volume, that is the sum of the volumes of all the compartments, has to be loaded (Bss).[4] The problem is that the drug cannot be injected immediately into these compartments but the entire amount of drug has to pass through the central compartment. For remifentanil:Vss = 5121 + 9852 + 5420 = 20 393 ml, Css = 5 ng/ml and Bss = 5 · 20393 = 101 965 ng = 102 µg /70 kg = 1.46 µg/kg. Peak blood concentration: Bss/Vc = 101 965/5121= 20 ng/ml.
For fentanyl:Vss = 7350 + 33940 + 275625 = 316915 ml, Css = 2.5 ng/ml and Bss = 2.5 · 316915 = 792287.5 ng = 792 µg/70 kg = 11.31 µg/kg. Peak blood concentration: Bss/Vc = 792287.5/7350 = 107 ng/ml.

This massive dose will bring the concentration close to the desired concentration but will certainly cause serious side effects. Notice that in the case of fentanyl there is still a period where the blood concentration is lower then the 'target' concentration because from the high concentration in the central compartment drug will be eliminated immediately. From a pharmacokinetic point of view remifentanil has a unique position because of its high clearance. For all other anaesthetic drugs it must be concluded that the approach as suggested for non-anaesthetic drugs to create a stable blood concentration with a single bolus and infusion rate, will not be appropriate. This has everything to do with the (side) effects of the anaesthetic drugs that do not allow us to administer massive bolus doses. To optimise the loading or induction dose another important concept of anaesthetic pharmacokinetics has to be introduced.

The effect of the anaesthetic drug usually is not propagated in the blood but somewhere at the site where the receptors for the drug exist. The model assumes immediate mixing but in practice there is a small delay between the blood concentration and the observed effect, probably due to the fact that the rise in concentration at the receptor site is not as fast as in the central compartment. The consequence of this is that the relationship between the concentration and the effect is not time-independent anymore, or in other words the concentration cannot be directly related to the effect irrespective of time. To overcome this problem a hypothetical compartment is connected to the central compartment (Figure 6). This is not a real pharmacokinetic compartment and by definition it has no volume. It is called the effect compartment. The only parameter that describes the effect compartment is the k_{e0}. This parameter again can be expressed as a half-life: the $t\frac{1}{2}_{ke0}$. ($t\frac{1}{2}_{ke0}$ = ln(2)/k_{e0}). Not only different drugs have different k_{e0}s but also different pharamacokinetic models for the same drug will have different k_{e0}s because the concept of the effect compartment is to a degree a 'patch' on the static compartmental model and is therefore part of a set of pharmacokinetic parameters.

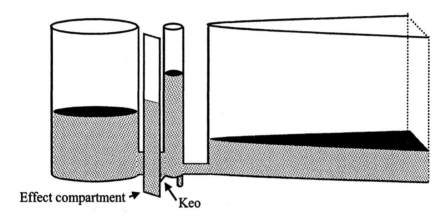

Effect compartment ↗   ↖ Keo

Figure 6. The effect compartment connected to the 3-compartment model.

The importance of the effect compartment is most apparent after an increase in the blood concentration. The effect compartment has less importance with a decrease in the blood concentration because a decrease is less immediate and the effect concentration will stay closer to the blood concentration. Nevertheless, even with decreasing blood concentration clinical effect has a better relationship with the effect site concentration.[5] The concept of the effect compartment explains why drug requirements are reduced when the infusion rate at induction is reduced, or why side effects in some dosing schemes are more evident than in others. With a fast infusion rate, even after switching off the infusion, the concentration in the effect compartment will rise as long as there is a concentration gradient between blood concentration and effect site concentration. Consequently, side effects will be more pronounced. With the lower infusion rate the effect will wear off much quicker and clinically these differences in infusion rates may lead to different conclusions about the pharmacodynamic properties of the drug. The lower boundary of the infusion rate is determined by the infusion rate that will give the desired concentration at steady state (see above). The upper boundary of course is the bolus where the infusion rate is supposed to reach infinity. As pointed out above, trying to load the steady state volume via the central compartment will lead to considerable side effects. Therefore, the effect compartment concept must be the starting point for defining the optimal loading dose. When the plasma concentration is stable as with Target Controlled Infusion, the effect compartment concentration (C_{eff}) will approach the central compartment concentration (C_1) dependent on the $t\frac{1}{2}_{ke0}$ only. After one half-life the effect site concentration will be 50% of that in C_1, after 2 half-lives 75% and after 3 half-lives 87.5% and so on. So with TCI, the delay in effect only is dependant on the value of the $t\frac{1}{2}_{ke0}$ and independent of other pharmacokinetic parameters.

When a bolus is given the effect compartment concentration also will rise dependent on the concentration gradient between V_1 and C_{eff}. The point where C_1 equals C_{eff} is called the peak effect, the time after the bolus is called the time to peak effect. The more flat the first part of the C_1 decay curve is, the less the difference will be between the initial peak plasma concentration and C_{eff}. With most drugs, again with remifentanil as an exception, the first part of the decay curve is dependent mainly on the distribution. So the time to peak effect after a bolus is dependent on the $t\frac{1}{2}_{ke0}$ and the distribution process. The ratio (Fce) of the peak plasma concentration to the peak effect concentration is fixed but only for the first bolus administration when the initialdrug concentration in all the compartments is zero.

Table 2. The times and ratios to peak effect of various anaesthetics.

	Ratio of peak plasma concentration/peak effect concentration	Time to peak effect(mm:ss))
Propofol	2.7	4:00
Midazolam	1.75	13:10
Thiopentone	2.73	1:40
Fentanyl	8.5	3:40
Alfentanil	1.58	3:00
Sufentanil	5.67	6:00
Remifentanil	3.34	1:30

Table 1 shows these ratios for the different anaesthetic drugs. With this ratio the initial bolus (Beff) that creates a specific target effect concentration (Ce_T) can be calculated through; $Beff = Fce \cdot Ce_T \cdot V$. For remifentanil: $3.34 \cdot 5 \cdot 5122 = 85537.4$ ng = 85.5 µg /70 kg = 1.22 µg/kg. For fentanyl: $8.5 \cdot 2.5 \cdot 7350 = 156187.5$ ng = 156 µg/70 kg = 2.23 µg/kg. The results are shown in Figure 7. With the use of pharmacokinetic data it is possible to define the initial dose and the final infusion rate, but between begin and end it is impossible to calculate exactly the necessary infusion rates to maintain a constant concentration without the help of a computer. While for one drug a single bolus and infusion rate may be sufficient to maintain the blood concentration constant, other drugs may need frequent adjustments to compensate for the diminishing effect of distribution. We may assume that the approach suggested above, loading the steady state volume (Bss) at once, has the best change of reducing the necessity of infusion adjustments during maintenance. It is obvious that the closer the optimal loading dose in relation to the effect (Beff) is to this Bss, the more likely a single infusion rate after the loading dose will result in a stable blood concentration.

When applying a loading dose followed by a maintenance infusion rate, ideally the infusion should start at the moment the effect concentration equals the blood concentration; the time to peak effect. In a clinical situation this is not very practical. If, for some reason, the start of the infusion pump is delayed then the rapidly declining blood concentration may render unacceptable low effect site concentrations. Starting the infusion simultaneously with the bolus dose will either lead to an overshoot in the effect concentration or, when the loading bolus is adjusted to compensate for the infusion, give a minimal delay in the time to peak effect. In Table 2 infusion schemes are presented that will result in an effect site concentration within 6% of the desired target effect concentration. To obtain the appropriate infusion rate for a specific desired effect site concentration the values need to be multiplied by the desired concentration. The loading bolus in this table is corrected for the immediate start of the first infusion and is therefore lower than the loading dose for the effect concentration described previously.

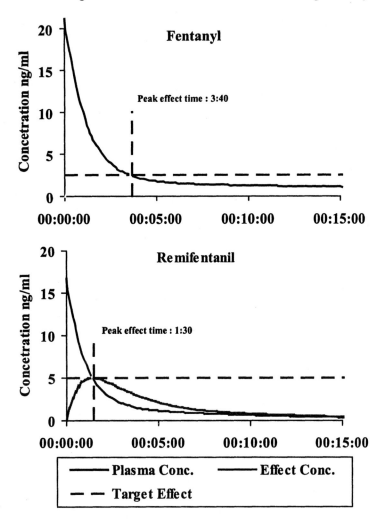

Figure 7. Plasma and effect site concentration of fentanyl and remifentanil as the result of a bolus calculated to obtain a specific effect site concentration.

Table 2. Bolus and infusion rates and times of initiation of the infusion rate, optimised to obtain an effect concentration within 6 % of the target concentration with as few infusion rate changes as possible. Values should be multiplied by the required target concentration/target ration in the table.

	Target	Bolus	Rate 1	Rate 2	Rate 3	Rate 4	Rate 5
Propofol[12]	1 µg/ml	0.44	2.75 0	2.2 0:21:00	1.86 01:35:00	1.64 07:45:00	
Midazolam[13]	100 ng/ml	57	93 0	71 01:30:00	57 04:00:00	43 09:30:00	
Thiopentone[14]	10 µg/ml	1.5	23 0	17 00:04:00	11 00:12:00	6.7 00:30:00	4.5 01:15:00
Fentanyl[15]	1 ng/ml	0.79	1.74 0	1.3 00:45:00	0.92 2:15:00	0.62 04:40:00	0.52 12:15:00
Alfentanil[16]	10 µg/ml	1.36	7.79 0	5.21 00:13:00	3.36 00:40:00	3.07 04:00:00	
Sufentanil[17]	0.1 µg/ml	0.08	0.125 0	0.096 01:45:00	0.088 7:00:00		
Remifentanil[9]	1 µg/ml	0.177	2.7 0	2.2 00:08:30			

Infusion rate is in µg/kg/h for midazolam, fentanyl, alfentanil, sufentanil and remifentanil and in mg/kg/h for propofol and thiopentone.

5. TARGET CONTROLLED INFUSION

It is unlikely that all the patients in theatre need the same blood concentration during the whole surgical procedure. Surgical stimulation will vary and different intra-operative events require different drug concentrations.[6,7] The approach outlined above will only allow a stable blood concentration that is predefined, but will not allow using the pharmacokinetic properties of the drug to change the blood concentration when necessary. By connecting a computer that is programmed to calculate the state of the pharmacokinetic model in real time, it is possible to maintain the target concentration very accurately and change the target concentration as required. Several experimental target controlled infusion systems are available but few commercial systems. However, more systems will become clinically available in the near future.

As stated above, in the clinical situation the goal during intravenous anaesthesia is to assure a specific anaesthetic effect not a specific blood concentration. Changing the blood concentration without accepting an overshoot in the central compartment will delay the time to maximum effect. Because the blood concentration is kept constant, the simple half-life rule can be applied to the effect site concentration: after one $t\frac{1}{2}_{keo}$ the effect site concentration is 50% of the blood concentration, after another $t\frac{1}{2}_{keo}$ this is 75% and so on. Please note the difference with the time to peak effect. Unless an initially higher target concentration is selected the induction by TCI will be slower than by bolus induction. The advantage of Target Controlled Infusion, however, is that information on the effect site concentration is available. A correlation between the effect site concentration and the clinical effect both during induction, maintenance and termination of anaesthesia has been shown in many studies.

It is of course possible to let the computer calculate an infusion scheme that will allow a fast increase in the effect site concentration.[8] By applying this so called effect site controlling TCI, the time to maximal effect is the same as the time to peak effect after a bolus administration. Every increase in the target effect site concentration will result in an overshoot in the blood concentration followed by a period of no infusion to allow blood and brain to equilibrate. Thereafter, 'normal' blood compartment TCI, to keep the blood concentration stable, is applied. When the target is lowered the infusion is stopped until the effect concentration equals the target. At this time, the blood concentration will be below the target concentration. The blood concentration will be increased until the target is reached and from then on 'normal' blood concentration target controlled infusion is continued. Experimental systems are available that feature this type of control. However, because the consequences of controlling a 'virtual' effect site concentration is not yet well investigated, it will probably take a while before these systems will become commercially available.

From a pharmacokinetic point of view the usefulness of Target Controlled Infusion has been challenged for the application and administration of ultra fast drugs such as remifentanil. Indeed, with a well-designed bolus and infusion scheme a stable blood concentration may easily be established. However, discontinuation of the infusion, for example when the syringe is changed, will give a fast decrease in the blood concentration. It will take quite a while before a restart of the infusion will re-establish the same blood concentration as before the interruption of the infusion. Target controlled infusion also makes the online use of covariates of pharmacokinetic data sets possible. For remifentanil a 3-compartment model is available with parameters adjusting the infusion rate to age and lean body mass. Blood concentration differences between subjects using this data set may be as much as 100% with the dosage based on mg/kg being equal.[9] In addition, the $t\frac{1}{2}_{ke0}$ associated with this data set is age dependent in such a way that an elderly patient has almost a twice as long a $t\frac{1}{2}_{ke0}$ than a younger patient.

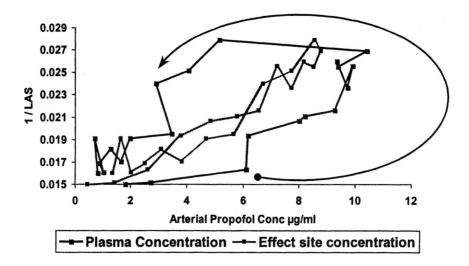

Figure 8. Experimental data from one subject showing the relationship between the effect (Level of anaesthesia score measured with auditory evoked potentials = LAS) and the measured plasma and theoretical effect concentration. The arrow indicates the direction of the hysteresis.

6. DETERMINATION OF THE T½K$_{E0}$

The k$_{e0}$ can be considered as a link parameter between the pharmacokinetics and pharmacodynamics. What is often not realized is that this parameter influences possible dosing strategies in theatre as outlined above. The k$_{e0}$ is most often associated with a specific pharmacokinetic data set and it partly compensates for the shortcomings of the static 3-compartment model. Determination of this parameter is completely different form the other pharmacokinetic parameters.[10] The volume of the effect compartment is virtually zero. If the k$_{e0}$ is measured in an individual a continuous measurement of the effect is desirable. By plotting the blood concentration against effect a phase difference between blood and effect becomes visible. This is called a hysteresis loop (Figure 8). The k$_{e0}$ is now modelled such that the hysteresis loop collapses. The collapsed loop describes the theoretical concentration in the effect compartment. One of the issues in the derivation of the k$_{e0}$ is the modelling of the blood concentrations. The time frame in which the hysteresis loop is studied is usually different from the timeframe of which the pharamacokinetic data are derived. The measured blood concentrations may not be fitted well by the pharmacokinetic model for reasons outlined above. A non-parametric approach could be selected whereby no assumption is made on the pharmacokinetic model and the sample points be connected by a straight line. Although the derived parameter probably may more accurately describe the phase difference between the blood concentration and the effect, it isolates the k$_{e0}$ from the pharmacokinetic model and makes it therefore less usable.

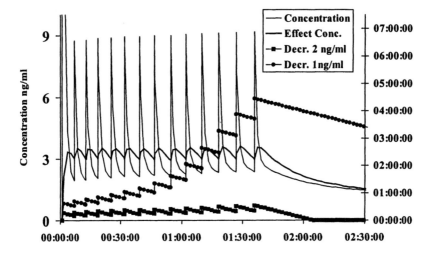

Figure 9. A pharmacokinetic analysis of a clinical application of intravenous anaesthesia. Fentanyl is given in repeated boluses. The theoretical patient responds exactly when the effect site concentration is below 3 ng/ml. The decrement times are shown corresponding to a decrement of the effect site concentration to 2 and 1 ng/ml.

7. THE CONTEXT-SENSITIVE DECREMENT TIME

The complexity of the pharmacokinetic models makes the classical parameters like the elimination half-life useless in the evaluation of the duration of effect of a drug. The context-sensitive decrement time has been introduced[11] to describe the decay of the drug concentration in a more clinical valuable way. Figure 9 illustrates a few of the practical dilemmas and possibilities. Fentanyl is given in this example in such a way that the effect site concentration always stays above 3 ng/ml. There is an increase in the time interval between the required boluses when the size of the bolus dose remains the same. The blood concentration fluctuates significantly whereas the fluctuations in the effect site concentration are less pronounced. The disadvantage of the multiple bolus dosing technique therefore lays not so much in the occurrence of side effects but in the fact that from time to time the patient may respond to a surgical stimulation. The idea of the bolus dosing technique is that the distance in time between the concentration for adequate analgesia and the concentration at awakening is reduced. This is only partially true. With a computer program the time required to decrease the concentration to a specific lower concentration can be calculated (Tivatrainer Simulation Software, Gutta BV, Aerdenhout the Netherlands, www.eurosiva.org). If the new concentration is e.g. 2 ng/ml the decrement time hardly increases even after prolonged anaesthesia. If this patient however, e.g. requires 1 ng/ml for adequate ventilation then this may take several hours after anaesthesia.

8. INTRA-INDIVIDUAL VARIABILITY IN PHARMACOKINETICS

Usually pharmacokinetics are derived from a group of volunteers or relative healthy patients in a controlled and standardized environment. Often in theatre, extremes in haemodynamic states are seen. It has been demonstrated that the cardiac output influences the distribution pharmacokinetics of some drugs used in anaesthesia. For other drugs not only a pharmacodynamic interactions has been demonstrated but also pharmacokinetic interactions, most likely based on the fact that the intravenous drugs used in anaesthesia directly or indirectly alter the haemodynamic state of our patients. Even when a stable concentration is created, the free and bound fraction of the drug may be altered by the addition of another substance. Metabolic pathways through cytochrome P450 may be altered by other drugs. From a pharmacokinetic point of view, potent drugs with a relative high clearance and a small distribution volume should be the most successful in these patients. This, because these agents allow rapid adjustments to the individual needs of these patients. Indeed the clinical experience is that with drugs as for example propofol and remifentanil, even after many hours of anaesthesia in sometimes haemodynamic unstable conditions, the anaesthetic state stays predictable and controllable.

9. CONCLUSION

This chapter offers insight in the determination of the pharmacokientics of anaesthetic agents. Furthermore, it provides some background on the clinical application of novel pharmacokinetic parameters. It furthermore provides insight in the power of computer simulation as an educative tool.

10. REFERENCES

1. J.A. Kuipers, F.Boer, E.Olofsen, J.G.Bovill and A.G.Burm, Recirculatory Pharmacokinetics and Pharmacodynamics of Rocuronium in Patients: The Influence of Cardiac Output. *Anesthesiology*; **94**: 47-55 (2001).
2. W.L.Chiou, The phenomenon and rationale of marked dependence of drug concentration on blood sampling site: implications in pharmacokinetics, pharmacodynamics, toxicology and therapeutics (Part I) *Clin Pharmacokinet*; **17**:175-99 (1989).
3. D.R.Stanski, F.G.Mihm, M.H.Rosenthal and S.M.Kalman, Pharmacokinetics of high-dose thiopental used in cerebral resuscitation *Anesthesiology* **53**: 169–71 (1980
4. R.N.Boyes, D.B.Scott, P.J.Jebson, M.J.Godman and D.G.Julian, Pharmacokinetics of lidocaine in man. *Clin Pharmacol Ther*; **12**:105-15; (1971)
5. P.O.Mitenko and R.I.Olgilvie. Rapidly achieved plasma concentrations plateaus with observations on theophylinne kinetics. *Clin Pharmacol Ther*;**13**:329-35 (1971).
6. T.Kazama, K.Ikeda, K.Morita and Y.Sanjo, Awakening Propofol Concentration with and without Blood-effect Site Equilibration after Short-term and Long-term Administration of Propofol and Fentanyl Anesthesia, *Anesthesiology* **88**:928-34 (1998).
7. J.Vuyk, T.Lim, F.H.M. Engbers, A.G.Burm, A.A.Vletter and J.G.Bovill, The pharmacodynamic interaction of propofol and alfentanil during lower abdominal surgery in women, *Anesthesiology* **83**(1): 8-22 (1995)
8. S.L.Shafer and K.M.Gregg KM. Algorithms to rapidly achieve and maintain stable drug concentrations at the site of effect with a computer controlled infusion pump, *J Pharmacokineti Biopharm* **20**:147-167 (1992).
9. C.F. Minto, Th.W.Schnider, T.D.Egan, E.Youngs, H.J.Lemmens,P.L.Gambus, V.Billard, J.F.Hoke, K.H.Moore, D.J.Hermann, K.T.Muir, J.W.Mandema and S.L.Shafer. Influence of age and gender on the pharmacokinetics and pharmacodynamics of remifentanil: I. Model development, *Anesthesiology* **86**: 10-23 (1997).
10. M. White, M.J.Schenkels and F.H.M.Engbers, Effect-site modelling of propofol using auditory evoked potentials, *Br J Anaesth* **82**(3): 333-910 (1999).
11. M.A.Hughes, P.S.A.Glass and J.R.Jacobs, Context-sensitive half-time in multicompartment pharmacokinetic models for intravenous anesthetic drugs. *Anesthesiology*;76:334-341 (1992).
12. J.F.Coetzee, J.B.Glen, C.A.Wium and L.Boshoff, Pharmacokinetic Model Selection for Target Controlled Infusions of Propofol. *Anesthesiology* **82**: 1328-1345 (1995).
13. K. Zomorodi, A. Donner, J. Somma, J. Barr, R. Sladen, J. Ramsay, E. Geller, S.L. Shafer, Population pharmacokinetics of midazolam administered by target controlled infusion for sedation following coronary artery bypass grafting. *Anesthesiology* **89** (6): 1418-29 (1998).
14. D.R. Stanski and P.O.Maitre, Population pharmacokinetics and pharmacodynamics of thiopental:the effect of age revisited. *Anesthesiology* **72**:412-422 (1990).
15. P.O.Maitre, S.Vozeh,J.Heykants, D.A. Thomson and D.R.Stanski, Population pharmacokinetics of alfentanil: the average dose-plasma concentration relationship and interindividual variability in patients, *Anesthesiology* **66**:3-12 (1987).
16. S.L. Shafer, J.R. Varvel, Pharmacokinetics, pharmacodynamics, and rational opioid selection. *Anesthesiology* **74** (1): 53-63 (1991).
17. J.G. Bovill, P.S. Sebel, C.L. Blackburn, C.L. Oei-Lim, J.J. Heykants, The pharmacokinetics of sufentanil in surgical patients, *Anesthesiology* **61** (5): 502-6 (1984).

BASIC CONCEPTS OF RECIRCULATORY
PHARMACOKINETIC MODELLING

Marije Reekers, Fred Boer and Jaap Vuyk[*]

1. INTRODUCTION

The science or art of pharmacokinetic analysis embodies the description of the time-dependant concentration changes of a drug. Pharmacokinetic models may be used to predict the behaviour of the drug in individuals, preferably under various circumstances. In the practice of anaesthesia pharmacokinetics can be studied on the work floor. Differences in pharmacokinetics between individuals are observed on a daily basis. Factors responsible for the interindividual variability are being studied extensively and more data become available in time. From these data the significance of demographic factors such as age and gender become increasingly apparent. Other factors like weight or lean body mass may be substitute parameters for physiologically based variations in pathways of distribution and elimination. Obesity e.g. may be considered as a disproportionate increase in adipose tissue mass. Peripheral blood flow must increase to supply this extra tissue. As organ-specific blood flow remains equal, cardiac output will increase. The surplus of fatty tissue will act as an extra depot for lipid-soluble drugs like thiopental. As a consequence, peak-concentrations are expected to decrease, whereas the terminal half-life and steady state volume of distribution will increase.[1] Physiological parameters such as cardiac output, flow and tissue distribution have a more direct relationship with pharmacokinetic parameters like distribution volumes and clearances. Inclusion of a parameter like cardiac output into a pharmacokinetic model may improve the accuracy of the model, especially with respect to fast acting drugs like intravenous anaesthetics. The influence of changes in cardiac output on the pharmacokinetics of anaesthetic agents is under research. The largest impact of a change in the cardiac output on the behaviour of drugs can be expected in compounds showing a flow-limited

---

[*] Marije Reekers, Fred Boer and Jaap Vuyk, Department of Anaesthesiology P5-38, Leiden University Medical Center, 2300 RC Leiden, The Netherlands

distribution and/or clearance such as thiopental,[1] lidocaine,[2] alfentanil[3] and propofol.[4] Pulmonary uptake can also be of influence on the early-phase distribution of a substance. These influences will be described in more detail further on in this chapter.

Another factor of influence on drug behaviour is the mode of administration. A rapid intravenous bolus injection will be characterized by a set of pharmacokinetic parameters different from parameters derived after a prolonged intravenous infusion as is used in devices for computer controlled infusion.[5, 6] Prolonged infusion of a drug with a rapid clearance and extensive distribution, such as propofol, may be better characterised by a 3-compartment model, whereas for a bolus injection a 2-compartment model may suffice. In a study published by Schnider and colleagues is shown that propofol concentrations after a bolus injection were not adequately described by the pharmacokinetic model derived from blood samples taken during a propofol infusion in the same patients.[7] Mainly the first 10 minutes after bolus injection were significantly biased with an overestimation at minute 2 and 4 and a subsequent underestimation of the actual propofol concentration. Tailoring of the pharmacokinetic model to the drug, the type of administration and phase of interest (early-phase or steady-state) is very important.

2. SELECTING A PHARMACOKINETIC MODEL

A large variety of pharmacokinetic models exists ranging from very abstract to naturalistic.[8] The commonly used models are linear and time-invariant (Figure 1). Empirical models describe the relationship between input, the drug dose, and output, the plasma concentration, in a mathematical form without reference to a physiological or pharmacological explanation. Empirical models treat the human body as a black box. The key to this method is the fitting procedure. Compartmental models are most frequently applied, consisting of 2 or 3 compartments. These compartments may have a physiological (plasma, tissue) basis but are derived purely mathematically.

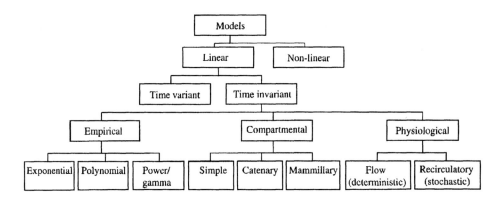

Figure 1. A taxonomy of pharmacokinetic models. Reproduced from J. Kuipers, Pharmacokinetic modelling of anaesthetics: The role of cardiac output. Ph.D. Thesis, with permission.

Compartmental models are based on the assumption of instantaneous mixing of the drug after a bolus injection within the central compartment. Distribution and elimination occur solely from the central compartment. Other compartments serve as "peripheral" compartments, with "slow" equilibration constants, from which the drug is redistributed. By assuming complete initial mixing within the central compartment, which is actually not justified, the compartmental model becomes limited when pulmonary uptake or the process of initial mixing in the first minutes after injection are studied.

3. THE DEVELOPMENT OF RECIRCULATORY MODELS

In the process of the pharmacokinetic evaluation of concentration-time data, analysis is frequently performed by fitting data to a 2- or 3- compartmental model. However, for some anaesthetic agents this may not be the best model suited. More and more drugs are introduced that exhibit a very rapid initial distribution resulting in the propagation of a clinical effect before complete mixing has occurred. Ignoring the mechanism of initial mixing may lead to large deviations in the estimation of the volume of the central compartment.[9] Other drugs such as fentanyl and meperidine,[10] sufentanil,[11] propofol,[12, 13] ketamine[14] and lidocaine[15,16] are known to undergo substantial pulmonary uptake. Furthermore, in fast acting compounds the distribution appears to be flow dependant.[17] Including a flow parameter such as cardiac output into the model is therefore strongly desired.[1] Taking these factors into consideration suggests that examination of early phase pharmacokinetics based exclusively on a conventional compartmental model, is insufficient[18] and provides inaccurate data.

One solution to the issues mentioned is the system dynamics approach as described by van Rossum.[19] This approach shows new possibilities by calculation of so-called body transfer functions. The transport function of the body (closed loop) is considered a stochastic process characterized by a density function of total body residence times. The relationship between the body transit time distribution and the body residence distribution is determined by the feedback-loop arrangement, the cardiac output and the extraction ratio. The cardiac output is included as a very important haemodynamic variable in this model.[20]

Other models allowing recirculation have been introduced, constructed as catenary compartmental models with different compartments linked in a serial manner. In a study by Avram and colleagues, this model of concurrent disposition of ICG and thiopental allowed to analyse intravascular mixing by computing the recirculation of the intravascular marker ICG, combined with a peripheral compartment for thiopental.[21] Further development led to recirculatory models using ICG as a marker for the intravascular compartment.[22] Finally, a combination of recirculatory compartments and peripheral slow and fast tissue compartments was developed that made the recirculatory model more physiologically based.[23]

For any study drug the complete recirculoratory model can be built on the basis of a model for ICG. Since the distribution of ICG is limited to the intravascular space, the ICG model describes the passage through the central and peripheral blood compartments. The central compartments are by definition located between the venous point of injection and the arterial point of sampling. The central intravascular part of the model, representing the flow through heart and lungs, is best described by two compartments. Hereby, modelling of pulmonary uptake and redistribution is allowed. Since the mean transit time of one compartment is shorter than that of the other compartment, they are identified as the fast central and the slow central compartment. Peripheral compartments are described similarly. The compartments for ICG are considered to represent the effect of dispersion of ICG in the vascular tree. In the model this dispersion is simulated by so-called tanks-in-series, being very small consecutive compartments from which the drug is cleared exponentially . Parallel pathways can differ in the number of tanks in series and the proportion of the blood flow to the respective compartments.

For the test drug peripheral tissue compartments are added to the ICG model. These tissue compartments are similar to the compartments of other catenary models. The tissue compartments are coupled to the peripheral vascular compartments such that the slow vascular compartment is coupled to the slow tissue compartment. If the drug undergoes significant pulmonary uptake a pulmonary tissue compartment may be added[21] (see Figure 2).

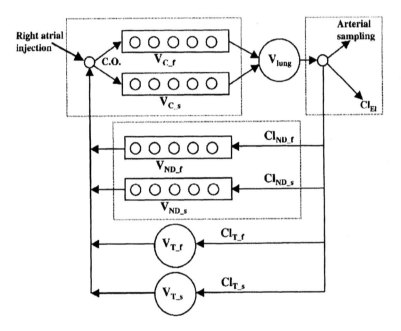

Figure 2. Recirculatory pharmacokinetic model used for analysis of indocyanine green and simultaneously injected drug (modified from Krejcie et al.[23]). The parts in the dashed boxes represent the recirculatory model for indocyanine green, the intravascular part of the model. These intravascular compartments are represented by a rectangle with five compartments, but the actual number of compartments may vary and has no physiological background, The concept of these compartments in series is only used to be able to describe the data properly. The intravascular model consists of a central part, receiving all of the cardiac output, divided in a slow (V_{c_s}) and a fast (V_{c_f}) central compartment and a peripheral part, divided in a slow (V_{ND_s}) and a fast (V_{ND_f}) peripheral compartment. The simultaneously injected drug distributes into organs and therefore, three tissue compartments are added to the intravascular indocyanine green model; the lung compartment (V_{lung}) and a slow (V_{T_s}) and a fast (V_{T_f}) peripheral tissue compartment. The sum of the peripheral clearances equals the cardiac output. Reproduced from J. Kuipers, Pharmacokinetic modelling of anaesthetics: The role of cardiac output. Ph.D. Thesis, with permission.

4. RECIRCULATORY MODELLING IN PRACTICE

Recirculatory models for different compounds such as thiopental,[21] halothane,[24] alfentanil,[3, 25] propofol,[13] and rocuronium[26] have been described. As a marker for the intravascular compartment ICG was used. To adequately measure the recirculation of ICG the sampling frequency must be high; the process of initial mixing is complete within five minutes. The quality of model fitting is therefore highly dependant on the amount of blood samples taken within the first minutes after the bolus dose administration. From these data the first-pass concentration curve of ICG can be determined, described by two parallel pathways consisting of Erlang functions, represented by a number of tanks in series. A representation of such a model is depicted in Figure 2. The parameters derived from this model can now be further combined with peripheral compartments to represent distribution and elimination as described above. Constructing such a model is possible using the SAAM II program. It consists of a numerical mode and a compartmental mode. The latter allows for the construction of a model on a canvas where the program attaches the formulas. The solver function of the program computes the parameters in an iterative way with fixed or relative weights (SAAM II manual). The statistics performed on the parameters are calculation of standard deviation, fractional standard deviation and representation of a correlation matrix, covariance matrix or the residual sum of squares. Other statistical tests described are the one sample runs test to check for random scatter around the fit. The group of Krejcie uses the IDENT2 program to check for identifiability and estimability of the parameter.[27]

5. RESULTS

As an example of differences in pharmacokinetic outcome using conventional 2-compartment modelling compared to recirculatory modelling, a short representation will be given of the results from a study performed by Kuipers and colleagues regarding the pharmacokinetics of rocuronium in patients.[26] In this study a recirculatory model has been used based on arterial ICG concentrations collected with a rapid sampling device. In addition, cardiac output was determined by dividing the dose of ICG by the area under the first-pass ICG concentration-time curve. Rocuronium had been selected as a model drug because of its fast onset of action. The effect of rocuronium could be quantified easily and reliably and be expected to be linked to cardiac output based on its dependency on the blood flow through the muscles. In addition, the effect measurements were included in a PK-PD model to determine the k_{e0} of rocuronium using compartmental modelling parameters and recirculatory modelling parameters. The recirculatory model, used to analyse indocyanine green and rocuronium pharmacokinetics and the rocuronium pharmacodynamics, was built like the model in Figure 2, with the exclusion of the lung compartment and with the addition of an effect compartment placed after the arterial sampling site. The effect compartment was not included in the recirculatory system. The sum of the clearances through the parallel fast and slow non-distributive circuits for ICG equals the cardiac output. Rocuronium data were evaluated by addition of a fast and slow peripheral distributive compartment to the ICG model. The ratio between fast and slow peripheral clearances were set equal in ratio for ICG and rocuronium, but the absolute values were allowed to differ. The pharmacokinetic data could well be fitted using recirculatory pharmacokinetics, whereas the two-compartment model showed large uncertainty regarding the drug behaviour in the first minutes. A pharmacokinetic-pharmacodynamic analysis could be done using recirculatory pharmacokinetics as well. Some of the parameters determined by the recirculatory model and the two-compartment model can be seen in Table 1.

Table 1. Pharmacokinetic and pharmacokinetic-dynamic parameters of rocuronium determined by a recirculatory model and a 2-compartment model (mean and SD). For abbreviations see legend of figure 2. The unit of k_{e0} is (min^{-1}), of EC_{50} is $(\mu g/l)$.

		V_C	V_{ss}	V_T	Cl_{EL}	V_1	V_2	Cl_{12}	k_{e0}	EC_{50}
Recirculatory	mean	1.52	17.29	14.77	0.45				0.129	876
	SD	0.40	4.82	4.85	0.11				0.036	118
2-compartment	mean		10.50		0.50	6.76	3.73	0.43	0.239	684
	SD		3.54		0.14	1.69	1.98	0.20	0.104	97

Reproduced from J. Kuipers, Pharmacokinetic modelling of anaesthetics: The role of cardiac output. Ph.D. Thesis, with permission.

The results showed correlation between cardiac output and the central volume of ICG and rocuronium. The clearances correlated significantly with cardiac output as well. The values of k_{e0} and EC_{50} obtained with the compartmental model were significantly different from the values estimated based on the recirculatory model. The k_{e0} determined using the compartmental model was nearly doubled and the EC_{50} approximately 22 % lower compared to those determined on the basis of the recirculatory approach. The k_{e0} of rocuronium showed correlation with cardiac output, although the correlation estimated from the recirculatory model was much stronger. This could well be explained by the difference in accuracy of fitting in the first minutes. It is known that by selecting a model, i.e. a 2- or 3-compartment model, the initial drug concentration may be either seriously underestimated or overestimated. In contrast, the recirculatory model was capable of accurately describing the front-end kinetics.[28] The correlation between cardiac output and effect site-equilibration time could be observed clinically as well. The patient with the lowest cardiac output (2.4 L/min) showed 90% twitch depression after 2.5 minutes, whereas the patient with the highest cardiac output (5.0 L/min) needed only 1.5 minutes for near-complete relaxation. In the context of a rapid sequence induction this means that not only the dose of muscle relaxant, but also the physiological status of the patient needs consideration. This supports the need for more accurate characterization of pharmacokinetic and pharmacodynamic parameters in the early phase when using fast-acting agents.

6. CONCLUSIONS

With the introduction of an increasing number of compounds exhibiting a rapid, flow dependant distribution and a rapid onset of effect before complete initial mixing, it becomes increasingly important to look at alternatives in pharmacokinetic modelling. At present, the most frequently used approach is the conventional 2- or 3-compartment model. This model is based on the assumption of complete mixing in the central compartment upon bolus-injection of the compound. This means that recirculation, flow-dependant distribution or pulmonary uptake are not taken into account. The introduction of recirculatory modelling as described by Krejcie et al.[23] has provided a tool to model these situations. Disadvantages of recirculatory modelling are innate to the small time frame in which the processes take place. First of all, it is necessary to administer a marker for the intravascular space (ICG) in combination with the compound of interest. Secondly, in order to have sufficient data to model the first-pass circulation of ICG, the sampling frequency must be high; every few seconds. Besides the practical implications of this methodology, it implies that the quality of the fit is highly dependant on the number of data points within the first three minutes. Accurate modelling of early-phase pharmacokinetics is very important, since the better the understanding of the behaviour of a drug in a "standard" situation (read "healthy subject"), the easier to predict the outcome when parameters change. Extending the knowledge in this field may lead to a better prediction of drug behaviour in e.g. elderly patients or in patients with an altered cardiovascular state. The development of techniques to measure cardiac output in a non or minimal invasive way, preferably on a beat-to-beat basis, may lead to fine-tuning of the pharmacokinetics of intravenous anaesthetics on a patient-basis. In addition, it has also been shown that recirculatory modelling can be used in pharmacokinetic-pharmacodynamic modelling. This may yield to large differences in the estimation of k_{e0} and EC_{50} compared to conventional approaches, as has been shown in the paragraph above. Drugs with a rapid distribution and a rapid mode-of-onset are widely dependant on the quality of modelling in the early-phase after administration, determining the accuracy in the estimation of PK-PD parameters. In clinical practice this may have direct implications, e.g. in the case of a rapid sequence induction. Taking the drug and patient characteristics into consideration may therefore lead to improvement of the safety of administration of anaesthetics.

7. REFERENCES

1. D. R. Wada, S. Bjorkman, W. F. Ebling, H. Harashima, S. R. Harapat, and D. R. Stanski, Computer simulation of the effects of alterations in blood flows and body composition on thiopental pharmacokinetics in humans, *Anesthesiology* **87**, 884-899 (1997).
2. J. A. Kuipers, F. Boer, A. de Roode, E. Olofsen, J. G. Bovill, and A. G. Burm, Modeling population pharmacokinetics of lidocaine: should cardiac output be included as a patient factor?, *Anesthesiology* **94**, 566-573 (2001).
3. T. K. Henthorn, T. C. Krejcie, and M. J. Avram, The relationship between alfentanil distribution kinetics and cardiac output, *Clin. Pharmacol. Ther.* **52**, 190-196 (1992).
4. G. L. Ludbrook and R. N. Upton, A physiological model of induction of anaesthesia with propofol in sheep. 2. Model analysis and implications for dose requirements, *Br. J. Anaesth.* **79**, 505-513 (1997).
5. E. Gepts, F. Camu, I. D. Cockshott, and E. J. Douglas, Disposition of propofol administered as constant rate intravenous infusions in humans, *Anesth. Analg.* **66**, 1256-1263 (1987).
6. J. Vuyk, F. H. Engbers, A. G. Burm, A. A. Vletter, and J. G. Bovill, Performance of computer-controlled infusion of propofol: an evaluation of five pharmacokinetic parameter sets, *Anesth. Analg.* **81**, 1275-1282 (1995).
7. T. W. Schnider, C. F. Minto, P. L. Gambus, C. Andresen, D. B. Goodale, S. L. Shafer, and E. J. Youngs, The influence of method of administration and covariates on the pharmacokinetics of propofol in adult volunteers, *Anesthesiology* **88**, 1170-1182 (1998).
8. G. T. Tucker, Pharmacokinetic models - different approaches, in: *Quantitation, Modelling and Control in Anaesthesia*, edited by H. Stoeckel (Georg Thieme Verlag, Stuttgart, 1985), pp 54-63.

9. W. L. Chiou, Potential pitfalls in the conventional pharmacokinetic studies: effects of the initial mixing of drug in blood and the pulmonary first-pass elimination, *J. Pharmacokinet. Biopharm.* **7**, 527-536 (1979).

10. D. L. Roerig, K. J. Kotrly, E. J. Vucins, S. B. Ahlf, C. A. Dawson, and J. P. Kampine, First pass uptake of fentanyl, meperidine, and morphine in the human lung, *Anesthesiology* **67**, 466-472 (1987).

11. F. Boer, J. G. Bovill, A. G. Burm, and R. A. Mooren, Uptake of sufentanil, alfentanil and morphine in the lungs of patients about to undergo coronary artery surgery, *Br. J. Anaesth.* **68**, 370-375 (1992).

12. Y. L. He, H. Ueyama, C. Tashiro, T. Mashimo, and I. Yoshiya, Pulmonary disposition of propofol in surgical patients, *Anesthesiology* **93**, 986-991 (2000).

13. J. A. Kuipers, F. Boer, W. Olieman, A. G. Burm, and J. G. Bovill, First-pass lung uptake and pulmonary clearance of propofol: assessment with a recirculatory indocyanine green pharmacokinetic model, *Anesthesiology* **91**, 1780-1787 (1999).

14. T. K. Henthorn, T. C. Krejcie, C. U. Niemann, C. Enders-Klein, C. A. Shanks, and M. J. Avram, Ketamine distribution described by a recirculatory pharmacokinetic model is not stereoselective, *Anesthesiology* **91**, 1733-1743 (1999).

15. C. Post and D. H. Lewis, Displacement of nortriptyline and uptake of 14C-lidocaine in the lung after administration of 14C-lidocaine to nortriptyline intoxicated pigs, *Acta Pharmacol. Toxicol. (Copenh)* **45**, 218-224 (1979).

16. T. C. Krejcie, M. J. Avram, W. B. Gentry, C. U. Niemann, M. P. Janowski, and T. K. Henthorn, A recirculatory model of the pulmonary uptake and pharmacokinetics of lidocaine based on analysis of arterial and mixed venous data from dogs, *J. Pharmacokinet. Biopharm.* **25**, 169-190 (1997).

17. R. N. Upton and Y. F. Huang, Influence of cardiac output, injection time and injection volume on the initial mixing of drugs with venous blood after i.v. bolus administration to sheep, *Br. J. Anaesth.* **70**, 333-338 (1993).

18. D. P. Vaughan and I. Hope, Applications of a recirculatory stochastic pharmacokinetic model: limitations of compartmental models, *J. Pharmacokinet. Biopharm.* **7**, 207-225 (1979).

19. J. M. van Rossum, J. E. de Bie, G. van Lingen, and H. W. Teeuwen, Pharmacokinetics from a dynamical systems point of view, *J. Pharmacokinet. Biopharm.* **17**, 365-392 (1989).

20. M. Weiss, Hemodynamic influences upon the variance of disposition residence time distribution of drugs, *J.Pharmacokinet. Biopharm.* **11**, 63-75 (1983).

21. M. J. Avram, T. C. Krejcie, and T. K. Henthorn, The relationship of age to the pharmacokinetics of early drug distribution: the concurrent disposition of thiopental and indocyanine green, *Anesthesiology* **72**, 403-411 (1990).

22. T. C. Krejcie, T. K. Henthorn, C. A. Shanks, and M. J. Avram, A recirculatory pharmacokinetic model describing the circulatory mixing, tissue distribution and elimination of antipyrine in dogs, *J. Pharmacol. Exp. Ther.* **269**, 609-616 (1994).

23. T. C. Krejcie, T. K. Henthorn, C. U. Niemann, C. Klein, D. K. Gupta, W. B. Gentry, C. A. Shanks, and M. J. Avram, Recirculatory pharmacokinetic models of markers of blood, extracellular fluid and total body water administered concomitantly, *J. Pharmacol. Exp. Ther.* **278**, 1050-1057 (1996).

24. M. J. Avram, T. C. Krejcie, C. U. Niemann, C. Klein, W. B. Gentry, C. A. Shanks, and T. K. Henthorn, The effect of halothane on the recirculatory pharmacokinetics of physiologic markers, *Anesthesiology* **87**, 1381-1393 (1997).

25. J. A. Kuipers, F. Boer, E. Olofsen, W. Olieman, A. A. Vletter, A. G. Burm, and J. G. Bovill, Recirculatory and compartmental pharmacokinetic modeling of alfentanil in pigs: the influence of cardiac output, *Anesthesiology* **90**, 1146-1157 (1999).

26. J. A. Kuipers, F. Boer, E. Olofsen, J. G. Bovill, and A. G. Burm, Recirculatory pharmacokinetics and pharmacodynamics of rocuronium in patients: the influence of cardiac output, *Anesthesiology* **94**, 47-55 (2001).

27. J. A. Jacquez and T. Perry, Parameter estimation: local identifiability of parameters, *Am. J. Physiol.* **258**, E727-E736 (1990).

28. T. C. Krejcie and M. J. Avram, What determines anesthetic induction dose? It's the front-end kinetics, doctor!, *Anesth. Analg.* **89**, 541-544 (1999).

RECIRCULATORY PHARMACOKINETICS.

Which covariates affect the pharmacokinetics of intravenous agents?

Thomas K. Henthorn[*]

1. INTRODUCTION

When drugs are administered by rapid intravenous (IV) infusion or bolus, drug concentrations in the arterial blood rise and fall in a damped oscillatory pattern before achieving the monotonic decline characterized by traditional pharmacokinetic models. Thus, analyses that do not account for this phenomenon misspecify drug concentrations in the first minutes after drug administration.[1] In order to capture the kinetic behaviour in the first minutes after rapid drug administration, recirculatory pk models have been developed that, essentially, put a 'front end' on traditional pharmacokinetic models.[2] This 'front end' incorporates first-pass/pulmonary-uptake and permits formalized examination of intercompartmental drug clearance in terms of blood flow and drug diffusion.

2. PHARMACOKINETICS-PHARMACDYNAMICS FOLLOWING IV BOLUS

Pharmacokinetic-pharmacodynamic studies are undertaken to predict future dose-response relationships and examine possible mechanisms of interindividual variability in dose-response. With peak effect occurring at approximately 90 seconds after bolus administration for such drugs a propofol, etomidate, thiopental, alfentanil, remifentanil and even rocuronium, the kinetics and dynamics surrounding this period need to be well characterized in order to have a useful predictive or meaningful mechanistic model. Typically, studies are designed with the opposite in mind; to avoid sampling during early onset and offset of effect, following a bolus dose, so as to avoid data that do not fit

[*] Thomas K. Henthorn, Department of Anesthesiology, University of Colorado Health Sciences Center, Denver, USA.

Advances in Modelling and Clinical Application of Intravenous Anaesthesia
Edited by Vuyk and Schraag, Kluwer Academic/Plenum Publishers, 2003

simplistic compartmental models. Another approach is to incorporate high-resolution arterial blood sampling in the pharmacokinetic arm and a continuous measure of effect for the pharmacodynamic arm, but in a continuous infusion design that tends to smooth out the fluctuations.[3] However, neither the "don't look – don't tell" approach of limited sampling nor the blunting effect of a steady infusion provide Pharmacokinetic-dynamic analyses that contain information useful to predict bolus administration events and bolus administration in anaesthesia practice shows no sign of going away anytime soon.   In addition the field of engineering tells us that an instantaneous input yields the maximum information about the system being studied, if only we have the tools to collect the data and the models with which to analyse them.

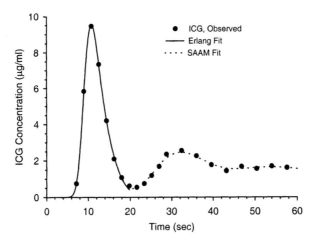

Figure 1. Arterial blood indocyanine green (ICG) concentration histories for the first 60 sec (illustrating the first- and second-pass peaks). The closed circles represent ICG concentrations, the solid line is defined by the first-pass model (Stewart-Hamilton C.O. principle) and the dashed line is the fitted recirculatory model (see figure 2).

Early bolus administration studies pointing to V_1, k_{e0}, or the early distribution Cl_1 were flawed as the concept of V_1 assumes instantaneous mixing throughout the compartment and the value of k_{e0} is dependent on the value of V_1 making k_{e0} (or $T_{1/2Ke0}$) a parameter that really should not be compared between studies.[4] What is needed is an analysis technique that examines the mixing process itself and a better way to characterize the pkpd link. This chapter will deal with a modelling methodology that addresses the former question with the advent of the recirculatory pharmacokinetic model and will examine how physiologic covariates affect this more physiologically-based model.

3. PHARMACOKINETICS OF INTRAVASCULAR MIXING

The most direct way to understand the recirculatory 'front end' of a pharmacokinetic model is to consider the pharmacokientics of an intravascular marker such as indocyanine green (ICG). This way we can limit our concern to events that describe the mixing and recirculation of blood and ignore tissue distribution. The arterial ICG concentration history following a nearly instantaneous central venous bolus is shown in Figure 1. The first seven concentrations and the solid line of best fit represent nothing more than the first-pass and forms the basis of the Stewart-Hamilton indicator-dilution cardiac output principle in which the ICG dose divided by the first-pass AUC equals the cardiac output (or the Cl_E from the non-recirculating system). In Figure 2 this first-pass portion would encompass the central venous injection site, the heart-lung segment and the arterial tree extending to points temporally equivalent to the arterial sampling site. Recirculating blood (and ICG) to this portion of the system results in the characteristic damped oscillation. On a more technical note, the presence and nature of the time delays is critical to this behaviour as well. Interestingly, the first recirculatory peak is caused by initial recirculation of only a minority of the peripheral blood flow. If it were all of the blood, a much larger second peak would be seen. Thus, the circulation needs to be viewed in terms of two peripheral blood circuits, one with a short time constant (low blood volume relative to blood flow) and one with a long time constant (large blood volume relative to its blood flow) in order to characterize the complete arterial blood ICG concentration history. This pharmacokinetic model of the circulation is consistent with physiologic models in which the slow peripheral circuit is thought to represent mainly the splanchnic circulation and the fast most of the rest.[5] Niemann, et al. demonstrated the effect of propranolol on the slow (splanchnic) circulation of healthy human volunteers.[6]

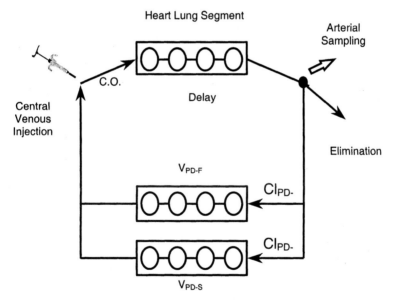

Figure 2. The model for the recirculatory pharmacokinetics of indocyanine green (ICG)[6]. The central circulation, defined by the delay elements of the heart-lung segment receives all of cardiac output (C.O.). The delay elements are represented generically by rectangles surrounding four compartments although the actual number of compartments needed varied between two and thirty in any given delay. Beyond the central circulation, the C.O. distributes to numerous circulatory pathways which lump, on the basis of their blood volume to blood flow ratios (MTTs), into fast (Cl_{PD-F}, V_{PD-F}) and slow (Cl_{PD-S}, V_{PD-S}) peripheral blood circuits. The elimination clearance (Cl_E) of ICG is modeled from the arterial sampling site without being associated with any particular peripheral circuit (with permission).

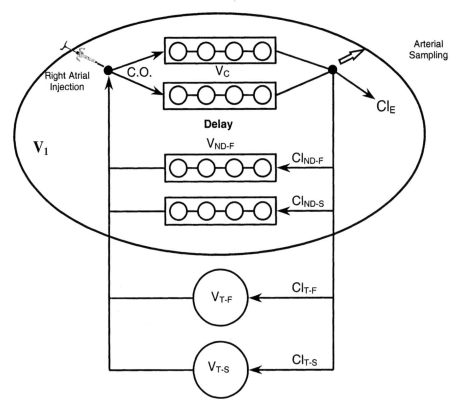

Figure 3. Multicompartment recirculatory pharmacokinetic model[2]. V_{T-F} and V_{T-S} are the fast and slow compartments of a three-compartment model whereas the delay elements included within the dotted circle are the expanded components of its V_1 which account for the first pass and the recirculation of drug back to the central circulation without appreciable tissue exchange (pharmacokinetic shunt).

4. INTRAVASCULAR MIXING AND DRUG DISTRIBUTION

When we move beyond an intravascular marker to a drug, the recirculatory model requires additional compartments in order to characterize the drug's distribution to tissues. Fortunately, these additions are nothing more than the peripheral compartments of traditional pk models. The main difference is that these tissue compartments are connected as parallel circuits in the recirculatory model (Figure 3). In addition, the intercompartmental clearances become components of the overall cardiac output. The preservation of the cardiac output in a recirculatory model becomes a major foundation in our ability to examine how physiological covariates affect the pharmacokinetics.

To summarize, a recirculatory model is a pharmacokinetic model (as opposed to a physiologic model) as it is a model arterial drug concentration versus time data (blood flow data *per se* is not collected or used). However, a recirculatory model has elements of a physiologic model in that 1) cardiac output is retained, 2) tissue distribution is modelled by compartments in parallel circuits, and 3) the model delineates disproportionate distribution of cardiac output. Perhaps the best way to think about the recirculatory model is as a 3-compartment model with a complex V_1. V_1 includes the delay through the heart-lung segment (1st pass) and the quick recirculation through a peripheral circuit in which there is little or no exchange of drug with tissue. This rapid recirculation of drug has variously been called a pharmacokinetic shunt or non-distributive blood flow. It may represent flow to tissues with little distributive capacity (relative to blood flow) such as kidney, skin and brain, or it may be the manifestation of distribution that is not flow-limited, i.e., where distribution is diffusion-limited. The latter is certainly the case for the hydrophilic muscle relaxants. In either case, changes in the proportion of cardiac output that makes up this quick non-distributive circuit directly affects the early blood drug concentrations and, thus, the exposure of the effect site to drug.

5. INTERCOMPARTMENTAL CLEARANCE AND CARDIAC OUTPUT

In proof of the dependence of intercompartmental clearance on cardiac output, Kuipers et al. showed a significant correlation between tissue distribution clearance of alfentanil and cardiac output in a recirculatory model.[7] This provided a more clear explanation for this relationship than was previously able to be shown by Henthorn et al., in which alfentanil pharmacokinetics were analysed with a traditional 3-compartment pharmacokinetic model.[8]

6. PHYSIOLOGIC COVARIATES AND PHARMACOKINETIC PARAMETERS

To study the effects of specific physiological covariates on drug distribution, the concept of a surrogate lipid-soluble drug marker has been advanced.[9] The main reasons for using a surrogate pharmacokinetic marker is that some anaesthetic drugs are known to have physiologic effects (e.g., thiopental and propofol), which can complicate study design, and administering these drugs may obtund subjects in a conscious-subject study design. Antipyrine is a lipid-soluble drug that distributes to tissue in a flow-limited fashion. It also has no discernable effects on physiology or consciousness. Avram et al. have recently demonstrated that the pharmacokinetics of antipyrine closely resembles those of thiopental.[9] In a study of the recirculatory kinetics of antipyrine performed in conscious dogs treated with vasoactive drugs, Krejcie et al. found that treatment with phenylephrine approximately doubled the antipyrine AUC from 0-3 minutes, while isoproterenol halved it over control.[10] The increase in AUC with phenylephrine was a direct result of an increased fraction of the cardiac output going through the non-distributive circuit. In contrast, the lower AUC for isoproterenol-treated dogs was a result of a much larger fraction of cardiac output going to tissues that rapidly equilibrated antipyrine with blood. Presumably, had a drug acting on the central nervous system been administered instead of antipyrine, a much greater peak effect would have been seen in the phenylephrine-treated subjects versus control and a lesser one in the those treated with isoproterenol. Thus we begin to appreciate how kinetic events during the mixing phase are related to the cardiac output and its distribution and how they may directly affect observed pharmacodynamics.

The fact that phenylephrine caused a disproportionate preservation of non-distributive blood flow nicely points out that changes in tissue blood flow are not simply proportional to cardiac output as others have assumed. Avram et al. showed a similar effect on $AUC_{0-3\ min}$ following treatment with isoflurane that was also caused by the combined effects of a decreased cardiac output and preservation of the non-distributive blood flow.[11]

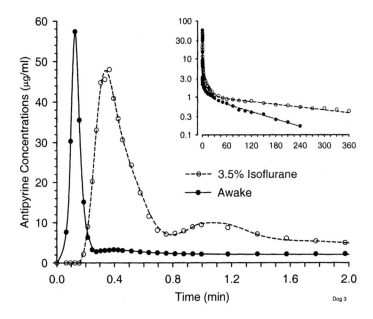

Figure 4. Arterial blood antipyrine concentration versus time profile for the first 2.0 min and for 360 min, or to the limit of detection (*inset*), after right atrial injection in one dog when it was awake (closed circles) and when it was anesthetized with 3.5% isoflurane (open circles). The circles represent measured antipyrine concentrations, and the lines represent concentrations predicted by the recirculatory models. Note the greatly increased area under the curve for the first 2 minutes when 3.5% isoflurane is administered. From Avram et al., Anesthesiology 2000;92:1757-1768.

7. PHYSIOLOGIC COVARIATES AND PHARMACODYNAMIC COVARIATES

Kuipers et al. have used a recirculatory approach to examine a pharmacokinetic-dynamic model for rocuronium.[7] They demonstrated a strong correlation between the k_{e0} and cardiac output ($r^2=0.7$, $P < 0.001$). However, they did not explore the relationship among cardiac output, non-distributive clearance, AUC during the mixing phase and peak effect. It would be interesting to ·see whether rocuronium behaves kinetically as a hydrophilic agent such as inulin or more like the lipophilic antipyrine.

8. CONCLUSION

In summary, a recirculatory model not only completely describes the concentration-time profile from the moment of intravenous injection, it is able to incorporate central blood volume, pulmonary uptake, and cardiac output into a quasi-physiologic pharmacokinetic model. Because of these attributes, the recirculatory approach allows a more comprehensive examination of pharmacokinetic events during the onset of drug effect after rapid intravenous administration. Studies using this approach have demonstrated that changes in cardiac output disproportionately affect non-distributive clearance (or blood flow), causing larger increases in AUC_{0-3min} than would be predicted by a decreased cardiac output alone. The k_{e0} of the muscle relaxant rocuronium in a recirculatory pkpd model is strongly correlated with cardiac output, indicating that k_{e0} is affected by muscle blood flow. Thus, a recirculatory approach is likely to prove increasingly useful for the delineation of the mechanisms underlying interindividual differences in peak drug responses after rapid intravenous administration.

9. REFERENCES

1. D.M. Fisher, (Almost) everything you learned about pharmacokinetics was (somewhat) wrong! *Anesth Analg* **83**, 901-3 (1996).
2. T.C. Krejcie, M.J. Avram. What determines anesthetic induction dose? It's the front-end kinetics, doctor! *Anesth Analg* **89**, 541-4 (1999).
3. K.B. Johnson, S.E. Kern, E.A. Hamber, S.W. McJames, K.M. Kohnstamm. T.D. Egan, Influence of hemorrhagic shock on remifentanil: a pharmacokinetic and pharmacodynamic analysis, *Anesthesiology* **94**, 322-32 (2001).
4. C.F. Minto, T.W. Schnider, K.M. Gregg, T.K. Henthorn, S.L. Shafer, Using the maximum effect site concentration to combine pharmacokinetics and pharmacodynamics, *Anesthesiology* (in press).
5. P. Caldini, S. Permutt, J.A. Waddell, R.L Riley, Effect of epinephrine on pressure, flow, and volume relationships in the systemic circulation of dogs, *Circulation Research* **34** (5), 606-23 (1974).
6. C.U. Niemann, T.K. Henthorn, T.C. Krejcie, C.A. Shanks, C. Enders-Klein, M.J. Avram, Indocyanine green kinetics characterize blood volume and flow distribution and their alteration by propranolol, *Clin Pharmacol Ther* **67**, 342-50 (2000).
7. J.A. Kuipers, F. Boer, E. Olofsen, J.G. Bovill, A.G.L. Burm, Recirculatory Pharmacokinetics and Pharmacodynamics of Rocuronium in Patients: The Influence of Cardiac Output, *Anesthesiology* **94**, 47-55 (2000).
8. T.K. Henthorn, T.C. Krejcie, M.J. Avram. The relationship between alfentanil distribution kinetics and cardiac output, *Clin Pharmacol Ther* **52**, 190-6 (1992).
9. M.J. Avram, T.C. Krejcie, T.K. Henthorn, The concordance of early antipyrine and thiopental distribution kinetics, *J Pharmacol Exp Ther* (in press).
10. T.C. Krejcie, Z. Wang, M.J. Avram, Drug-induced hemodynamic perturbations alter the disposition of markers of blood volume, extracellular fluid, and total body water, *J Pharmacol Exp Ther* **296**, 922-30 (2001).
11. M.J. Avram, T.C. Krejcie, C.U. Niemann, C. Enders-Klein, C.A. Shanks, T.K. Henthorn, Isoflurane alters the recirculatory pharmacokinetics of physiologic markers, *Anesthesiology* **92**, 1757-68 (2000).

RESPONSE SURFACE MODELLING OF DRUG INTERACTIONS

Charles Minto and Jaap Vuyk[*]

1. INTRODUCTION

In every day clinical practice anaesthesiologists administer drugs based on rough estimations of the patient's needs. These rough estimations are based on a basic understanding of the pharmacokinetics and pharmacodynamics of the drugs used and the patient's variables that influence these. A proper assessment of the pharmacokinetics and dynamics of a drug in an individual patient is important because side effects of anaesthetic agents are serious. Inappropriately low drug concentrations during general anaesthesia will lead to nociception and/or an insufficient level of unconsciousness whereas inappropriately high drug concentrations lead to undesired cardiovascular and/or ventilatory depression. Next to the pharmacokinetics and dynamics of single agents, anaesthetic agents also affect each other's distribution and elimination and effect at the receptor site. Pharmacokinetic interactions cause blood drug concentrations to change by 10-15% and are therefore of less importance compared to the pharmacodynamic interactions that may shift concentration-effect curves of the second agent by up to 400%.[1,2] The modelling of pharmacodynamic interactions has been an area developing very rapidly over the past 10-20 years and its current status is discussed in this chapter.

2. PHARMACODYNAMIC MODELLING OF SINGLE AGENTS

Before discussing the analysis of drug interactions a short description of the analysis of the action of single agents is appropriate. The most commonly used pharmacodynamic

---

[*] Charles Minto and Jaap Vuyk, Department of Anaesthesia and Pain Management, University of Sydney, Australia and Department of Anaesthesiology P5-38, Leiden University Medical Center (LUMC), 2300 RC Leiden, The Netherlands

Advances in Modelling and Clinical Application of Intravenous Anaesthesia   35
Edited by Vuyk and Schraag, Kluwer Academic/Plenum Publishers, 2003

model to describe the concentration-effect relationship of anaesthetic agents is the sigmoid E_{max} model:

$$E = E_{max} \bullet \frac{C^\gamma}{C^\gamma + EC_{50}{}^\gamma}$$

where E is the effect, E_{max} is the maximum effect; EC_{50} is the concentration that evokes 50% of the maximum effect and γ a dimensionless parameter describing the slope of the sigmoidal concentration-effect curve. When given as single agent the relationship between the concentration of a drug in the blood and the effect can be described on the basis of 4 modalities. These are potency, efficacy, slope and variability. Potency reflects the sensitivity of the organ or tissue to the drug, and is defined by the location of the curve on the x-axis of the concentration-effect relationship. Potency is often described in terms of the EC_{50} or the MAC, the median effective concentration of intravenous and inhalational anaesthetic agents. With this parameter the effectiveness of different agents with respect to a specific effect, and the effectiveness with which a single agent exerts various effects can be determined. Efficacy, or maximum efficacy, is the (maximum) effect E_{max} that a drug can produce. With E_{max} one may differentiate between full agonists, partial agonists and antagonists. Full agonists induce the full effect often when only a fraction of the receptors is occupied, partial agonists produce only a fraction of the maximum possible effect with all receptors occupied and antagonists produce no effect at all. In the presence of a full agonist the addition of a partial agonist will produce antagonistic effects. The competition for receptors causing agonist molecules to be replaced by the partial agonist that only produces a fraction of the effect of the full agonist is responsible for this phenomenon. The dimensionless parameter γ is related to the mechanism of action of the drug, e.g. receptor binding. The steepness of a curve describes the concentration range between almost no effect and maximum effect. The higher γ the steeper the concentration-effect curve. Finally, in a pooled data analysis, the interindividual variability in concentration-effect relationships is reflected by the variance and the standard error of the EC_{50} or the MAC reflects the precision of the EC_{50} estimate.

3. TERMINOLOGY OF DRUG INTERACTIONS

In general 4 classes of drug interactions can be defined.[3] Zero-interaction is said to occur when the effect of the combination of two drugs is exactly the sum of the effects of the individual agents. This is more often referred to as an additive interaction or when only one of the agents is effective the interaction may be called inert. This occurs when two agents do not really interact but simply provide their action next to one another without influence. Inhalational anaesthetic agents generally exhibit an additive interaction. Consequently, 0.5 MAC of nitrous oxide combined with 0.5 MAC of isoflurane gives a mixture with a potency of 1 MAC. When the effect of the combination is greater than that expected based on the concentration-effect relationships of the individual agents, the interaction is said to be synergistic. Supra-additivity or potentiation are often used as synonyms for synergism. In this case one needs relatively less of the combination to obtain a certain effect compared to when one of the agents is given as single agent. Finally, an infra-additive interaction is said to occur when the effect of the combination is less than the sum of the effects of the individual agents. One then needs relatively more of the combination of agents to obtain a certain effect compared to when one of the agents is given as single agent. This type of interaction may be observed when an agonist and partial agonist are combined e.g. alfentanil and nalbuphine. Lastly, antagonism considers the situation when the effect of the combination is less than that of one of its constituents, e.g. the combined effect of alfentanil and naloxone is less than that of alfentanil alone.

4. METHODS OF PHARMACODYNAMIC INTERACTION MODELLING

Many methods have been developed over the years to characterize the nature and magnitude of pharmacodynamic interactions. Some of these methods are differentiating between types of interaction on a qualitative basis; others do so with a more quantitative mathematical approach. The basis of modern interaction modelling can be found in the fractional analysis and isobolographic analysis.[4] These 2 analytical techniques can be viewed as more or less one, of which fractional analysis offers the more mathematical solution of the graphically oriented isobolographic analysis. Over the past two decades response surface modelling has evolved from isobolographic analysis as a step further in the full description of pharmacodynamic drug interactions.[5] Next to these, interactions at a dose-response relationship level have, amongst others, also been evaluated using parallel line assays[6] or through a method described by Plummer et al.[7,8] Parallel line assay is based on the assumption that the interaction between two drugs is additive when combining increasing doses of one drug to a fixed dose of a second drug causes parallel displacement of the dose-response curve. A non-parallel displacement then is indicative of a non-additive (synergistic or infra-additive) interaction. Along this line, the method by Plummer et al. also quantifies a deviation from additivity. Because isobolographic analysis and response surface modelling with their current mathematical justification form the front-end of pharmacodynamic interaction analysis the remainder of this chapter will deal with these analytical techniques.

4.1. Fractional and Isobolographic Analysis

The classical isobolographic approach, as already used in the late 19th century, is based on a qualitative graphical analysis. The methodology of isobolographic analysis is best explained on the basis of an example.[3,4] When studying drug A and B e.g. for their hypnotic power when combined one may study, next to the agents when given alone, various concentrations of drug A and B and study the concentrations at which loss of consciousness occurs. In this way one may determine various pairs of A-B concentration combinations (c_A, c_B) that all exert the same effect: loss of consciousness. By drawing a line through these iso-effective combinations an isobole is constructed. Furthermore, a line is drawn through the single agent effect concentrations associated with this effect (C_A, C_B). This line is called the line of additivity. Isobolographic analysis now learns that the location of the isobole simply determines the nature of the interaction (Figure 1). The line of additivity is characterized as a straight line. In fractional analysis additivity is

characterized as:
$$\frac{c_A}{C_A} + \frac{c_B}{C_B} = 1$$

Isobolographically below and left of the line of additivity, synergism is present associated with a concave-up shaped isobole. This is characterized in fractional analysis as:

$$\frac{c_A}{C_A} + \frac{c_B}{C_B} < 1$$

Lastly, data above and right of the line of additivity are associated with an infra-additive interaction. This is characterized by a concave-down isobole and is referred to by fractional analysis by the equation:

$$\frac{c_A}{C_A} + \frac{c_B}{C_B} > 1$$

Isobolographic analysis has some inherent features. The interaction between two agents may not be univariate. Interactions may be additive at low concentrations and supraadditive at higher concentrations. Secondly an isobole just gives information on a single effect level, e.g. on the EC_{50}, or EC_{95}. As such the isobolographic analysis can be viewed as the act of determining 2-dimensional iso-effective slices within the greater 3-dimensional response surface.

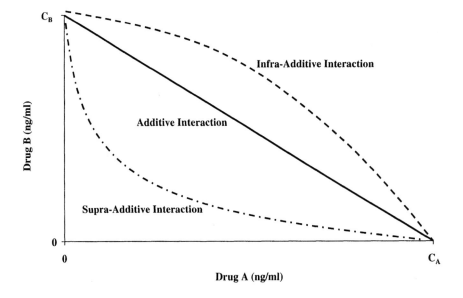

Figure 1. Isoboles for drug A and B when given as sole agents (C_A and C_B) or when given in combination to induce loss of consciousness. The figure displays the various shapes isoboles may have and the nature of the interaction associated with these shapes.

Numerous methods have been described to demonstrate statistically significant deviation from additivity. For studies with only one or two studied concentration-combinations of the drugs tested the *t*-test has been used to evaluate the distance of the studied concentration combination (c_A, c_B) from the line of additivity. Another method useful in the case of only one or two studied combinations, is to determine the 95% confidence intervals for the line of additivity and (c_A, c_B) may then be judged to be either in- or outside these limits to decide on whether the combination exerts either an additive or nonadditive interaction, using the method described by Tallarida et al.[6,9,10]

For studies with multiple concentration combinations of drugs A and B the analysis of the nature of the interaction becomes more complex. In the presence of response/no response data this often is dealt with using logistic regression analysis. In a study on the intraoperative interaction between propofol and alfentanil e.g. Vuyk et al.[11] determined by logistic regression modelling the probability of a response or no response to various surgical events, as a function of the measured blood propofol and alfentanil concentrations.[11,12] A logistic regression was performed twice for each stimulus to explore both the possibility of an additive as well as of a non-additive interaction. The possibility of an additive interaction between propofol and alfentanil was examined by the following

equation:
$$\pi = \frac{e^{\beta_0 + \beta_1 C_{prop} + \beta_2 C_{alf}}}{1 + e^{\beta_0 + \beta_1 C_{prop} + \beta_2 C_{alf}}}$$

The possibility of a non-additive interaction between propofol and alfentanil was

examined by equation:
$$\pi = \frac{e^{\beta_0 + \beta_1 C_{prop} + \beta_2 C_{alf} + \beta_3 C_{prop} C_{alf}}}{1 + e^{\beta_0 + \beta_1 C_{prop} + \beta_2 C_{alf} + \beta_3 C_{prop} C_{alf}}}$$

where π is the probability of (no) response; C_{prop} is the blood propofol concentration; C_{alf} is the blood remifentanil concentration; and β_0, β_1, β_2 and β_3 are the coefficients describing the shape of the curve. The interaction parameter β_3 is equivalent to Berenbaum's interaction index (with β_3 is 0: the result is a straight line suggesting additivity, with $\beta_3 \neq 0$ the result is a curved line suggesting non-additivity). To determine the nature of the interaction the likelihood ratio test was used to assess the significance of incorporating an interaction term in the logistic regression model. Compared to the analysis described above this methodology has the advantage that one does not need to determine the C_A or C_B of the individual agents. In other words, to determine the shape and place of the isobole one doesn't need to determine where it crosses the x- and y-axis. However mathematical disadvantageous of this method are present as well. If only one

drug is present the equation then writes as:
$$\pi = \frac{e^{\beta_0 + \beta_1 C_{prop}}}{1 + e^{\beta_0 + \beta_1 C_{prop}}}$$

This is inconsistent with the single drug model that is described by the equation:
$$\pi = \frac{e^{\beta_0 + \beta_1 \log C_{prop}}}{1 + e^{\beta_0 + \beta_1 \log C_{prop}}}$$

Furthermore, when both drugs are absent, the model then still predicts a drug effect

according to the equation:
$$\pi = \frac{e^{\beta_0}}{1 + e^{\beta_0}}$$

5. RESPONSE SURFACE MODELLING

As mentioned above, the isobolographic method is limited to only a single level of effect (e.g. only the EC_{50}). To describe the complete set of levels of effect ($EC_{01} - EC_{99}$) one may construct in the 3rd dimension all the other iso-effect lines thus creating a surface of iso-effect lines, the so called response surface. The response surface methodology thus differs from isobolographic analysis in the amount of information offered by the result, it also differs in its analytical approach. Whereas with fractional and/or isobolographic analysis a set of studied concentration combinations is compared with a set with no interaction (the line of additivity) during response surface modelling all data are fitted at once and interaction parameters are then estimated.

Basically, the response surface modelling method, as reported since 1988 by Greco et al.[13] Carter et al.[14] and recently in the anaesthetic literature, by Minto et al.[5] is founded on two basic concepts. First, there is the notion that the combination of the two drugs studied should be regarded as one new drug with its own unique properties, with the concentration-effect relation $E = f(CA/C_{50,A} + CB/C_{50,B}; \Psi)$, where the parameter vector Ψ controls the properties of the interaction and specifically how it deviates from pure additivity. Second, Ψ is assumed to depend only on the ratio of the concentrations of the two administered drugs. These two concepts are crucial because they allow for a greatly reduced number of parameters necessary to describe a surface and thus allow these to be estimated from a study of reasonable size. A proper choice of Ψ and f may further reduce the number of parameters while describing the concentration-effect relation in the range measured.

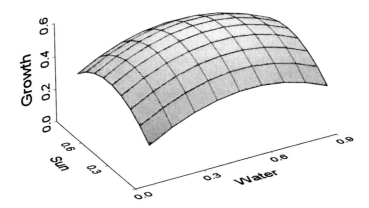

Figure 2. A hypothetical response surface with water, sun and growth on the 3 axes.

The name response surface methodology (RSM) has been given to the statistical methodology concerned with the design of studies to estimate response surfaces, the actual estimation of response surfaces, and the interpretation of the results. Response surface methodology is generally employed for two principal purposes: to provide a description of the response pattern in the region of the observations studied, and to assist in finding the region where the optimal response occurs (i.e., where the response is at a maximum or a minimum). In Figure 2, a polynomial function has been fit to hypothetical data showing the effects of water and sunshine on plant growth. The fitted response surface showed can be used to determine the optimal amount of sun and water for plant growth. The use of polynomial response functions to approximate complex response surfaces is common in many experimental situations. A description of methods used to estimate and evaluate a fitted response surface, and of tests used to decide whether interaction effects are found in Neter *et al.*,(17) and a full description by Box and Draper.[18]

5.1. Experimental Design

A large variety of experimental designs have been developed for estimating response surfaces efficiently.[14] The "ray" design studies the response of two variables present in a number of fixed ratios. In the case of two drugs, each ratio can be considered as a single drug, which permits an analysis based on the same principles as that associated with single drug experiments. The "full factorial" design studies the response of all combinations of two variables at a number of different levels ("fractional factorial" designs are also employed). In the case of two drugs, the different levels usually represent different doses.[19-21] The "central composite design" was developed to provide enough treatment combinations to permit the estimation of the parameters in a quadratic predictive model, while using considerable fewer treatment groups. When there are three variables, they should be (1) studied alone, (2) studied in three pairs, and (3) studied in the triple combination.[15]

Short et al. evaluated by computer simulation various trial designs. These included maintaining drug A at a semi-steady constant concentration while varying drug B (the slices design), maintaining drug A constant while varying drug B in 50% of the patients while maintaining drug B constant and varying drug A (the crisscross design) and the radial design that allowed, by zero-order infusion of both drugs, to "cut" radial slices through the response surface. In this study these authors concluded that the crisscross trial design was most robust in discriminating the correct order of the interaction term with the least number of patients.

5.2. Modelling a Response Surface

Many different approaches have been used to model drug interactions.[3,4] A major strength of response surface approaches is that they can help explain the similarities and differences among other approaches used to study drug interactions.[13] A response surface is a mathematical equation or the graph of that equation that relates a dependent variable (such as a drug effect) to inputs (such as two drug concentrations). A response surface illustrating a synergistic interaction for the hypnotic effect of two drugs illustrated in figure 4.

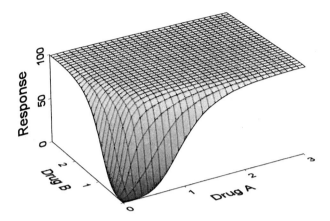

Figure 4. A response surface between drug A and B.

5.3. The Optimal Response

In many experimental situations, response surfaces are used to determine optimal response conditions. Although the optimal conditions are readily determined from Figure 2 (the highest point), these are not so easily determined in Figure 4. Either drug alone or any ratio of the two drugs is capable of achieving the maximum effect (if this is the goal). Furthermore, in general the optimum cannot be determined without considering the pharmacokinetic and side effect profiles of the individual drugs. Consequently, in future studies, to allow us to define the optimal combination of 2 drugs, applicable in clinical practice the interaction between two agents should be studied not only for the desired effects but also for the side effects.

On the basis of isobolographic analysis some progress has been made in this direction. For the propofol-opioid combinations, Vuyk et al., while taking into consideration both the pharmacokinetics and dynamics of propofol and the opioids, determined the various optimal propofol-opioid concentrations associated with intraoperative adequacy of anaesthesia and the most rapid possible return to consciousness thereafter.[16] The optimal propofol concentrations changed with the opioids used showing that not only pharmacodynamic issues were involved but differences in the pharmacokinetics of the opioids affected the optimal intraoperative propofol concentration. In the near future we expect that more and more data will become available that take into consideration both the pharmacokinetics and dynamics of the agents combined considering both the desired effect as the side effects in a final determination of the optimal concentration combination.

6. REFERENCES

1. J.Vuyk, Pharmacokinetic and pharmacodynamic interactions between opioids and propofol, *J.Clin.Anesth.* **9**, 23S (1997).

2. J.Vuyk, Drug interactions in anaesthesia, *Minerva Anestesiol.* **65**, 215 (1999).

3. M.C.Berenbaum, Concepts for describing the interaction of two agents, *Radiat.Res.* **126**, 264 (1991).

4. M.C.Berenbaum, What is synergy?, *Pharmacol.Rev.* **41**, 93 (1989).

5. C.F.Minto, T.W.Schnider, T.G.Short, K.M.Gregg, A.Gentilini, and S.L.Shafer, Response surface model for anesthetic drug interactions, *Anesthesiology* **92**, 1603 (2000).

6. R.J.Tallarida, F.Porreca, and A.Cowan, Statistical analysis of drug-drug and site-site interactions with isobolograms, *Life Sci.* **45**, 947 (1989).

7. J.L.Plummer and T.G.Short, Analysis of effects of drug combinations, *Br.J.Anaesth.* **68**, 114 (1992).

8. J.L.Plummer and T.G.Short, Statistical modeling of the effects of drug combinations, *J.Pharmacol.Methods* **23**, 297 (1990).

9. R.J.Tallarida, Statistical analysis of drug combinations for synergism, *Pain* **49**, 93 (1992).

10. R.J.Tallarida, Drug synergism: its detection and applications, *J.Pharmacol.Exp.Ther.* **298**, 865 (2001).

11. J.Vuyk, T.Lim, F.H.Engbers, A.G.Burm, A.A.Vletter, and J.G.Bovill, The pharmacodynamic interaction of propofol and alfentanil during lower abdominal surgery in women, *Anesthesiology* **83**, 8 (1995).

12. J.Vuyk, F.H.Engbers, A.G.L.Burm, A.A.Vletter, G.E.Griever, E.Olofsen, and J.G.Bovill, Pharmacodynamic interaction between propofol and alfentanil when given for induction of anesthesia, *Anesthesiology* **84**, 288 (1996).

13. W.R.Greco, G.Bravo, and J.C.Parsons, The search for synergy: a critical review from a response surface perspective, *Pharmacol.Rev.* **47**, 331 (1995).

14. W.H.Carter and R.A.Carchman, Mathematical and biostatistical methods for designing and analyzing complex chemical interactions, *Fundam.Appl.Toxicol.* **10**, 590 (1988).

15. T.G.Short, J.L.Plummer, and P.T.Chui, Hypnotic and anaesthetic interactions between midazolam, propofol and alfentanil, *Br J Anaesth* **69**, 162 (1992).

16. J.Vuyk, M.J.Mertens, E.Olofsen, A.G.Burm, and J.G.Bovill, Propofol anesthesia and rational opioid selection: determination of optimal EC50-EC95 propofol-opioid concentrations that assure adequate anesthesia and a rapid return of consciousness, *Anesthesiology* **87**, 1549 (1997).

17. J. Neter , Wasserman W, Kutner MH. Applied Linear Statistical Models. Irwin: Third Edition. Section 9.4 (Response Surface Methodology) in Chapter 9 (Polynomial Regression).

18. G.E.P. Box, Draper NR. Empirical Model-Building and Response Surfaces. John Wiley & Sons, 1987

19. C.J. Zablocki. Matrix study of irbesartan with hydrochlorothiazide in mild-to-moderate hypertension. *Am J Hypertension.***12**, 797-805 (1999).

20. J. Scholze, Zilles P, Compagnone D.,Verapamil SR and trandolapril combination therapy in hypertension - a clinical trial of factorial design. *Brit J Clin Pharm* **45**, 491-5 (1998).

21. J.L. Pool, Cushman WC, Saini RK, Nwachuku CE, Battikha JP. Use of the factorial design and quadratic response surface models to evaluate the fosinopril and hydrochlorothiazide combination therapy in hypertension. *Am J Hypertension* **10**, 117-23 (1997).

AGE RELATED CHANGES OF THE PK-PD OF INTRAVENOUS ANAESTHETICS

Thomas W. Schnider and Charles F. Minto[*]

1. INTRODUCTION

It is clinical common sense that the dose of anaesthetics must be reduced in the elderly. The therapeutic window of most hypnotics, opiates and muscle relaxants is wide. The most serious side effects of the newer therapeutics are hypotension and bradycardia. These adverse effects are often due to overdosing, but even with appropriate dosing for the desired effect, such as hypnosis, haemodynamic changes can be observed. At the end of anaesthesia the desired intra-operative effect becomes an undesired effect if it is not terminated in a timely manner. That is, prolonged sedation and residual muscle relaxation can harm the patient in the postoperative period. Prolonged analgesia is not a concern of opiate administration but respiratory depression, which is clinically irrelevant in the ventilated patient, becomes a serious side effect during the recovery period.

Dosing recommendations of anaesthetics are nearly uniformly based on weight. Theoretically this dosing approach is based on the notion that drug distribution is linearly correlated with weight. In other disciplines, for instance oncology, dosing is based on body surface area. Weight and body surface area are covariates of drug distribution and elimination. In the past, whether to dose proportional to weight or to body surface area was based more on tradition than on scientific reasons.[1] There are other covariates, which should be explored and probably included into dosing.

There are many physiological changes with age affecting the pharmacology of anaesthetics. Body composition, cardiovascular changes and hepatic and renal changes in the elderly influence the pharmacokinetics of drugs. Other factors that mandate dose adjustment, are protein binding and end organ sensitivity. Age related changes of PK/PD of intravenous anaesthetics are of scientific interest. In many studies different age groups

[*] Thomas W. Schnider and Charles F. Minto, Department of Anaesthesiology, St Gallen, Switzerland and Department of Anaesthesia and Pain Management, University of Sydney, Australia.

have been investigated and it was possible to conclude that age indeed affects PK/PD. Of more clinical interest is how to include the covariate age rationally into dosing. Do we have to use age for dose adjustment or should we dose according to cardiac output, renal function or protein binding?

In this review we will look from a general point of view on how aging affects the pharmacology of intravenous anaesthetics, how systematic covariate analysis helps to use the covariates for dosing and specific drugs will be discussed.

2. PHYSIOLOGIC CHANGES WITH AGE

Total body water is decreased in the elderly as a result of a reduction in muscle mass and an increase in body fat, particularly in older women. These changes obviously might affect the distribution of drugs. It is impossible to predict how these changes of body composition affect the kinetics of drugs in the elderly. The increased body fat suggests that the total volume of distribution is larger and the terminal half-life is longer. Simulation studies[2] based on compartmental models have shown that from the changes of single model parameters it is not possible to predict the influence on the time course of the concentration. The decreased total body water might be responsible for higher concentration after bolus administration or rapid infusions.

Cardiac output typically decreases with increasing age but it seems to be well preserved in healthy individuals. Some left ventricular hypertrophy is common in the elderly. It has to be emphasized that arteriosclerosis is pathologic that is it is not present in the healthy elderly patients. There is a big variability in the physical condition among elderly patients. The population of elderly volunteers selected for drug studies is very dissimilar from the dehydrated patients with arteriosclerosis presenting for emergency laparotomy.

To some extent all anaesthetics decrease cardiac performance[3-7] to which the elderly are more sensitive because of their reduced cardiac reserve. Therefore they are more prone to the hypotensive effects of anaesthetics. Renal blood flow and kidney mass decrease with age. Renal function is reduced and the ability to excrete drugs declines. Of the drugs used for anaesthesia, pancuronium is eliminated predominately by the kidney.[8] Since there are many alternatives to pancuronium there are good reasons to avoid pancuronium in the elderly.

Hepatic blood flow decreases with age due to a decline of the liver mass. The intrinsic hepatic capacity is reduced in proportion to the decrease in liver mass. Most intravenous drugs used in anaesthesia are metabolised in the liver. Anaesthesia per se also decreases liver blood flow. This has been shown for different anaesthetics.[9,10] It can be assumed that this reduction in liver blood flow is responsible for the reduced maintenance doses of drugs that are rapidly cleared by the liver (e.g. propofol). For capacity limited drugs the influence on the dose is less marked and only due to the reduced functional capacity in the elderly.

Plasma protein binding also affects the pharmacokinetics and the pharmacodynamic of intravenous anaesthetics. Acidic drugs tend to bind to albumin and basic drugs bind to α_1-acid glycoprotein. Albumin is decreased in the elderly whereas α_1-acid glycoprotein is increased. Since only the unbound fraction of a drug is pharmacologically active and available for metabolism and excretion, protein binding might have an important impact on the time course of effect of anaesthetic drugs.[11]

The sensitivity of the end-organs to anaesthetic drugs is generally increased. This change is partially due to changes in the receptor mediated responses of the autonomic nervous system,[12] the cardiovascular system[13] and the peripheral and the central nervous system.[14]

Although the normal aging process alters drug pharmacokinetics and pharmacodynamics, this brief outline on the physiological changes occurring in the elderly tells that the physiology and not the pharmacokinetic and pharmacodynamic parameters per se, change with age. Over the years a lot of effort has been invested into pharmacokinetic and pharmacodynamic investigations of age effects with respect to the parameters of PK/PD models. The findings of these studies are often inconsistent. The study design and the analysis and modelling methodology have a major impact on the results. Furthermore, because of marked interindividual differences between healthy subjects of the same age, a statistical significant age effect cannot be detected if the age range of the investigated population is not big enough. Chronological age often does not reflect biological age and therefore an 80 years old marathon runner might be physiologically younger than a 60-year-old inactive smoker.

3. SPECIFIC AGE EFFECTS ON DIFFERENT ANAESTHETICS

The age effect has been investigated in the past most often by comparing different age groups. From most of these age-controlled studies it can be inferred that the elderly are more sensitive to the effects and to the side effects of anaesthetics. Only more recent investigations have been aimed at quantifying these differences. From what is known about the physiological changes with age it is obvious that the pharmacokinetic changes lead to higher concentrations in the elderly and because of the increased sensitivity of the central nervous system lower drug concentrations are needed for a comparable effect in the elderly. Only well designed studies with appropriate effect measures and adequate drug concentration monitoring can differentiate between pharmacokinetic and pharmacodynamic reasons for the age effect. The results of different studies often seem to be conflicting. Often, if no age effect can be detected, covariates other than age are not well controlled or the range of age studied is not big enough. The consequence of both is that an investigation cannot detect a difference because of a lack of power. Based on the hypnotics thiopental and propofol and the opioids alfentanil and remifentanil, we will discuss the influence of age on these specific substances. These drugs have been investigated extensively also with the focus on age effects.

3.1. Thiopental

Less thiopental is required for induction in the elderly than in younger patients. Chrstiansen reported that the dose for induction in a group of 60-70 yr patients of both gender was 70% of the value reported for a group of younger men and women between 20 and 40 yr.[15,16] Homer and Stanski[17] used the electroencephalogram (EEG) as the measure of thiopental effect. The dose producing burst suppression on the EEG decreased linearly with age (10.4 mg/kg at age 20 yr, and 4.4 mg/kg at age 80 yr). Because they administered lower infusion rates in the elderly than in the young the result may have been biased. During a slow infusion the difference between the blood concentration and the concentration at the effect site is smaller than during a fast infusion because of the lag time. Because of the time lag for equilibration more drug is in the body when a given effect concentration (or effect) is reached. Gentry[18] has demonstrated that the infusion rate of thiopental affects the dose-response relationship. The same has been shown for other hypnotics as well.[19] The analysis approach of Homer and Stanski also included an effect compartment. With this analysis method the measures of drug concentration and the electroencephalographic effect measure were analysed combined. It enabled the investigators to differentiate between pharmacodynamic and pharmacokinetic effects. Whereas they detected an age effect on the pharmacokinetics they observed no age related changes of the pharmacodynamics. Therefore, the effect site concentration required to produce a particular effect does not change with age. The decreased dose requirement in the elderly was attributed to a marked decrease in the initial distribution volume of thiopental with advancing age (29.8 litres at age 20 yr, and 2.9 litres at age 80 yr). In another investigation Avram et al.[20] administered indocyanine green concurrently with thiopental in order to develop a model designed to describe thiopental's early drug distribution as precisely as possible. They found a decrease in the rapid intercompartmental clearance in the elderly, but no change in the central volume of distribution. They also found an increase in the total volume of distribution with age due to an increase in the volume of the slowly equilibrating compartment. The lack of agreement with Homer and Stanski's earlier work was thought to be the result of differences in experimental design and the difficulties inherent in accurate description of early drug distribution processes.

Stanski and Maitre[21] re-examined the influence of age on thiopental pharmacokinetics and EEG pharmacodynamics using a population pharmacokinetic model. They analysed the data from a larger group of patients and volunteers. A 3-compartment population model was fitted to their data. They also found a decreased rapid intercompartmental clearance between the age of 35 and 80 yr. This 27% decrease between the age of 35 and 80 yr was attributed to the decrease in the rapid intercompartmental clearance. They could not describe the data from the infusion studies and the bolus dose studies together. In contrast to the earlier investigation of Homer and Stanski they found no age related decrease in thiopental's initial distribution volume. The equilibration half time ($t_{1/2} k_{e0}$) was significantly correlated with age but because of a low coefficient of determination ($R^2 = 0.11$) this was considered insignificant. The potency of thiopental was independent of age in this study as in the previous study by Stanski.

Avram et al.[22] further investigated age effects of thiopental induction dose requirements. Clinical and surrogate effect measures (EEG) were used in this study comprising 60 patients. The dose related potency of thiopental increased with increasing age for the clinical endpoint and for the EEG endpoint. These results did not enable the differentiation between pharmacokinetic and pharmacodynamic effects but confirmed that the elderly need less drug for induction.

Since that time, the influence of age on the pharmacokinetics and pharmacodynamics of thiopental has not been further evaluated. The exact reason for age differences in thiopental requirements remain unclear. The earlier finding of a reduced initial distribution volume could not be confirmed and is probably wrong. It also remains unclear whether the elderly really is more sensitive to the effects of thiopental.

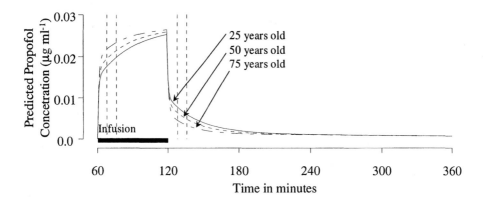

Figure 1. Time course of concentrations during and after a 60-minute infusion starting at time 60 min predicted with the parameters of Schnider et al. In the elderly the concentration increases faster during the infusion but also decreases more rapidly after termination of the infusion (Reprinted with permission).

3.2. Propofol

The initially recommended induction dose of propofol of 2 – 2.5 mg/kg has marked haemodynamic side effects in the elderly. Steib et al.[23] compared a dose of 1 mg/kg propofol with a 2 mg/kg induction dose of thiopental and found similar haemodynamic effects between the two agents. They concluded that propofol could be used to induce anaesthesia in elderly high-risk patients without deleterious cardiovascular effects. An early pharmacokinetic study by Kirkpatrick et al.[24] investigated an iv bolus of propofol 2.5 mg/kg in the young (18-35 yr) and 2.0 mg/kg in the elderly (65-80 yr). They reported that the propofol concentrations were higher in the elderly immediately following injection, and attributed this to a 25% smaller initial volume of distribution in the elderly than in the young (19.6 L versus 26.3 L). Additionally, they reported a 20% lower clearance in the elderly than in the young (1.44 L/min versus 1.79 L/min). However, these age-related pharmacokinetic differences are insufficient to explain the magnitude of the dose reduction observed in the elderly. Scheepstra et al.[25] administered an initial dose of 1.5 mg/kg of propofol over 20-40 seconds to a group of young (25-39 yr) and elderly (66-80 yr) patients. After 1 min, 5out of 18 young patients and 15 out of 19 elderly patients had lost the eyelash reflex. If unconsciousness was not obtained after 1 min, additional 20 mg boluses were given to a total of 2.2 mg/kg and 1.7 mg/kg in the young and elderly groups, respectively. However, this study may not have accurately characterized the differences between the two groups, because propofol peak effect site concentrations occur later than 1 min after the bolus dose. Peacock et al.[26] examined the total induction dose of propofol in young and elderly subject using slow iv infusions, rather than iv bolus administration, and found that the elderly required a 44% smaller induction dose than the young. These early studies with propofol in the elderly indicated that the dose of propofol must be reduced in the elderly particularly for haemodynamic reasons. There was evidence that pharmacokinetic differences are responsible for this increased sensitivity to propofol but additional pharmacodynamic effects could be suspected.

The pharmacokinetics of propofol has been described in many studies.[27-33] Though there are only few studies, which formally investigated the effect of age. With a population pharmacokinetic model Schnider et al.[34] analysed arterial concentration data obtained from 24 healthy volunteers aged 21-81 yr, who received a bolus dose of propofol, followed one hour later by a 60-min infusion in 2 sessions. No age effect on the central volume of distribution or metabolic clearance was detected. However, a significant reduction in the size of the rapidly equilibrating peripheral compartment and the rapid intercompartmental clearance in the elderly was found. These pharmacokinetic parameters predict a more rapid increase in concentration at the beginning of an infusion and a more rapid decrease in concentration after the end of an infusion (Figure 1). In contrast to the model currently used in the commercially available target controlled infusion device (TCI),[30] the central compartment was not correlated with weight. Recently, Schüttler and Ihmsen[35] analysed 4112 samples of 270 individuals aged 2-88 years using a population pharmacokinetic model of previously published data from five research groups. This data set consisted of arterial and venous concentration data collected after either administration by iv bolus or iv infusion. The final covariate model comprised 18 estimated parameters. In this model weight was a significant covariate for all parameters but V_3 and age was a significant parameter for the central volume and the metabolic clearance. The parameter sets of Schnider and Schuttler give conflicting results with regard to predicting context-sensitive decrement-times.[36]Figure 2 shows the 80% decrement-times predicted with the parameters of Marsh et al., Schüttler and Inhmsen and Schnider et al. for a 75 yr old person (height 175 cm, weight 70 kg). Since the parameters of Marsh are only weight scaled (V_1 proportional to weight), the curve remains the same for different ages and different weights or heights. The predicted context-sensitive decrement-times are remarkably different, particularly for infusion rates of more than 1 hour.

To separate the pharmacokinetic from the pharmacodynamic effects, studies with simultaneous measurement of drug concentration and drug effect are necessary. Schnider et al. investigated the influence of age on clinical and EEG effects of propofol in a PK/PD study in volunteers.[37] A logistic regression analysis was performed of the concentration data after an infusion of 1 h duration together with the assessment of the sleep / no sleep response. The C_{50} for this relationship was 50% less in a 75 yr old compared with a 25 yr old (1.25 µg/ml versus 2.35 µg/ml). Analysis of the EEG data also detected a greater sensitivity in the elderly, but the $t_{1/2keo}$ (2.19 min) was not affected by age. Animal studies with propofol suggest that aging induces functional alterations of neurotransmitters.[38,39] Based on these results it can be inferred that the increased brain sensitivity contributes to the decreased dose requirement in the elderly.

Kazama et al.[40] compared the speed of onset of EEG and haemodynamic effects in elderly and younger patients. They used a target controlled infusion to rapidly attain and maintain 4 sequentially increasing, randomly selected plasma propofol concentrations from 1 to 12 µg/ml in 41 patients aged 20-85 yr. The target concentration was maintained for about 30 min. Bispectral index (BIS) and systolic blood pressure were used as measures of effect. They found no age-related differences in the $t_{1/2keo}$ for the EEG effect. The half-times for the plasma-effect site equilibration for BIS were approximately 2.3 min in all age groups. However, the half-times for the effect on systolic blood pressure increased with age (from 5.68 min in the 20-39 yr age group to 10.22 min in the 70-85 yr age group). Importantly, the C_{50} for the haemodynamic effect was 55% less (2.09 µg/ml in the 20-39 yr age group versus 4.61 µg/ml in the 20-39 yr age group). Thus, with a constant plasma concentration, in the elderly the systolic blood pressure decreases to a greater degree, but more slowly. In another investigation Kazama et al.[41] evaluated the optimal propofol plasma concentration during upper gastrointestinal endoscopy in young, middle-aged and in elderly patients. The concentration needed to suppress somatic response decreased with increasing age.

Several investigators explored induction of anaesthesia with propofol. As with other anaesthetic drugs, the applicability of compartmental models to the initial part of the concentration time data is limited. For propofol in sheep Ludbrook[42] showed that models derived from low infusion rate and small dose data only poorly predicted data from high infusion rates and big doses. Upton et al.[43] found that the initial arterial concentrations of propofol after iv administration are inversely related to cardiac output in the sheep. Thus, changes in cardiac output during induction may be an important factor in determining propofol dose requirements. Adachi et al.[44] also found cardiac output a significant determinant of induction dose together with age and weight.

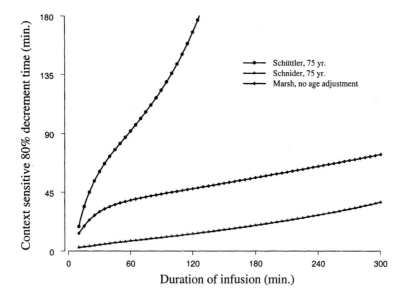

Figure 2. Context sensitive 80 % decrement times of propofol predicted for a 75 yr. old, 175 cm tall and 70 kg heavy person. Since the parameters of Marsh et al. are only weight scaled i.e. V_1 is proportional to weight, the curve is the same for any age, weight or height. There is a big discrepancy in the prediction between the parameters of Schüttler and Ihmsen and the parameters of Schnider et al.

All pharmacokinetic studies that investigated an adequate range of ages, found age dependence of the kinetics. However the extent of the difference varies. Some of the difference might be due to differences in study design and in particularly in infusion schemes. Since infusion rates and dilution of propofol have an impact on induction dose,[19] and the initial part of the concentration-time relationship is sometimes better described with a physiological model[45], traditional compartmental model parameters must differ between studies. As Krejcie and Avram[46] pointed out, the front-end kinetics might be responsible for some of the discrepancy.

However, all available data indicate that the elderly are significantly more sensitive to the EEG, sedative and haemodynamic effects of propofol than the young. The message for the clinician is straightforward: reduce the dose of propofol and inject the reduced dose more slowly in the elderly. With adequate monitoring and adaptation of the dose, even old patients with compromised cardiac reserve can be anaesthetised with propofol.[47]

3.3. Fentanyl

In an early study, Bentley et al.[48] administered 10 μg/kg fentanyl to a group of young (<50 yr) and elderly patients (>60 yr). Fentanyl concentrations were significantly higher in the older patient group. The volumes of distribution were similar, but the clearance was reduced in the elderly (265 ml/min vs. 991 ml/min) and the terminal elimination half-life was longer (945 min vs. 265 min). However, the sampling duration was only 420 min, so the estimate of the terminal half-life in the elderly may be unreliable. Scott and Stanski[49] compared the pharmacokinetic parameters of a compartmental model of younger patients with the parameters of older patients. They found no significant difference and concluded that not the pharmacokinetics but the pharmacodynamics are responsible for the decreased requirement of opiate in the elderly. The IC_{50} (concentration necessary for 50% of inhibition) for an EEG effect decreased by 50% from age 20 to age 85 yr, but no age-related change in the $t_{1/2ke0}$ was observed.

3.4. Alfentanil

As a newer opiate, alfentanil has been the subject of many studies. Helmers et al.[50] compared the pharmacokinetics of 15 elderly patients with the pharmacokinetics of 9 younger subjects. They found a lower clearance in the elderly subject than in the young subjects. Scott and Stanski[49] found that the elimination half-life of alfentanil increased with increasing age, but did not find an age-related change in the clearance of alfentanil. Lemmens et al.[51] tried to explain the inclusive results of the alfentanil pharmacokinetics by a gender effect. They showed that the effects of age on the pharmacokinetics of alfentanil are different between women and men. Maitre et al.[52] analysed the data of 4 previously published studies with a population pharmacokinetic approach to estimate the influence of age on the pharmacokinetics of alfentanil. For this big data set the clearance was found to decrease above the age of 40 yr. In an evaluation of the accuracy of the parameters the authors found good performance.[53] Though in a prospective evaluation of the parameters, Raemer et al.[54] with a target controlled infusion system found that they were consistently biased whereas Scott's[49] pharmacokinetic parameters performed well, suggesting that clearance does not decrease in the elderly. As for fentanyl, Scott and Stanski[49] observed a 50% decrease in alfentanil's C_{50} (EEG effect) from age 20 to age 85 yr, but no age-related change in the $t_{1/2ke0}$. Using clinical endpoints Lemmens et al.[55,56] could not confirm an increased sensitivity to alfentanil in the elderly. Lemmens et al.[56] found that the total alfentanil dose was decreased by approximately 50% in elderly subjects, and suggested that pharmacokinetic differences may be responsible.

3.5. Remifentanil

The effect of age on the pharmacokinetics and pharmacodynamics of remifentanil was investigated in specifically designed volunteer studies before its introduction into clinical practice. Minto and colleagues[57,58] administered remifentanil by constant rate infusion of 3 μg/kg/min to 35 healthy individuals between 40 and 85 years old. With the data of this study and 3 studies in younger subjects (20–39 yr)[59,60] age adjusted pharmacokinetic and pharmacodynamic models were developed. They found that from the age of 20 to 80 yr the central volume decreased by 20%, the clearance decreased by 30%, the C50 (EEG effect) halved and the $t_{1/2keo}$ doubled. The covariate adjusted model performed better than the simple model (without covariates) when evaluated prospectively in 15 other volunteers. Minto explored the influence of age on dose requirements by computer simulations[57] with the models and found that the that bolus doses should be halved and infusion rates decreased to one third in the elderly compared with the young to achieve the same EEG effect. The simulations also suggested that the variability in the recovery times should increase with age. Furthermore, the onset of drug effect is slower in the elderly. In a young patient the peak drug effect can be expected about 90 seconds after a bolus injection whereas in the elderly it takes about 2-3 minutes until the maximal effect is achieved. In a smaller study with 24 patients of ages between 18 and 60 yr, Westmoreland et al.[61] did not find an age effect on the pharmacokinetics. The shorter 1-min infusion and the smaller age range may have limited the power for detection of an age effect. In a prospective evaluation of the age adjusted models of Minto et al., Drover and Lemmens[62] found good model performance. However,they could not detect an effect of age on any clinical pharmacodynamic endpoint. The models of Minto et al. formed the basis for the age adjusted dose recommendations in the package insert of remifentanil.

4. CONCLUSION

The elderly patient generally needs smaller bolus doses for induction of anaesthesia and lower infusion rates for maintenance of the anaesthetic effect. The reason for these lower requirements is either an increased concentration or an increased sensitivity of the end organ. For clinical purposes this distinction is not always important. The seemingly conflicting results of some of the pharmacokinetic and pharmacodynamic studies are partially due to differences in study design and analysis methods and sometimes due to not ideal endpoints. Whether the central compartment of a 3-compartment model is smaller in the elderly might be irrelevant when the time course of the concentration during an infusion is of interest. It might be better to assess onset characteristics on the basis of time to peak effect and recovery by calculating relevant decrement times.[63]

Even extensive covariate analysis (e.g. weight, height, ASA status, age and cardiac output) can only account for some of the interindividual variability observed. Therefore, any dose recommendation will only be optimal for the *average* patient. Our patient, who will never be an "average patient" needs to be dosed individually. Titration to the desired effect is probably more important than finding the right "single shot" dose. In order to minimize the haemodynamic side effects in the elderly, we should start by giving less drug, we should give it more slowly and we should wait longer to allow for the effect to reach its peak. Pharmacokinetic and pharmacodynamic studies have increased our understanding of the variability of the drug response. The results may also help to select drugs with a better side effect profile in the elderly. Beyond guidelines for the initial dose, the selection and timing of an appropriate dose and the subsequent titration of dose to effect remains part of the art of anaesthesia.

5. REFERENCES

1. M.J. Ratain, Body-surface area as a basis for dosing of anticancer agents: science, myth, or habit? *Science* **16**, 2297-2298 (1998).
2. E.L. Youngs, Shafer SL, Pharmacokinetic parameters relevant to recovery from opioids, *Anesthesiology* **81**, 833-842 (1994).
3. J. Sprung, Ogletree-Hughes ML, Moravec CS: The effects of etomidate on the contractility of failing and nonfailing human heart muscle, *Anesth Analg* **91**, 8-75 (2000).
4. B.E. Filner, Karliner JS: Alterations of normal left ventricular performance by general anesthesia. *Anesthesiology* **45**, 610-21 (1976).
5. F. Kehl, Kress TT, Mraovic B, Hettrick DA, Kersten JR, Warltier DC, Pagel PS, Propofol alters left atrial function evaluated with pressure-volume relations in vivo, *Anesth Analg* **94**, 1421-6 (2002).
6. B. Preckel, Ebel D, Mullenheim J, Frabetadorf J, Thamer V, Schlack W, The direct myocardial effects of xenon in the dog heart in vivo, *Anesth Analg* **94**, 545-51 (2002)
7. H.P. Gelissen, Epema AH, Henning RH, Krijnen HJ, Hennis PJ, den Hertog A, Inotropic effects of propofol, thiopental, midazolam, etomidate, and ketamine on isolated human atrial muscle, *Anesthesiology* **84**, 397-403 (1996).
8. L. Berntman, Rosberg B, Shweikh I, Yousef H, Atracurium and pancuronium in renal insufficiency, *Acta Anaesthesiol Scand* **33**, 48-52 (1989).
9. S. Gelman, Fowler KC, Smith LR, Liver circulation and function during isoflurane and halothane anesthesia, *Anesthesiology* **61**, 726-30 (1984).
10. P.F. Wouters, Van de Velde MA, Marcus MA, Deruyter HA, Van Aken H, Hemodynamic changes during induction of anesthesia with eltanolone and propofol in dogs, *Anesth Analg* **81**, 125-31 (1995).
11. H.J. Lemmens, Burm AG, Bovill JG, Hennis PJ, Gladines MP, Pharmacodynamics of alfentanil. The role of plasma protein binding, *Anesthesiology* **76**, 65-70 (1992).
12. M.D. Tasch, Priebe HJ, The autonomic nervous system and geriatric anesthesia. The aged cardiovascular risk patient, *Int Anesthesiol Clin* **26**, 143-51 (1988).
13. H.J. Priebe, The aged cardiovascular risk patient, *Br J Anaesth* **85**, 763-78 (2000).
14. M. Naguib, Flood P, McArdle JJ, Brenner HR, Advances in neurobiology of the neuromuscular junction: implications for the anesthesiologist, *Anesthesiology* **96**, 202-31 (2002).
15. J.H. Christensen, Andreasen F, Jansen JA, Pharmacokinetics and pharmacodynamics of thiopentone, A comparison between young and elderly patients, *Anaesthesia* **37**, 398-404 (1982).
16. J.H. Christensen, Andreasen F, Jansen JA, Influence of age and sex on the pharmacokinetics of thiopentone, *Br J Anaesth* **53**, 1189-95 (1981).
17. T.D. Homer, Stanski DR, The effect of increasing age on thiopental disposition and anesthetic requirement, *Anesthesiology* **62**, 714-724 (1985).
18. W.B. Gentry, Krejcie TC, Henthorn TK, Shanks CA, Howard KA, Gupta DK, Avram MJ, Effect of infusion rate on thiopental dose-response relationships. Assessment of a pharmacokinetic-pharmacodynamic model, *Anesthesiology* **81**, 316-24 (1994).
19. T. Kazama, Ikeda K, Morita K, Kikura M, Ikeda T, Kurita T, Sato S, Investigation of effective anesthesia induction doses using a wide range of infusion rates with undiluted and diluted propofol, *Anesthesiology* **92**, 1017-28 (2000).
20. M.J. Avram, Krejcie TC, Henthorn TK, The relationship of age to the pharmacokinetics of early drug distribution: the concurrent disposition of thiopental and indocyanine green, *Anesthesiology* **72**, 403-411 (1990).
21. D.R. Stanski, Maitre PO, Population pharmacokinetics and pharmacodynamics of thiopental: the effect of age revisited, *Anesthesiology* **72**, 412-422 (1990).
22. M.J. Avram, Sanghvi R, Henthorn TK, Krejcie TC, Shanks CA, Fragen RJ, Howard KA, Kaczynski DA, Determinants of thiopental induction dose requirements, *Anesthesia and Analgesia* **76**, 10-17 (1993).
23. A. Steib, Freys G, Beller JP, Curzola U, Otteni JC, Propofol in elderly high risk patients. A comparison of haemodynamic effects with thiopentone during induction of anaesthesia, *Anaesthesia* **43** Suppl: 111-4 (1988).

24. T. Kirkpatrick, Cockshott ID, Douglas EJ, Nimmo WS: Pharmacokinetics of propofol (diprivan) in elderly patients. *Br. J. Anaesth* **60**, 146-150 (1988).
25. G.L. Scheepstra, Booij LH, Rutten CL, Coenen LG, Propofol for induction and maintenance of anaesthesia: comparison between younger and older patients, *Br J Anaesth* **62**, 54-60 (1989).
26. J.E. Peacock, Spiers SP, McLauchlan GA, Edmondson WC, Berthoud M, Reilly CS, Infusion of propofol to identify smallest effective doses for induction of anaesthesia in young and elderly patients, *Br J Anaesth* **69**, 363-7 (1992).
27. J.M. Bailey, Mora CT, Shafer SL, Pharmacokinetics of propofol in adult patients undergoing coronary revascularization. The Multicenter Study of Perioperative Ischemia Research Group, *Anesthesiology* **84**, 1288-1297 (1992).
28. E. Gepts, Jonckheer K, Maes V, Sonck W, Camu F, Disposition kinetics of propofol during alfentanil anaesthesia, *Anaesthesia* **43**, Suppl: 8-13 (1988).
29. E. Gepts, Camu F, Cockshott ID, Douglas EJ, Disposition of propofol administered as constant rate intravenous infusions in humans, *Anesthesia and Analgesia* **66**, 1256-1263 (1987).
30. B. Marsh, White M, Morton N, Kenny GN, Pharmacokinetic model driven infusion of propofol in children. *Br. J. Anaesth* **67**, 41-48 (1991).
31. B.K. Kataria, Ved SA, Nicodemus HF, Hoy GR, Lea D, Dubois MY, Mandema JW, Shafer SL, The pharmacokinetics of propofol in children using three different data analysis approaches, *Anesthesiology* **80**, 104-122 (1994).
32. A. Shafer, Doze VA, Shafer SL, White PF, Pharmacokinetics and pharmacodynamics of propofol infusions during general anesthesia, *Anesthesiology* **69**, 348-356 (1988).
33. I. Murat, Billard V, Vernois J, Zaouter M, Marsol P, Souron R, Farinotti R, Pharmacokinetics of propofol after a single dose in children aged 1-3 years with minor burns. Comparison of three data analysis approaches, *Anesthesiology* **84**, 526-32 (1996).
34. T.W. Schnider, Minto CF, Gambus PL, Andresen C, Goodale DB, Shafer SL, Youngs EJ, The influence of method of administration and covariates on the pharmacokinetics of propofol in adult volunteers, *Anesthesiology* **88**, 1170-1182 (1998).
35. J. Schuttler, Ihmsen H, Population pharmacokinetics of propofol: a multicenter study, *Anesthesiology* **92**, 727-38 (2000).
36. J. Vuyk, Schnider T, Engbers F, Population pharmacokinetics of propofol for target-controlled infusion (TCI) in the elderly, *Anesthesiology* **93**, 1557-60 (2000).
37. T.W. Schnider, Minto CF, Shafer SL, Gambus PL, Andresen C, Goodale DB, Youngs EJ, The influence of age on propofol pharmacodynamics, *Anesthesiology* **90**: 1502-16 (1999).
38. Y. Wang, Kikuchi T, Sakai M, Wu JL, Sato K, Okumura F, Age-related modifications of effects of ketamine and propofol on rat hippocampal acetylcholine release studied by in vivo brain microdialysis, *Acta Anaesthesiol Scand* **44**, 112-7 (2000).
39. H. Keita, Lasocki S, Henzel-Rouelle D, Desmonts JM, Mantz J, Aging decreases the sensitivity of the GABA carrier to propofol and etomidate, *Br J Anaesth* **81**, 249-50 (1998).
40. T. Kazama, Ikeda K, Morita K, Kikura M, Doi M, Ikeda T, Kurita T, Nakajima Y, Comparison of the effect-site k(eO)s of propofol for blood pressure and EEG bispectral index in elderly and younger patients, *Anesthesiology* **90**, 1517-27 (1999).
41. T. Kazama, Takeuchi K, Ikeda K, Ikeda T, Kikura M, Iida T, Suzuki S, Hanai H, Sato S, Optimal propofol plasma concentration during upper gastrointestinal endoscopy in young, middle-aged, and elderly patients, *Anesthesiology* **93**, 662-9 (2000).
42. G.L. Ludbrook, Upton RN, Grant C, Martinez A, A compartmental analysis of the pharmacokinetics of propofol in sheep, *J Pharmacokinet Biopharm* **27**, 329-38 (1999).
43. R.N. Upton, Ludbrook GL, Grant C, Martinez AM, Cardiac output is a determinant of the initial concentrations of propofol after short-infusion administration [see comments], *Anesth Analg* **89**, 545-52 (1999).
44. Y.U. Adachi, Watanabe K, Higuchi H, Satoh T, The determinants of propofol induction of anesthesia dose, *Anesth Analg* **92**, 656-61 (2001).
45. R.N. Upton, Ludbrook GL, A model of the kinetics and dynamics of induction of anaesthesia in sheep: variable estimation for thiopental and comparison with propofol, *Br J Anaesth* **82**, 890-9 (1999).
46. T.C. Krejcie, Avram MJ, What determines anesthetic induction dose? It's the front-end kinetics, doctor! *Anesth Analg* **89**, 541-4 (1999).
47. I.E. Leonard, Myles PS, Target-controlled intravenous anaesthesia with bispectral index monitoring for thoracotomy in a patient with severely impaired left ventricular function, *Anaesth Intensive Care* **28**, 318-21 (2000).
48. J.B. Bentley, Borel JD, Nenad RE, Jr., Gillespie TJ, Age and fentanyl pharmacokinetics. *Anesth Analg* **61**, 968-71 (1982).

49. J.C. Scott, Stanski DR, Decreased fentanyl and alfentanil dose requirements with age. A simultaneous pharmacokinetic and pharmacodynamic evaluation, *J Pharmacol Exp Ther* **240**: 159-166 (1987).
50. H. Helmers, Van Peer A, Woestenborghs R, Noorduin H, Heykants J, Alfentanil kinetics in the elderly, *Clin Pharmacol Ther* **36**: 239-43 (1984).
51. H.J. Lemmens, Burm AG, Hennis PJ, Gladines MP, Bovill JG, Influence of age on the pharmacokinetics of alfentanil. Gender dependence, *Clin Pharmacokinet* **19**, 416-22 (1990).
52. P.O. Maitre, Vozeh S, Heykants J, Thomson DA, Stanski DR, Population pharmacokinetics of alfentanil: the average dose- plasma concentration relationship and interindividual variability in patients, *Anesthesiology* **66**, 3-12 (1987).
53. P.O. Maitre, Ausems ME, Vozeh S, Stanski DR, Evaluating the accuracy of using population pharmacokinetic data to predict plasma concentrations of alfentanil, *Anesthesiology* **68**, 59-67, (1988).
54. D.B. Raemer, Buschman A, Varvel JR, Philip BK, Johnson MD, Stein DA, Shafer SL, The prospective use of population pharmacokinetics in a computer- driven infusion system for alfentanil, *Anesthesiology* **73**, 66-72 (1990).
55. H.J. Lemmens, Burm AG, Bovill JG, Hennis PJ, Pharmacodynamics of alfentanil as a supplement to nitrous oxide anaesthesia in the elderly patient, *Br J Anaesth* **61**, 173-9 (1988).
56. H.J. Lemmens, Bovill JG, Hennis PJ, Burm AG, Age has no effect on the pharmacodynamics of alfentanil, *Anesth Analg* **67**, 956-60 (1988).
57. C.F. Minto, Schnider TW, Shafer SL, Pharmacokinetics and Pharmacodynamics of Remifentanil. II Model Application, *Anesthesiology* **86**, 24-33 (1997).
58. C.F. Minto, Howe C, Wishart S, Conway AJ, Handelsman DJ, Pharmacokinetics and pharmacodynamics of nandrolone esters in oil vehicle: effects of ester, injection site and injection volume, *J Pharmacol Exp Ther* **281**, 93-102 (1997).
59. T.D. Egan, Lemmens HJ, Fiset P, Hermann DJ, Muir KT, Stanski DR, Shafer SL, The pharmacokinetics of the new short-acting opioid remifentanil (GI87084B) in healthy adult male volunteers, *Anesthesiology* **79**, 881-892 (1993).
60. T.D. Egan, Minto CF, Hermann DJ, Barr J, Muir KT, Shafer SL, Remifentanil versus alfentanil: comparative pharmacokinetics and pharmacodynamics in healthy adult male volunteers, *Anesthesiology* **84**, 821-833 (1996).
61. C.L. Westmoreland, Hoke JF, Sebel PS, Hug CCJ, Muir KT, Pharmacokinetics of remifentanil (GI87084B) and its major metabolite (GI90291) in patients undergoing elective inpatient surgery, *Anesthesiology* **79**, 893-903 (1993).
62. D.R. Drover, Lemmens HJ, Population pharmacodynamics and pharmacokinetics of remifentanil as a supplement to nitrous oxide anesthesia for elective abdominal surgery, *Anesthesiology* **89**, 869-877 (1998).
63. T.W. Schnider, Shafer SL, Evolving clinically useful predictors of recovery from intravenous anesthetics, *Anesthesiology* **83**, 902-905 (1995).

CLINICAL APPLICATION OF PHARMACOKINETIC AND PHARMACODYNAMIC MODELS

Valerie Billard[*]

1. INTRODUCTION

Anaesthesiologists have a special interest in pharmacology, maybe even more than other physicians who prescribe drugs and often follow narrow approved dosing guidelines. Anaesthetic drugs can be administered in a wide dose range, with relative under dosage (awareness, muscle tension or pain) adequate dosage and relative over dosage (late recovery, side effects) all being observed within the approved dose range. The art, or the science, of the anaesthetist is to choose both the drug and the dose in order to achieve an adequate level of anaesthesia as fast as possible and maintain it just as long as necessary in any individual patient. Pharmacokinetic and pharmacodynamic modelling helps to achieve these clinical goals by differentiation within the dose-effect relationship into a dose-concentration relationship and a concentration-effect relationship. Clinically, kinetic-dynamic modelling can be used to adjust the dose to a desired level of effect at any time through target-controlled delivery systems.

2. PK/PD MODELLING OF THE DOSE-EFFECT RELATIONSHIP

Pharmacokinetic and dynamic models basically consist of sets of mathematical equations that link the dose of a drug to the corresponding concentration in the blood and its effects in time. Models generally are developed by administration of a known dose of a drug and consecutive measurement of the blood concentration and its effect over time.

---

[*] Valerie Billard, Service d'Anesthésie, Institut Gustave Roussy 39, Rue C. Desmoulins 94805, Villejuif, France

Advances in Modelling and Clinical Application of Intravenous Anaesthesia
Edited by Vuyk and Schraag, Kluwer Academic/Plenum Publishers, 2003

57

These concentration-time and concentration-effect data then are fitted using a priori chosen models like the 2- or 3-compartments mamillary models in the case of pharmacokinetic modelling and the sigmoid E_{max} model regarding pharmacodynamic modelling (Figure 1, top).

From mathematical models…

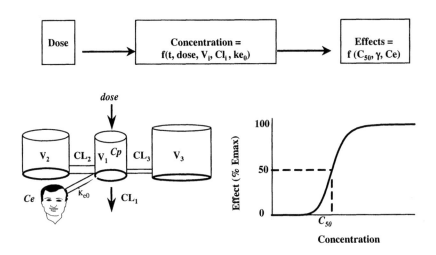

… to clinical use.

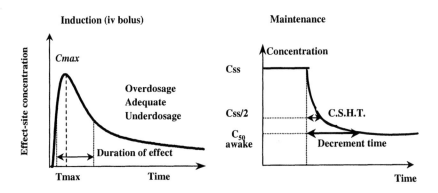

Figure 1. An overview of the relationship between pharmacokinetic and pharmacodynamic parameters as derived through scientific observation and the application of these data in computer simulation and clinical practice.

These parameters obtained from PK-PD studies then may be used to predict the blood concentrations and associated effects for other patients at different times after different doses.[1] This generally is a patient-naïve process and thus assumes that the most important factors in the dose-effect relationship are drug related and not patient related. This assumption is essential because most of the patients to whom we give anaesthesia come along only once. It is not useful to measure blood concentrations and define a pharmacokinetic parameter set during a first session and call a patient for surgery as a second session, or to wait for a real steady-state to allow the surgeon to do his job. Fortunately, clinically the above-mentioned assumption is, within limits, often true for anaesthetic drugs.

3. RATIONAL CHOICE OF DRUGS AND DOSES

The first application of PK-PD models is to compare dose-concentration-effect relationships between drugs in order to choose the best drug for a specific procedure or patient group. Interpretation of pharmacokinetic parameters (Figure 1, top) is difficult and may induce interpretation errors.[2] To support this process pharmacokinetic parameters may be incorporated into simulation software programmes that display the time course of the blood drug concentration for any given drug and dose (Table 1). These programmes are easy to use for anaesthesiologists, other specialists, medical students and anaesthesia nurses to evaluate their actions in clinical practice and may help them to achieve a stable and adequate anaesthetic level. Most of the software programmes used are based on published 2- or 3-compartment models together with an additional compartment describing the effect-site[3] and display the predicted drug concentration in plasma and effect-site for any given dose. Simulation programs are wonderful tools for pharmacology education. Their clinical application may be separated into 3 areas; an area that deals with delay and duration of action after a short period of administration (induction, short cases), that deals with optimisation of recovery after long-term use and an area that deals with adjustment of the administration of agents to specific groups of patients.

3.1. Use of PK models for induction or short term procedures

The pharmacokinetic models that incorporate the effect-compartment may be used to evaluate the time from an intravenous bolus dose to its maximal effect (Tmax, Figure 1 bottom)[4]. This indicates the time period for a bolus to be anticipated before the maximum effect is available. For example, it illustrates why remifentanil or alfentanil are suitable for response suppression to strong and short duration stimuli like intubation, endoscopy, or bone fracture repositioning (Figure 2). It also shows the decay in the blood and effect site concentrations after a bolus, suggesting that fentanyl and sufentanil better be given by repeated bolus dosing, whereas alfentanil and remifentanil may better be administered by continuous infusion for procedures longer than a few minutes. Finally, simulating the time course of the effect-site concentration after a bolus dose shows how increasing the dose may shorten the onset but increase the duration of action. This has been widely used for choosing the size of the dose of muscle relaxants. This resulted in the classical selection of the dose for muscle relaxants of twice the ED_{95} for intubation as the optimal balance between a short onset to intubation and a reasonable duration of action to avoid postoperative residual blockade. But everybody knows that the dose may be doubled for a rapid sequence intubation.

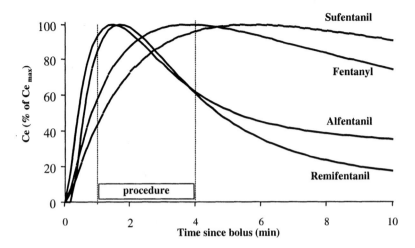

Figure 2. Computer simulation of the time to peak effect after a bolus dose of fentanyl, alfentanil, sufentanil and remifentanil.

3.2. Optimising recovery after long time administration

At medical school the duration of action was taught to be constant for each anaesthetic drug, and was related to the elimination of the drug from the body. PK-PD modelling, however, shows that adequate anaesthesia is achieved above a given threshold concentration, while recovery takes place below another concentration ("the MAC awake" or its intravenous equivalent EC_{50} for return to consciousness). At recovery a substantial amount of drug is still present in the body. The time span from the anaesthesia maintenance concentration to the recovery concentration depends on the height of the respective concentrations and the decay of the drug in the body, which is governed by redistribution, and the clearance of the drug and the duration of administration.

The influence of the drug characteristics and the infusion duration on the recovery is best illustrated by the concept of the context-sensitive half-time (CSHT, Figure 1) described 10 years ago.[5] The context-sensitive half-time is the time required for the plasma concentration to decrease by 50 % after termination of the infusion of a drug. It increases markedly with the duration of infusion when the drug accumulates early in the body as for fentanyl. Conversely, it is low and insensitive to infusion duration when a drug does not accumulate and is eliminated rapidly like remifentanil does. This concept explains why remifentanil is especially suitable for prolonged infusion when a fast recovery is desired. For example in severe COPD or obese patients. Alfentanil and sufentanil may be suitable for long infusion when intermediate delay of recovery is possible and fentanyl continuous infusion may be less suitable when postoperative ventilation is absolutely undesirable. It can also explain why propofol is suitable for maintenance of anaesthesia and thiopental is not.

The context-sensitive half-time gives an estimate of the time to recovery only when the maintenance concentration is twice the recovery concentration; clinically this is often not true. Therefore, the concept of the CSHT has been extended. Beside the time required for a 50% in concentration, the decrement time has been defined as the time after termination of infusion required to have the concentration fall by any percent[6] (Figure 3). This parameter, determined by computer simulation, is helpful clinically in the selection of the proper drug and the desired concentration for various effects reckoning with the consequences of this choice on the recovery time. This has been nicely described for the various opioids by Shafer et al. In case of minor surgery e.g. with little postoperative pain, a concentration above the recovery concentration by 20% may be sufficient. In that case, there is no difference between fentanyl, alfentanil or sufentanil regarding recovery time up to 120 minutes of surgery and any of the 4 opioids can be used (Figure 3, top). If the surgical stimulus is stronger, opioid concentration around twice the recovery concentration may be chosen, but the physician must be aware that postoperative mechanical ventilation may be necessary with fentanyl, and that sufentanil allows faster recovery than alfentanil up to 8 hours of infusion (Figure 3, middle). When analgesia is the main concern and postoperative sedation is not a problem as in cardiac surgery, opioid concentrations 4 fold above the recovery concentration may be applied. Simulation shows that after these high opioid concentrations recovery may be faster using alfentanil than sufentanil for surgery longer than 2 hours. This notion is not very much used in clinical practice! (Figure 3, bottom). Finally, the calculation of decrement time shows the specific behaviour of remifentanil compared to the other opioids. Remifentanil offers an advantage when rapid recovery is the main concern, but the fast disappearance of all the opioid effects must be anticipated especially when postoperative pain might be expected.

3.3. Adjusting to special populations

Another application of pharmacokinetic modelling is to evaluate the influence of variables as weight or age on the time course of concentration and effect. Unfortunately, most of the initial pharmacokinetic studies published on anaesthetic agents did not include obese patients or patients with extremes of age. Some did a classical analysis describing a set of parameters for young adults next to another set for the elderly. The use of these models is limited because for anaesthetics in patients with intermediate ages interpolation between models then is necessary and may be inaccurate.

The most useful models to incorporate in simulation software programmes express the physiological variables as a covariate of the model as determined by population pharmacokinetic analysis.[7-10] Models including physiological variables are very relevant in clinical practice because they show how much the dose should be modified in special populations of patients to achieve a desired concentration. This has been illustrated for remifentanil in Figure 4. Until now, only simple and constant variables like age, weight, gender or lean body mass have been included in simulation programmes for intravenous drugs. Varying parameters as cardiac output are included in simulation software for volatile agents as Gasman[TM]. For intravenous drugs, these physiological variables have rarely been determined in association with pharmacokinetic analysis and are only used in physiological models and rarely by routine physicians.

4. CLINICAL BENEFITS OF PHARMACODYNAMIC MODELLING

Pharmacodynamic models describe the mathematical relationship between the concentration of a drug and its effect, and the probability of effect for binary effects like response to incision or to verbal command. Pharmacodynamic modelling caused a change of mind in the past. Anaesthetists stopped to describe the effects of a drug as a function of the dose (since this relationship is changing every second) but started to control the concentration on one hand, and assess the corresponding response on the other hand. Then, they had to decide if the response was adequate, and if it was not, they adjusted the dose not as a final goal but in order to increase or decrease the concentration. This process improved the management of intravenous anaesthetics close to the delivery of volatile agents. Nobody cares about the number of millilitres of volatile agent given, but the dose delivered is adjusted to achieve a chosen end-tidal fraction and to maintain the level of anaesthesia considered to be adequate.

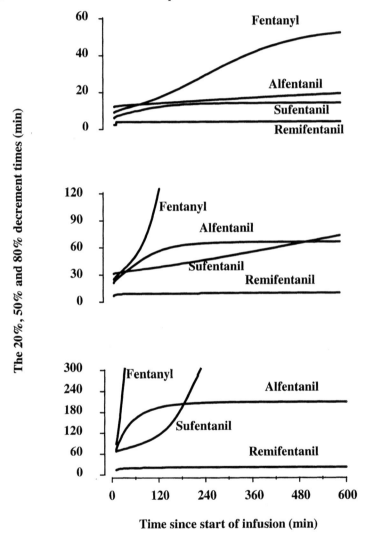

Figure 3. Computer simulation of the decay in the opioid blood concentration after termination of the infusion of up to 600 min to reach 20%, 50% or 80% of the initial concentration after termination of an infusion of fentanyl, alfentanil, sufentanil and remifentanil. With permission of S. Shafer, website, table 1.

Pharmacodynamic modelling allowed an insight in clinically important features of the concentration-effect relationship. Pharmacodynamic research revealed that the requirements differ with the effect considered. The opioid concentration necessary for intubation is higher than for incision[11] and the concentration of a muscle relaxant to block the diaphragm or the larynx is higher than to block the peripheral muscles of the hand.[12] That is why at any time of anaesthesia, the dose should be adjusted to achieve the adequate concentration for the current surgical procedure. The efficacy of a drug is influenced by physiological variables as age; for example the adequate concentrations are reduced by about 50% in elderly patients for all μ-opioids[13] and by 30% for propofol.[14] The time to equilibration between blood and effect site (brain) is longer in elderly for remifentanil.[13] Similarly, this is true for the haemodynamic effects of propofol.[15] These data suggest that induction in elderly patients should aim at lower concentration than in younger adults, and to achieve these less rapidly to avoid side effects.

The second major clinical interest in pharmacodynamic modelling has lead to the study of interactions between drugs. The most relevant interaction in anaesthesia is the synergism between hypnotics (intravenous or volatile) and opioids. This can be displayed as a 3 dimensional surface with on the x and y axes the drug concentrations and on the z-axis the effect.[16] Just as for the concentration-effect relationship of single agents, the concentration-effect relationship of combinations differs with the effect considered. Opioids reduce only moderately the concentration of the hypnotic necessary to induce loss of consciousness (30 to 50%).[17] They markedly reduce (60-85%) the concentration of the hypnotic needed to block motor response to surgical stimulation. The maximal synergism is observed when considering the haemodynamic response to noxious stimuli (up to 90% reduction).[18] It is important to note that potentiation also is present for side effects as hypotension[19] or respiratory depression.

For every surgical event and every type of response, several combinations of concentrations may provide adequate anaesthesia. To maintain a non-moving patient in haemodynamic stability, any point on the iso-effective curve is good. Below the curve, the patient may show signs of light anaesthesia, and above the curve signs of over dosage. If the level of noxious stimulation changes rapidly, it may be advantageous to shift the balanced anaesthesia to the faster responding drug. This is to the opioid side (Figure 5) with remifentanil of alfentanil, or to the hypnotic side with propofol, desflurane or sevoflurane. If fast recovery and discharge are the main concern, the balance better is shifted to the drug having the faster elimination.

These applications of drug interaction data have been nicely illustrated by Vuyk et al. who performed simulations of anaesthesia for gynaecologic surgery and recovery with opioids and propofol.[20] These authors concluded that when fentanyl is used, because of its decrement time being much longer than that of propofol, the fastest recovery would be obtained with an excess of propofol (see Figure 5). With alfentanil or sufentanil, agents that exhibit a decrement time similar to propofol, fastest recovery was achieved for a balanced combination.

Whereas, with remifentanil (fast decrement time compared to propofol whatever the duration of infusion), the fastest recovery was obtained with a high opioid-low propofol combination. In summary, pharmacodynamic modelling during balanced anaesthesia can help the anaesthetist to select the optimal strategy of drug administration.

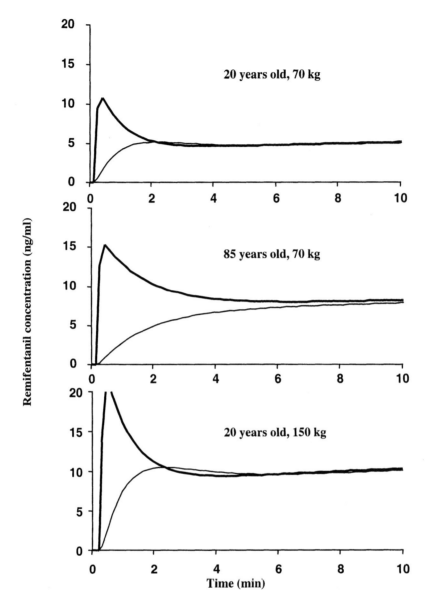

Figure 4. Computer simulation of the remifentanil plasma (bold lines) and effect site (thin lines) concentration in 3 patients with different characteristics who received intravenous remifentanil 1 μg/kg followed by 0.25 μg/kg/min. The pharmacokinetic data used in the simulation were adjusted on the basis of the pharmacokinetic parameter set by Minto et al.[8]

5. PK-PD MODELLING FOR DRUG ADMINISTRATION OPTIMISATION

Three clinical applications of PK-PD models have been used in anaesthesia to control the administration of the drug given. The first one, target controlled infusion, is already widely used in routine practice, at least for propofol. The others, Bayesian adjustment and closed loop control, are still limited to prototypes and research protocols but could come to the routine practice in the next future if the regulatory requirements are met.

5.1. Target controlled infusion

When pharmacodynamic models describe the adequate concentrations of all drugs for every surgical procedure, the anaesthetist may choose a concentration to achieve and maintain and have a dedicated software programme calculate the required dose. This is the basis of target-controlled infusion (TCI). Described more than 30 years ago,[21] this technique has been further developed during the last 20 years through several prototypes in Germany,[22,23] The Netherlands,[24] and USA.[25-28] Then, TCI has moved from the scientific scene into routine practice for propofol with the development by Zeneca of a dedicated medical device, the Diprifusor™ which was CE approved in 1996.[29, 30] Today, there is no need to define TCI. Several reviews have described this technique[31-33] and most of the anaesthetists in Europe either practice TCI or at least have been told about it (see chapter by Glen).

Propofol TCI has been widely used in routine practice. From anaesthesia for minor procedures,[34] to anaesthesia for cardiac surgery[36] where it has been very helpful for early extubation.[37] It has also been proposed for sedation during local or regional anaesthesia,[38] as well as for endoscopy or fiberoptic intubation when spontaneous ventilation is essential. TCI has shown several clinical benefits related to an improved adjustment of the drug effect over time. For propofol, TCI reduced the incidence of movements during surgery[39;40] and decreased the number of human interventions.[40,41] It didn't save drug dose[39,40,42] but shortened the time to discharge from the recovery room[41] and decreased the incidence of postoperative nausea and vomiting compared to manual infusion.[42] It has been described as easy to use with a minimal training, and most of the anaesthetists who used it for scientific studies continued to use it afterwards.[39]

For opioid administration, TCI improved haemodynamic stability because the opioid concentration could be titrated better at any surgical time.[25,43,44] TCI has also been proposed in ICU for propofol or midazolam sedation and reduces the interindividual variability of the sedation score.[45] TCI may target either the plasma (as the Diprifusor™ does), or the effect site.[46] Targeting the effect-site shortens the time to achieve the effect compared to a plasma targeting technique.[47] It is necessarily associated with an initial overshot of the plasma concentration that may theoretically be detrimental, but this risk has never been clinically demonstrated, and could likely be avoided by careful titration in fragile patients. Most of the simulation programs mentioned (Table 1) are capable of controlling a syringe pump in TCI mode and can target either the plasma or the effect site. However, all are systems not approved for clinical use apart from research with specific approval. To get CE approved for TCI, the device needs to be submitted to a risk and safety analysis, and the recommended target concentration needs to be added to the regulatory recommendations.[30]

5.2. Bayesian adaptation

Both pharmacokinetic and dynamic responses in an individual often differ from the model established in a population. When the population PK-PD model is coupled to a quantitative assessment of the concentration or effect in an individual, the model can be adjusted to this individual. This is known as the Bayesian approach. Bayesian techniques are well known to improve the administration of antibiotics and antineoplasic agents. But these drugs generally are given in repeated doses over longer periods of time. This setting thus allows for adjustments to plasma assays that need several hours to be performed. Conversely, adjustment of anaesthesia cannot wait for a classical drug assay since the result would show up far after the patient's recovery or discharge! One study described the theoretical benefit of the Bayesian approach to improve the kinetic model of alfentanil, but it was retrospective of nature.[48] The Bayesian technique thus may be clinically helpful for the improvement of kinetic models only if associated with fast assays, available in a few minutes. Another use of the Bayesian approach in anaesthesia would be to measure the effect and adjust the whole PK-PD population model according to this measurement. This could be done in real time for muscle relaxants[46,49] and for hypnotics using EEG parameters. The Bayesian adjustment could be controlled manually as in Stanpump or included in an automatic closed loop.

Table 1. Some of the simulation software programmes available. All can be used in conventional infusion and TCI mode. In TCI mode all are capable of targeting the plasma and the effect site, and some can target the EEG effect (Rugloop, next version) or the level of neuromuscular blockade (Stanpump).

Name	Author and request address	Drugs included and specific features
Stanpump	S.L. Shafer http://anesthesia.stanford.edu/pkpd	Most intravenous agents, run 1 pump Several models per drug Bayesian for NMBA
Stelpump	J. Coetzee http://anesthesia.stanford.edu/pkpd	Most intravenous agents, runs 2 pumps Few models per drug
Rugloop	M. Struys http://allserv.rug.ac.be/~mstruys	Most intravenous agents. Several models and drugs, also data management (Datex AS3, BIS, Anemon)
Tivatrainer	F. Engbers http://www.eurosiva.org	Hypnotics & opioids, 1 model and drug Including PD interaction model
Toolbox	L. Barvais lbarvais@ulb.ac.be	Most intravenous anaesthetic & vasoactive agents, runs several pumps Few models per drug
PAMO	X. Viviand xviviand@ap-hm.fr	Hypnotics & opioids Runs several pumps Several models per drug
Gasman	J. Philips http://www.gasmanweb.com	Volatile anaesthetic agents only Simulation only Adjustable cardiac output & ventilation

5.3. Closed-loop control

When the effect of a drug can be measured and the measured parameter automatically transmitted to the infusion controller software, the dose or the target concentration then may be adjusted by iterations to minimize the difference between the desired and observed effect, realizing a closed-loop. The adjustment could be done directly on the dose, using simple controllers as in industrial processes (Proportional, Proportional-Derivative, Proportional-Integral-Derivative) or by fuzzy logic controllers.[49] However, this technique needs repeated measurements during the procedure, and loss of the signal could result in inappropriate dose adjustments.

The second way to build a closed-loop system is to adjust not the dose but the pharmacokinetic or dynamic model according to the measured value. This has been described for hypnotics using, as a quantitative effect, spectral analysis of EEG,[50] BIS[51] or auditory evoked potentials.[52] In these studies, quite stable anaesthesia could be maintained. This methodology has also been proposed for the administration of muscle relaxants.[46] Theoretically, this approach is more robust than a closed loop adjusting the dose, because it can reduce the interindividual variability and adjust the model to each patient using very few measurements. Then, even if the measured effect is lost, the model is still adjusted to this patient, and the anaesthetic level should remain stable. However, the influence of the opioid and the surgical stimulation on the EEG parameters and subsequently on the adjustment of the model is difficult to describe and should be further studied before a routine use in clinical conditions.

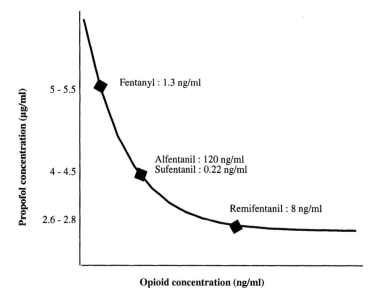

Figure 5. Propofol-opioid interaction for intraoperative adequacy of anaesthesia as adapted from Vuyk et al.[17,][20] Opioid concentration greatly diminishes propofol requirements for loss of consciousness. Similarly, with increasing propofol cooncentration less opioid is needed for adequate intraoperative anaesthesia

6. CONCLUSION

At this stage of pharmacology research, PK-PD modelling is an essential tool in the understanding of the behaviour of anaesthetic drugs in the body. At the bedside, PK-PD models may be used through simulation software programmes to display the predicted concentration and the effect and thus allow for a rational choice of the drug and the required dose. PK-PD models give to the anaesthetist the opportunity to widen his/her horizon and improve the insight into the dose-concentration–effect relationship. This will allow the anaesthesiologist to optimise the onset, stability and offset of the delivered anaesthetic in clinical practice, especially through target controlled infusion devices.

7. REFERENCES

1. E. Gepts, S.L. Shafer, F. Camu, D.R. Stanski, R. Woestenborghs, A. Van Peer, J.J.P. Heykants, Linearity of pharmacokinetics and model estimation of sufentanil, *Anesthesiology* **83**, 1194-240 (1995).
2. S.L. Shafer, D.R. Stanski, Improving the clinical utility of anesthetic drug pharmacokinetics. *Anesthesiology* **76**, 327-30 (1992).
3. L.B. Sheiner, D.R. Stanski, S. Vozeh, J. Ham, R.D. Miller, Simultaneous modeling of pharmacokinetics and pharmacodynamics: Application to d-tubocurarine, *Clinical Pharmacology and Therapeutics* **25**, 358-71 (1979).
4. S.L. Shafer, J.R. Varvel, Pharmacokinetics, pharmacodynamics and rational opioid selection. *Anesthesiology* **74**: 53-63 (1991).
5. M.A. Hughes, P.S.A. Glass, J.R. Jacobs, Context-sensitive half-time in multicompartment pharmacokinetic models for intravenous anesthetic drugs, *Anesthesiology* **76**, 334-41 (1992).
6. T.W. Schnider, S.L. Shafer, Evolving clinically useful predictors of recovery from intravenous anesthetics, *Anesthesiology* **83**, 902-5 (1995).
7. P.O. Maitre, S. Vozeh, J. Heykants, J.A. Thomson, D.R. Stanski, Population pharmacokinetics of alfentanil: average dose-plasma concentration relationship and interindividual variability, *Anesthesiology* **66**, 3-12 (1987).
8. C.F. Minto, T.W. Schnider, T.D. Egan, E. Youngs, H. Lemmens, P.L. Gambus, V. Billard, J.F. Hoke, K. Moore, D.J. Herman, K.T. Muir, J. Mandema, S.L. Shafer, Influence of age and gender on the pharmacokinetics and pharmacodynamics of remifentanil. I. Model development, *Anesthesiology* **86**, 10-23 (1997).
9. T.W. Schnider, C.F. Minto, P.L. Gambus, C. Andresen, D.B. Goodale, S.L. Shafer, E.J. Youngs, The influence of method of administration and covariates on the pharmacokinetics of propofol in adult volunteers, *Anesthesiology* **88**, 1170-82 (1998).
10. J. Schuttler, H. Ihmsen, Population pharmacokinetics of propofol: a multicenter study. *Anesthesiology* **92**, 727-38 (2000).
11. M.E. Ausems, C.C. Hug Jr, D.R. Stanski, A.G.L. Burm, Plasma concentrations of alfentanil required to supplement nitrous oxide anesthesia for general surgery, *Anesthesiology* **65**, 362-73 (1986).
12. F. Donati, B. Plaud, C. Meistelman, Vecuronium neuromuscular blockade at the adductor muscles of the larynx and adductor pollicis, *Anesthesiology* **74**, 833-7, (1991).
13. C.F. Minto, T.W. Schnider, S.L. Shafer, Pharmacokinetics and pharmacodynamics of remifentanil. II. Model application, *Anesthesiology* **86**: 240-244, (1997).
14. T.W. Schnider, C.F. Minto, S.L. Shafer, P.L. Gambus, C. Andresen, D.B. Goodale, E.J. Youngs, The influence of age on propofol pharmacodynamics, *Anesthesiology* **90**, 1502-16 (1990).
15. T. Kazama, K. Ikeda, K. Morita, M. Kikura, M. Doi, T. Ikeda, T. Kurita, Y. Nakajima, Comparison of the effect-site k(e0)s of propofol for blood pressure and EEG bispectral index in elderly and younger patients, *Anesthesiology* **90**, 1517-27 (1999).
16. C.F. Minto, T.W. Schnider, T.G. Short, K.M. Gregg, A. Gentilini, S.L. Shafer, Response surface model for anesthetic drug interactions, *Anesthesiology* **92**, 1603-16 (2000).
17. J. Vuyk, F. Engbers, A.G. Burm, A. Vletter, G.E.R. Griever, E. Olofsen, J.G. Bovill, Pharmacodynamic interaction between propofol and alfentanil given for induction of anesthesia, *Anesthesiology* **84**, 288-99 (1996).
18. T. Katoh, K. Ikeda, The effect od fentanyl on sevoflurane requirements for loss of consciousness and skin incision, *Anesthesiology* **88**, 18-24 (1998).
19. V. Billard, F. Moulla, J.L. Bourgain, A. Megnibeto, D.R. Stanski, Hemodynamic response to induction and intubation. Propofol/fentanyl interaction, *Anesthesiology* **81** (1994)

20. J. Vuyk, M.J. Mertens, E. Olofsen, A.G.L. Burm, J.G. Bovill, Propofol Anesthesia and Rational Opioid Selection: Determination of Optimal EC50-EC95 Propofol-Opioid Concentrations that Assure Adequate Anesthesia and a Rapid Return of Consciousness, *Anesthesiology* **87**, 1549-62 (1997).

21. E. Kruger-Thiemer, Continuous intravenous infusion and multicompartment accumulation, *Eur J Pharmacol.* **4**, 317-24 (1986).

22. H. Schwilden, A general method for calculating the dosage scheme in linear pharmacokinetics, *Eur J Clin Pharmacol.* **20**, 379-86 (1981).

23. J. Schuttler, H. Schwilden, H. Stoekel, Pharmacokinetics as applied to total intravenous anaesthesia. Practical implications, *Anaesthesia* **38** Suppl: 53-6 (1983).

24. M.E. Ausems, D.R. Stanski, C.C. Hug, An Evaluation of the Accuracy of Pharmacokinetic Data for the Computer Assisted Infusion of Alfentanil, *Br.J.Anaesth.* **57**, 1217-25 (1985).

25. J.M. Alvis, J.G. Reves, A.V. Govier, P.G. Menkhaus, C.E. Henling, J.A. Spain, E. Bradley, Computer-assisted Continuous Infusions of Fentanyl during Cardiac Anesthesia : Comparison with a Manual Method, *Anesthesiology* **63**, 41-9 (1985).

26. J.R. Jacobs, Analytical solution to the three-compartment pharmacokinetic model, *IEEE Trans.Biomed.Eng* **35**, 763-5 (1988).

27. S.L. Shafer, L.C. Siegel, J.E. Cooke, J.C. Scott, Testing Computer-controlled Infusion Pumps by Simulation, *Anesthesiology* **68**, 261-6 (1988).

28. P.O. Maitre, S.L. Shafer, A Simple Pocket Calculator Approach to Predict Anesthetic Drug Concentrations from Pharmacokinetic Data, *Anesthesiology* **73**, 332-6 (1990).

29. M. White, G.N.C. Kenny, Intravenous propofol anaesthesia using a computerised infusion system, *Anaesthesia* **45**, 204-8 (1990).

30. J.B. Glenn, The development of 'Diprifusor': a TCI system for propofol, *Anaesthesia* **53**, Suppl 1: 13-21 (1988).

31. V. Billard, J.B. Cazalaa, F. Servin, X. Viviand, Anesthésie intraveineuse à objectif de concentration, *Ann Fr Anesth Réan* **16**, 250-73 (1997).

32. E. Gepts, Pharmacokinetic concepts for TCI anaesthesia, *Anaesthesia* **53**, 4-12 (1998).

33. M.C. van den Nieuwenhuyzen, F.H. Engbers, J. Vuyk, A.G.L. Burm, Target-controlled infusion systems: role in anaesthesia and analgesia, *Clin Pharmacokinet.* **38**, 181-90 (2000).

34. S. Chaudri, M. White, G.N. Kenny, Induction of anaesthesia with propofol using a target-controlled infusion system, *Anaesthesia* **47**, 553 (1992).

35. K.R. Watson, SM.Shah, Clinical comparison of 'single agent' anaesthesia with sevoflurane versus target controlled infusion of propofol, *Br J Anaesth* **85**, 541-6 (2000).

36. L. Barvais, I. Rausin, J.B. Glen, S.C. Hunter, D. D'Hulster, F. Cantraine, A. D'Hollander, Administration of propofol by target-controlled infusion in patients undergoing coronary artery surgery, *Journal of Cardiothoracic and Vascular Anesthesia* **10**, 877-83 (1996).

37. P. Olivier, D. Sirieix, P. Dassier, N. D'Attellis, J.F. Baron, Continuous infusion of remifentanil and target-controlled infusion of propofol for patients undergoing cardiac surgery: a new approach for scheduled early extubation, *J Cardiothorac.Vasc.Anesth* **14**, 29-35 (2000).

38. C. Newson, G.P. Joshi, R. Victory, P.F. White, Comparison of propofol administration techniques for sedation during monitored anesthesia care, *Anesthesia & Analgesia* **81**, 486-91(1995).

39. D. Russell, M.P.Wilkes, S.C. Hunter, P. Hutton, G.N. Kenny, Manual compared with target-controlled infusion of propofol, *Br.J.Anaesth.* **75**, 562-6 (1995).

40. F. Servin. TCI compared with manually controlled infusion of propofol: a multicentre study, *Anaesthesia* **53** Suppl 1, 82-6 (1998).

41. C. Newson, G.P. Joshi, R. Victory, P.F. White, Comparison of propofol administration techniques for sedation during monitored anesthesia care, *Anesth.Analg.* **81**, 486-91 (1995).

42. S. Suttner, J. Boldt, C. Schmidt, S. Piper, B. Kumle, Cost analysis of target-controlled infusion-based anesthesia compared with standard anesthesia regimens, *Anesth.Analg.* **88**, 77-82 (1999).

43. M.E. Ausems, J. Vuyk, C.C. Hug Jr, D.R. Stanski, Comparison of a computer-assisted infusion versus intermittent bolus administration of alfentanil as a supplement to nitrous oxide for lower abdominal surgery, *Anesthesiology* **68**, 851-61 (1988).

44. V. Billard, A. Deleuze, C. Penot, C. Lohberger, F. Kolb, D. Elias, [Sufentanil in balanced anesthesia: need to predict concentrations for dose optimization], *Ann Fr Anesth Reanim* **18**, 237-42 (1999)

45. J. Somma, A. Donner, K. Zomorodi, R. Sladen, J. Ramsay, E. Geller, S.L. Shafer, Population pharmacodynamics of midazolam administered by target controlled infusion in SICU patients after CABG surgery, *Anesthesiology* **89**, 1430-43 (1998).

46. S.L. Shafer, Stanpump manual.

47. J.G. Bovill, Targetting the effect site, On the study and practice of intravenous anaesthesia, Edited by Vuyk J, Engbers F, Groen-Mulder S. Dordrecht, Kluwer Academic Publishers, pp 17-26 (2000).

48. P.O. Maitre, D.R. Stanski, Bayesian forecasting improves the prediction of intraoperative plasma concentrations of alfentanil, *Anesthesiology* **69**, 652-9 (1988).
49. V. Billard, P. Mavoungou, Computer-controlled infusion of neuromuscular blocking agents, On the study and practice of intravenous anaesthesia. Edited by Vuyk J, Engbers F, Groen-Mulder S. Dordrecht, Kluwer Academic Publishers, pp 159-72 (2000).
50. H. Schwilden, H. Stoeckel, J. Schüttler, Closed-loop feedback control of Propofol anaesthesia by quantitative EEG analysis in humans, *Br J Anaesth* **62**, 290-6 (1989).
51. E. Mortier, M. Struys, T. De Smet, L. Versichelen, G. Rolly, Closed-loop controlled administration of propofol using bispectral analysis, *Anaesthesia* **53**, 749-54 (1998).
52. G.N.C. Kenny, H. Mantzaridis, Closed-loop control of propofol anaesthesia, *Br J Anaesth* **83**, 223-8 (1999).

GENDER DIFFERENCES IN MORPHINE PHARMACOKINETICS AND DYNAMICS

Elise Sarton, Raymonda Romberg and Albert Dahan[*]

1. INTRODUCTION

The opioid system, composed of a family of structurally related endogenous peptides acting at μ-, δ- and κ-opioid receptors, μOR, δOR and κOR, is involved in responses to pain, stress, reward and emotion and has a modulatory influence on physiological functions such as the control of breathing, thermoregulation, nociception and the immune response.[1] The opioid system displays marked differences among individuals with respect to its pharmacological and physiological effects. Evidently, this is the cause of the large variable effects of opioids in the delivery of adequate analgesia in patients with acute and chronic pain. Animal studies, particularly those using inbred strains of mice and rats, show that this variability is related, in part, to genetic differences in pain sensitivity, in the analgesic potency of exogenously administrated opioids, and in the response of the endogenous opioid system to pain and stress.[2-4] Recent studies revealed the importance of sex-related differences in the analgesic/antinociceptive responses of opioids. For example, male rats are more sensitive to the antinociceptive properties of morphine compared to female animals.[5] Strain- and sex-differences are not restricted to the analgesic properties of opioids, but also involve other opioid-mediated behaviour, such as locomotor activity, respiration, learning, memory, and addiction. Prospective human studies on the interaction of sex and opioid effect are scarce. An overview of studies investigating gender and opioid effect is given in Table 1. Here we describe the effects of gender on morphine's pharmacokinetics and pharmacodynamics. The emphasis of this chapter will be on prospective placebo-controlled analgesic and respiratory studies.

[*] E. Sarton et al. Department of Anaesthesiology, Leiden University Medical Center, Leiden, The Netherlands

Advances in Modelling and Clinical Application of Intravenous Anaesthesia
Edited by Vuyk and Schraag, Kluwer Academic/Plenum Publishers, 2003

2. MORPHINE AND ITS MECHANISM OF ACTION

Morphine is the prototype μ-opioid receptor agonist. In humans, morphine remains the most valuable drug to alleviate acute and chronic pain, despite the occurrence of sometimes-serious acute and chronic adverse effects such as sedation, nausea, respiratory depression, tolerance and addiction. The involvement of the μOR in morphine-induced antinociception and respiratory depression has recently been shown.

Table 1. Effect of μ- and κ-opioids and placebo in men versus women

Authors	Year	Setting	Type*	End-point:	Greater/ faster in
Gordon *et al.*[9]	1995	morphine after molar extraction surgery	pro	pain relief	no difference
Gear *et al.*[10]	1996	pentazocine (κ-agonist) after molar extraction	pro	pain relief	women
Minto *et al.*[11]	1997	remifentanil effect on EEG in volunteers	pro	C_{50} of 95% spectral edge frequency	no difference
Drover & Lemmens [12]	1998	abdominal anesthesia with 66% N_2O in patients	pro	remifentanil concentration for adequate anesthesia	women
Miakowski & Levine [13]	1999	review of 18 studies on PCA morphine	retro	opioid consumption	men
Dahan *et al.*[14] Sarton *et al.*[15]	1989 1999	0.13 mg/kg morphine given to volunteers	po	effect on ventilatory CO_2 and hypoxic response	women
Gan *et al.*[16]	1999	recovery from alfentanil/propofol/N_2O anesthesia	retro	wake-up time	women
Butterworth *et al.*[17]	2000	post coronary artery surgery	pro	duration of postoperative intubation	women
Sarton *et al.*[18]	2000	0.13 mg/kg morphine given to volunteers	pro	opioid potency	women
Zacny [19]	2001	10 mg/kg morphine given to volunteers	retro	subjective effects	women
Averbuch & Katzper [20]	2001	placebo after molar surgery	retro	pain relief	no difference
Romberg *et al.*[21]	2002	0.3 mg/kg M6G	pro	opioid potency	women

* pro = prospective, retro = retrospective; M6G = morphine-6-glucuronide

Knockout mice lacking exon 2 of the μ-opioid receptor gene show no analgesic or respiratory responses to high dose morphine (up to 100 mg/kg) or its active metabolite, morphine-6-glucuronide (up to 40 mg/kg).[6-8] See also Figure 2. Interestingly, the mice without μOR's displayed higher resting breathing frequencies suggesting an inhibitory role for μ-opioid receptors and their endogenous ligands in respiratory rhythmogenesis. Furthermore, anaesthetic potency was less in the knockout mice relative to their wild type littermates (*i.e.*, mice with intact μOR's). Overall, these data suggest the μ-OR gene product is essential for generating morphine's antinociceptive and respiratory effects and suggest further the absence of involvement of δ- and κ-opioid receptors.

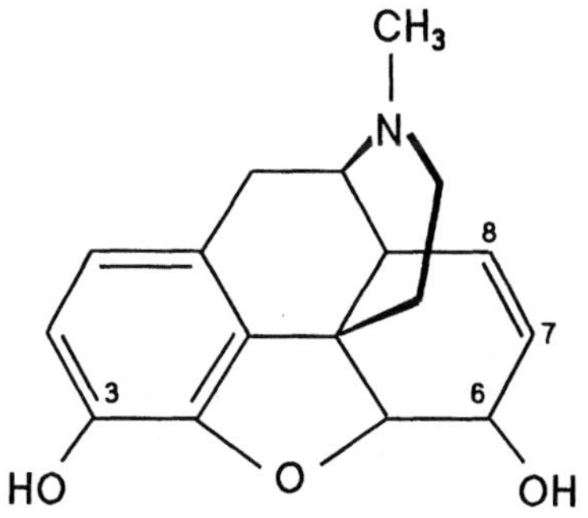

Figure 1. The structure formulation of morphine

However, some caution is needed before definite conclusions can be drawn. These knockout mice lacked the μOR gene throughout development. Functional compensations may have –partly— masked the phenotype resulting from the long-term absence of the gene. Furthermore, it may well be that δ-activity is dependent on functional μ-receptors.[22] Presently, the following morphine effects are thought to be related to exon 2 of the μ-opioid receptor: analgesia (spinal and supra-spinal), hyper-locomotion, reward, withdrawal, inhibition of gastro-intestinal transport, immunosuppression, increase of anaesthetic potency, hypothermia and respiratory depression. In humans, but not in mice and most rat strains, morphine is metabolised to the active opioid morphine-6-glucuronide (M6G) and the inactive compound morphine-3-glucuronide (M3G). Recent studies in exon 1 μOR knockout mice indicate that M6G acts at a splice variant of the μOR.[23] In this mouse strain, morphine is inactive while M6G and heroin show analgesic activity. Whether these findings are relevant to humans remains unknown.

3. ABSENCE OF GENDER DIFFERENCES IN THE PHARMACOKINETICS OF MORPHINE

Gender effects may have PK or PD grounds. We therefore initially assessed plasma morphine, M6G and M3G concentrations in 10 healthy and young men and 10 healthy and young women after intravenous morphine administration (bolus dose = 0.1 mg/kg followed by a continuous infusion of 0.03 mg/kg per h for 1-h).[18]

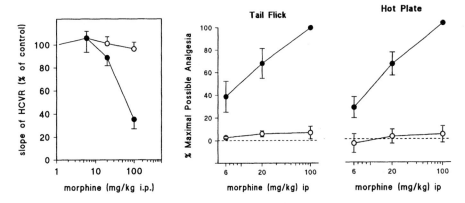

Figure 2. Effect of morphine on the slope of the hypercapnic ventilatory response (HCVR, left), and morphine pain responses (right) in the tail immersion and hot plate tests in μ-OR knockout mice (B) and their wild type littermates (•). Data from ref. 7

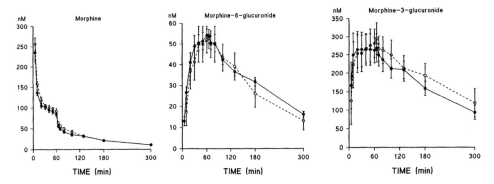

Figure 3. Morphine, morphine-6-glucuronide and morphine-3-glucuronide plasma concentrations after a bolus of 0.1 mg/kg and a continuous infusion of 0.03 mg/kg per h for 1-h in healthy men (closed symbols) and women (open symbols). Data from ref. 18.

The results of this study are given in figure 3, showing no difference between the concentration of the three tested compounds over time between men and women. A PK analysis was performed on the morphine *versus* time data using a three-compartmental model with rate constant k and weight normalized V_1 (analysis performed using a population approach with NONMEM). Inclusion of the covariate sex, age, weight or lean body mass did not improve the model fits ($P > 0.01$). The population parameters (± SE) and measures of interindividual variability (% CV or percentage coefficient of variation) are collected in table 2.

These findings indicate that gender differences after intravenous morphine are not related to differences in blood concentrations of morphine, M6G or M3G. Furthermore, the peak concentrations of M6G after a bolus or a short term infusion of morphine are relatively low (< 100 nM). Much higher concentrations of M6G are needed (> 1000 nM) for significant analgesic effects to occur.[21]

4. MORPHINE PHARMACODYNAMICS

4.1 Sex Differences in Morphine Analgesia: Occurrence and Mechanisms

We designed a prospective study to compare the analgesic effects of a bolus and short (1-h) infusion of morphine in healthy men and women by measuring the pain threshold and tolerance using an experimental pain model (electrical transcutaneous pain).[18] Also arterial blood concentrations of morphine were obtained allowing us to perform PK/PD modelling. The model we used consists of (1) a part that describes the pharmacokinetics (see above), (2) a part that describes the time lag between morphine plasma concentrations and effect-site concentrations, and (3) a part that translate the effect-site concentration into analgesic effect. Using thus approach we will get informed on the effect of gender on morphine's rate constant, $t\frac{1}{2}k_{e0}$, and potency parameter, C_{50}. We assumed that morphine was the sole cause of analgesic effect (and not M6G, see above), that complete analgesia is possible and further that morphine causes the attenuation of pain signal propagation or central pain signal processing.

Table 2. Morphine pharmacokinetic parameters of the 3-compartment model.

	Value	SE	% CV
V_1 (L/kg)	0.075	0.034	13
k_{10} (min^{-1})	0.300	0.115	12
k_{12} (min^{-1})	0.183	0.098	11
k_{21} (min^{-1})	0.087	0.055	20
k_{13} (min^{-1})	0.290	0.144	14
k_{31} (min^{-1})	0.013	0.002	18

The averaged currents inducing pain tolerance data are given in figure 4. It shows the greater effect of morphine in women, compared to men. The PK/PD analysis revealed that morphine's potency was greater in women ($P < 0.01$; Table 3), while its effect on $t\frac{1}{2}k_{e0}$ indicated a slower speed of onset and offset in women ($P < 0.01$; Table 3). Evidently, these findings have major clinical implications and confirm earlier (retrospective) findings on postoperative PCA morphine consumption in men and women (Table 1).

The mechanism of these differences remains obscure but is likely related to differences in opioid receptor density or affinity in brain sites involved in pain control.[24] These differences are possibly related to long term developmental and organizational effects of sex steroids that occur in prenatal and early postnatal life, causing differences in brain neurobiology and structure (sexual dimorphism) between men and women. Regulation of the μOR gene is dependent on specific dual promoter genes, one of which in turn is specifically stimulated by Sox 18 proteins (the distal promoter or DP). Sox proteins play an important role in the regulation of numerous developmental pathways, including the nervous system.[25] Furthermore, Sox proteins play a critical role in sex determination. Sox18 regulation could well mediate the observed sex differences in μ-opioid receptor expression. It is therefore possible that dual promoters could be a mechanism for sexually dimorphic gene regulation by Sox factors, to provide sex differences in pain responses and in the effectiveness of various analgesic agents that act on μOR's.[25]

4.2 Sex Differences in Morphine-induced Respiratory Depression

The influence of intravenous morphine on the control of breathing was assessed in 26 young healthy men and women.[14] In women, morphine reduced the slope of the ventilatory response to carbon dioxide whereas in men there was no significant effect. Morphine did increase the position of the ventilatory CO_2 response slope relative to the x-axis (apnoeic threshold) in men exclusively. The ventilatory response to acute isocapnic hypoxia was affected in women only (depression > 50%).

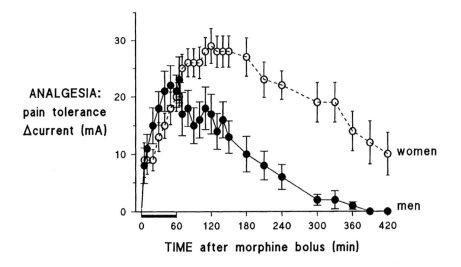

Figure 4. Gender differences in morphine analgesia after a bolus dose (0.1 mg/kg given at t = 0) and a continuous infusion of 0.03 mg/kg per h for 1-h (thick bar). Data were obtained in 10 men and 10 women and are presented as mean ± 95% confidence intervals. Note the greater analgesic responses in women compared to men (see also table 3). Similar results were obtained for pain threshold. The greater analgesic responses in women were due to greater morphine potency. Data are from ref. 18.

The effect of morphine was not dependent on the acute effect of sex hormones (progesterone, estradiol or testosterone) or the day of the menstrual cycle in women. We calculated that the factor sex contributed 80% to the observed differences in opioid effect in men and women, while 20% was related to sex-independent factors.

In a second study,[15] the site of the observed sex-differences in morphine-induced depression of the ventilatory response to carbon dioxide was assessed. Within the ventilatory control system, morphine may affect breathing at peripheral sites (peripheral chemoreceptors in the carotid bodies, phrenic nerve, diaphragm, intercostal muscles, lung) or central sites (suprapontine sites, central chemoreceptors, respiratory integrating centres, spinal cord). The ventilatory response to square wave changes in end-tidal PCO_2 was separated into a fast, peripheral component, and a slow, central component. The fast component arises at the peripheral chemoreceptors of the carotid bodies, the slow component at the central chemoreceptors. The data invariably showed that the site of morphine-induced differences in respiratory depression is within the peripheral chemoreflex loop (*i.e.*, the peripheral chemoreceptors, the sinus nerve, and sites within the brainstem involved in the processing of afferent peripheral input). Our findings agree with earlier studies showing sex differences in the physiologic adaptation to hypoxia of high altitude, which are related to sexual differences in catecholamine activity in certain areas of the afferent peripheral pathways.[26] Animals studies have shown the importance of *N*-methyl-D-aspartate (NMDA) receptors in the process of chemo afferent impulse transmission.[27] NMDA receptors may modulate μOR's, which is a sex-dependent process.[28] It is therefore well feasible that activated μ-OR's may interact with NMDA receptors in a different fashion in men and women in the peripheral afferent pathways activated by hypoxia and hypercapnia.

Table 3. Pharmacodynamic parameters of
morphine's analgesic effect in men and women.

	Men	Women
$t\frac{1}{2}k_{e0}$	1.6 h	4.8 h *
C_{50}	74 nM	40 nM *
γ	2.8	2.8
Baseline current**	40 mA	40 mA

* $P < 0.01$ (NONMEM)
** Baseline current is dependent on the frequency of the
noxious stimulation and the rate of rise of current in
time of the experimental noxious stimulation.

5. SIMULATION STUDIES: CLINICAL RELEVANCE

These findings have evident clinical importance. To explore these we performed some simulations using the PK and PD morphine data (Tables 2 and 3) and compared our findings with those from clinical studies in the literature. Initially, we mimicked a PCA device and aimed at equal analgesic levels in men and women (Figure 5).[18] Our simulation revealed the need for 20 to 40% greater morphine use (or consumption) in men compared to women. This equals the observations made by Miaskowski and Levine in postoperative patients.[13] In figure 6, we show a simulation of the analgesic effect of a bolus dose of morphine at time = 0 of 0.1 mg/kg followed after 4-h by a bolus dose of 0.05 mg/kg. Our data indicate that initially pain relief is better in men. This is not due to greater morphine potency in men (as defined by parameter C_{50}), but to a faster speed of onset (as defined by parameter $t\frac{1}{2}k_{e0}$). This observation is of importance and shows the need for assessing the time lag of opioid effect when studying sex differences.

Simulation of PCA morphine

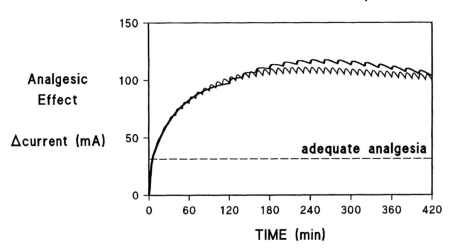

Analgesic Effect

Δcurrent (mA)

TIME (min)

Figure 5. Simulation of PCA morphine in men (thick line) and women (thin line). The simulation was performed using the data from tables 2 and 3, and was intended to obtain identical analgesic levels in men and women. The men used 33 mg of morphine over 7-h, the women only 24 mg over the same time span. Each simulation started with a bolus dose (men 12 mg; women 15.4 mg) followed by bolus doses of 0.5 mg at 10-min intervals in men, and bolus doses of 0.34 mg at 10-min intervals from time $t = 2$-h on. Data are from ref. 18.

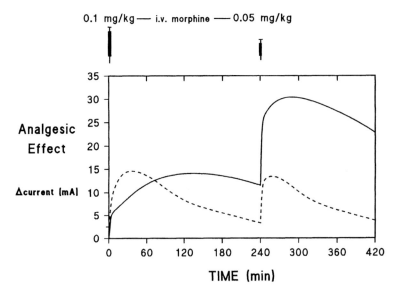

0.1 mg/kg — i.v. morphine — 0.05 mg/kg

Analgesic Effect

Δcurrent (mA)

TIME (min)

Figure 6. Simulation of the effect of a bolus dose of morphine at time $t = 0$ (0.1 mg/kg) followed by a bolus dose at time $t = 4$ h on pain tolerance in men (- - - -) and women (———). Note that during the initial hour, morphine analgesia is greater in men than in women despite the greater morphine potency in women (see text for explanation). This may be the cause of the greater morphine antinociception in males as is observed in certain animal studies.

6. CONCLUSIONS

Gender differences in morphine effect are related to its pharmacodynamics in conjunction with sex-related differences in endogenous pain inhibitory circuitry. In humans, morphine is more potent in women than men, causing greater analgesia and respiratory depression. These factors have to be taken into account when administrating morphine for pain relief. Consequently, there is the need for separate analgesic regimens for men and women directed at the ideal combination of optimal pain relief with minimal respiratory depression.

7. REFERENCES

1. B.L. Kieffer, Opioids: first lessons from knockout mice, *TIPS.* **20,** 19-26 (1999).
2. J.S. Mogil, S.P. Richards, L.A. O'Toole, M.L. Helms, S.R. Mitchell and J.K. Belknap, Geneteic sensitivity to hot-plate nociception in DBA/2J and C57BL/6J inbred mouse strains: possible sex-specific mediation by δ_2-opioid receptors, *Pain* **70,** 267-277 (1997).
3. J.S. Mogil, W.F. Sternberg, P. Marck, B. Sadowski, J.K. Belknap and J.C. Liebeskind, The gentics of pain and pian inhibition, *Proc. Natl. Acad. Sci. USA* **93,** 3048-3055 (1996).
4. H.R. Frischknecht, B. Siegfried and P.G. Wagner, Opioids and behavior: genetic aspects, *Experientia* **44,** 473-481 (1998).
5. T.J. Cicero, B. Nock and E.R. Meyer, Sex-related differences in morhine's antinociceptive activity: relationship to serum and brain morphine concentration, *J. Pharmacol. Exp. Ther.* **282,** 939-944 (1997).
6. H.W.D. Matthes, R. Maldonad, F. Somonin, O. Valverde, S. Slowe, I. Kitchen, K. Befort, A. Dierich, M. Lemeur, P. Dolle, E. Tzavara, E. Hanoune, B.P. Roques and B.L. Kieffer, Loss of morphine-induced analgesia, reward effect and withdrawal symptoms in mice lacing the μ-opioid-receptor gene, *Nature* **383,** 819-823 (1996).
7. A. Dahan, E. Sarton, L. Teppema, C. Olievier, D. Nieuwenhuijs, H.W.D. Matthes and B.L. Kieffer, Anesthesic potency and influence of morphine and sevoflurane on respiration in μ-opioid receptor knockout mice, *Anesthesiology* **94,** 824-832 (2001).
8. E. Sarton, L. Teppema, D. Nieuwenhuijs, H.W.D. Matthes and B.L. Kieffer, Opioid effect on breathing frequency and thermogenesis in mice lacking exon 2 of the mu-opioid receptor gene, *Adv. Exp. Med. Biol.* **499,** 399-404 (2001).
9. N.C. Gordon, R.W. Gear, P.H. Heller, S. Paul, C. Miaskowski and J.D. Levine, Enhancement of morphine analgesia by the GABA B agonist baclofen, *Neuroscience* **69,** 345-349 (1995).
10. R.W. Gear, C. Miaskowski, N.C. Gordon, S.M. Paul, P.H. Heller and J.D. Levine, Kappa-opioids produce significantly greater analgesia in women than in men, *Nat. Med.* **21,** 1248-1250 (1996).
11. C.F. Minto, T.W. Schnider, T.D. Egan, E. Youngs, H.J. Lemmens, P.L. Gambus, V. Billard, J.F. Hoke, K.H. Moore, D.J. Hermann, K.T. Muir, J.W. Mandema and S.L. Shafer, Influence of age and gender on the pharmacokinetics and pharmacodynamics of remifentanil. I. Model development, *Anesthesiology* **86,** 10-23 (1997).
12. D.R. Drover and H.J.M. Lemmens, Population pharmacodynamics and pharmacokinetics of remifentanil as a supplement to nitrous oxide anesthesia for elective abdominal surgery, *Anesthesiology* **89,** 869-877 (1998).
13. C. Miaskowski and J.D. Levine, Does opioid analgesia show a gender preference for females? *Pain Forum* **8,** 34-44 (1999).
14. A. Dahan, E. Sarton, L. Teppema and C. Olievier, Sex-related differences in the influence of morphine on ventilatory control in humans, *Anesthesiology* **88,** 903-913 (1998).
15. E. Sarton, L. Teppema and A. Dahan, Sex differences in morphine-induced ventilatory depression reside within the peripheral chemoreflex loop, *Anesthesiology* **90,** 1329-1338 (1999).
16. T.J. Gan, P.S. Glass, J. Sigl, P. Sebel, F. Payne, C. Rosow and P. Embree, Women emerge faster from general anesthesia with propofol/alfentanil/nitrous oxide faster than men, *Anesthesiology* **90,** 1283-1287 (1999).
17. J. Butterworth, R. James, R. Prielipp, J. Cerese, J. Livingston, D, Burnett and the CABG Benchmarking Database Participants. Female gender associates with increased duration of intubation and lenth of stay after coronary surgery, *Anesthesiology* **92,** 414-424 (2000).

18. E. Sarton, E. Olofsen, R. Romberg, J. den Hartigh, B. Kest, D. Nieuwenhuijs, A. Burm, L. Teppema and A. Dahan, Sex differences in morphine analgesia: an experimental study in healthy volunteers, *Anesthesiology* **93**, 1245-1254 (2000). See also: http:// www.anesthesiology.org.

19. J.P. Zacney, Morphine responses in humans: a retrospective analysis of sex differences, *Drug Alcohol Depend.* **63**, 23-28 (2001).

20. M. Averbuch and M. Katzper, Gender and the placebo analgesic effect in acute pain, *Clin. Pharmacol. Ther.* **70**, 287-291 (2001).

21. R. Romberg, E. Sarton, J. den Hartigh, E. Olofsen and A. Dahan, Pharmacokinetic/pharmacodynamic modelling of the analgesic effects of morphine-6-glucuronide in healthy men and women, Manuscript in preparation.

22. Matthes HW, C. Smadja, O. Valverde, JL. Vonesch, AS Foutz, E. Boudinot, M. Denavit-Sauble, C. Severini, L. Negri, B.P. Roques, R. Maldonado and B.L. Kieffer, Activity of the delta-opioid receptor is partially reduced, whereas activity of the kappa-receptor is maintained in mice lacking the mu-receptor, *J. Neurosci.* **18**, 7285-7295 (1998).

23. A.G.P. Schuller, M.A. King, J. Zhang, E. Bolan, Y.X. Pan, D.J. Morgan, A. Chang, M.E. Czick, E.M, Unterwald, G.W. Pasternak and J.E. Pintar. Retention of heroin and morphine-6β-glucuronide analgesia in a new line of mice lacking exon 1 of MOR 1, *Nat Neurosci* **2**, 151-156 (1999).

24. J-K. Zubieta, R.F. Dannals and J.J. Frost, Gender and age influences brain mu-opioid receptor binding measured by PET, *Am. J. Psychiatr.* **156**, 842-848 (1999).

25. H-J. Im, D. Smirnov, T. Yuhi, S. Raghavan, J.E. Olsson, G.E. Muscat, P. Koopman, H.H. Loh, Transcriptional modulation of mouse μ-opioid receptor distal promotor activity by Sox18, *Mol. Pharmacol.* **59**, 1486-1496 (2001).

26. T. Laitinen, J. Haitikainen, E. Vanninen, L. Niskanen, G. Geelen and E. Lansimies, Age and gender dependency of baroreflex sensitivity in healthy subjects, *J. Appl. Physiol.* **84**, 576-583 (1998).

27. R.C. Ang, B. Hoop and H. Kazemi, Role of glutamate as the central neurotransmitter in the hypoxic ventilatory response, *J. Pll. Physiol.* **72**, 1480-1487 (1992).

28. S. M. Lipa and M. Kavaliers, Sex differences in the inhibitory effect of NMDA antagonist MK-801, on morphine and stress-induced analgesia, *Brain Res. Bull.* **24**, 627-630 (1990).

INFLUENCE OF PROPOFOL ON THE
CONTROL OF BREATHING

Albert Dahan, Diederik J.F. Nieuwenhuijs and Erik Olofsen[*]

1. INTRODUCTION

The intravenous anaesthetic propofol is frequently used as mono-anaesthetic/sedative for a range of small surgical procedures in patients who breathe spontaneously or is combined with regional anaesthesia for larger surgical procedures. Like the inhalational anaesthetics, propofol has a considerable effect on the ventilatory control system, reducing the ventilatory responses to carbon dioxide and hypoxia; induction doses of propofol (1.5 to 2.5 mg/kg) cause the cessation of breathing activity when infused rapidly. These effects may be related to direct effects of propofol at peripheral (*e.g.*, peripheral chemoreceptors, lung, diaphragm) and/or central sites (*e.g.*, central chemoreceptors, respiratory centres, centres involved in blood pressure control) and/or to indirect effects at sites involved in the control of vigilance/arousal/wakefulness. For example, animal studies indicate that propofol causes an inhibitory effect on areas of the dorsomedial and ventrolateral medulla, which contain the central chemoreceptors and centres controlling pressor responses.[1]

To fully describe and understand the influences of propofol on cardiorespiratory control in humans, we performed a set of experiments on the effects of propofol on various cardiorespiratory and EEG parameters such as resting ventilation, resting end-tidal carbon dioxide concentration ($P_{ET}CO_2$), blood pressure and heart rate, bispectral index of the EEG (BIS) and the ventilatory responses to carbon dioxide and hypoxia, at our institution.[2-4] Experiments were performed in healthy volunteers enabling us to study pure metabolic or chemical control of breathing without the confounding influences of surgery, pain, stress, inflammation, and underlying disease, which occur in peri-operative patients. Here, we report the effects of propofol on the various respiratory variables and parameters. Taken into account the above, extrapolation to patients in pain should be

[*] A.Dahan et al. Department of Anaesthesiology, Leiden University Medical Center, Leiden, The Netherlands

Advances in Modelling and Clinical Application of Intravenous Anaesthesia
Edited by Vuyk and Schraag, Kluwer Academic/Plenum Publishers, 2003

81

done with care. Pain and stress cause a chemoreflex-independent tonic ventilatory drive, which may offset ventilatory depression from drugs (opioids, anaesthetics, sedatives) and sedation.

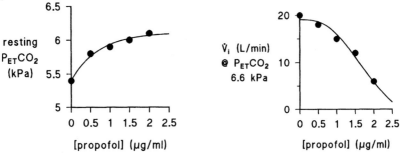

Figure 1. The influence of propofol on resting end-tidal carbon dioxide concentration (left) and on minute ventilation at a fixed end-tidal carbon dioxide concentration of 6.6 kPa or 50 mmHg (right). While the rise in resting $P_{ET}CO_2$ precludes large decreases in resting ventilation, the reduction of the slope of the hypercapnic ventilatory response by propofol causes the drop in ventilation at a fixed end-tidal PCO_2. These data are averages from 10 healthy male subjects.

2. RESTING VENTILATION AND $P_{ET}CO_2$

When low dose propofol (up to blood concentrations of 2000 ng/ml) is infused slowly, the rise in arterial carbon dioxide concentration precludes large changes in resting ventilation. At a fixed end-tidal CO_2 concentration the effect on minute ventilation is more outspoken (see Figure 1), with a C_{50} ranging from 1300 to 1500 ng/ml among subjects.[4]

3. THE STEADY-STATE VENTILATORY RESPONSE TO CARBON DIOXIDE

An increase in end-tidal CO_2 concentration above resting values causes an increase in minute ventilation in a linear fashion (see Figure 2). This relationship is best described as follows:[5]

$$V_i = G_{TOT} (P_{ET}CO_2 - B) \tag{1}$$

$$G_{TOT} = G_P + G_C \tag{2}$$

where B is the apnoeic threshold or extrapolated $P_{ET}CO_2$ at zero ventilation, and parameter G_{TOT} the slope of the hypercapnic ventilatory response curve (or CO_2 sensitivity). G_P and G_C denote the CO_2 sensitivities of the central and peripheral chemoreflex loops. While propofol does not affect the linear nature of this relationship, it causes a severe reduction of the slope of the response curve (G_{TOT}). At a propofol concentration of about 2000 ng/ml, parameter G_{TOT} is reduced by more than 50%. The control and propofol response curves pivot at a $P_{ET}CO_2$ of about 6 kPa. Consequently, the apnoeic threshold is reduced by propofol (Figure 2). In some subjects, propofol at doses < 500 ng/ml, causes excitatory respiratory behaviour with a small increase in slope of the

CO_2 response curve. This observation is in agreement with the excitatory EEG behaviour observed at low propofol concentrations. The effect of this excitatory behaviour on respiration was predominantly on tidal volume with no effect on breathing frequency.

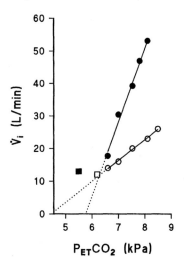

Figure 2. The influence of 2000 ng/ml propofol on the ventilatory response to carbon dioxide. Each circle represents a steady-state data point obtained at an elevated end-tidal PCO_2: closed circles are control data, open circles propofol data points. The squares denote resting data points (that is, without any inspired carbon dioxide). In this male subject, the value of G (see eqn. (1)) is reduced from 22 L/min per kPa to 6 L/min per kPa. Note the reduction in apnoeic threshold (= the intersection of the dotted lines and the *x*-axis).

4. THE DYNAMIC VENTILATORY RESPONSE TO CO_2

The dynamic ventilatory response to CO_2 can be broken up into a fast and a slow ventilatory component using a mathematical model of the ventilatory controller. The fast component is attributed to the peripheral chemoreflex loop, the slow component to the central chemoreflex loop.[5, 6] By studying this dynamic response, important information may be obtained about the function of the peripheral chemoreceptors at the carotid bodies with relative ease. For example, applying dynamic CO_2 inputs, we showed the selective effect of low dose inhalational anaesthetics on the peripheral chemoreceptors.[7-9] Since the peripheral chemoreceptors convey the hypoxic ventilatory response and play an important role in overcoming upper airway obstruction, we tested the effect of propofol on the dynamic ventilatory response to carbon dioxide in ten healthy volunteers. In this study, the end-tidal CO_2 input function consisted of a multi frequency binary sequence (MFBS), involving 13 steps into and 13 steps out of hypercapnia (duration about 24 min).[3] This input function increases the precision of the estimation of parameters related to the peripheral chemoreflex loop (without compromising precision of the estimation of central parameters) relative to step input functions.[3] Further, in order to cause a more potent and selective stimulus to the peripheral chemoreceptors, we performed experiments at the background of moderate hypoxia.

The results showed that sedative concentrations of propofol (mean BIS 67) caused depression of the dynamic response to CO_2, which was attributed to an exclusive effect within the central chemoreflex loop. In other words, the peripheral chemoreflex loop remained unaffected by propofol. This is an important observation, and contrasts sharply with our findings at sedative concentrations of halothane, isoflurane and sevoflurane.[7-10] We relate these differences to the distinct mechanisms by which the inhalational anaesthetics and propofol act. Apparently propofol has no molecular target within the peripheral chemoreflex loop, while some of the halogenated anaesthetics do. Most probably, the target of halothane (and the other inhalational anaesthetics) is the background K^+ channel in the carotid body chemoreceptor cell.[11] This channel is involved in tonic inhibition of cellular excitability and is probably an important link in the cascade leading to CO_2 and O_2 sensing at the carotid bodies. The molecular target of propofol within the central chemoreflex loop is probably the $GABA_A$ receptor system causing a net inhibitory effect on the respiratory neuronal network. Furthermore, the loss of wakefulness may also affect the central carbon dioxide sensitivity.

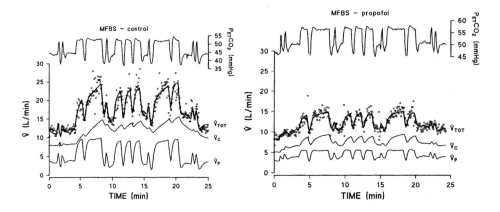

Figure 3. An example of the influence of 1200 ng/ml propofol on the dynamic ventilatory response to carbon dioxide against the background of mild hypoxia in one subject. Left: control response; Right: propofol response. The end-tidal carbon dioxide input function (top panels) consists of a multi-frequency binary sequence (MFBS) involving 13 step into and 13 steps out of hypercapnia and lasting altogether 23 min 28 s. The ventilatory response is dived into a fast component from the peripheral chemoreceptors (V_p) and a slow component from the central chemoreceptors (V_c). Each dot represents one breath. The thick line through the breaths is the data fit ($V_{TOT} = V_p + V_c$ + a trend term, which is not shown).

5. THE VENTILATORY RESPONSE TO HYPOXIC PULSES

The peripheral chemoreceptors are activated when perfused with blood of low P_aO_2. As a result, inspired minute ventilation increases abruptly. A peak response is obtained within 3-min. This is a life-saving chemoreflex, ensuring adequate delivery of oxygen to the brain and other vital organs. Note that the carotid bodies are strategically situated at the bifurcation of the carotid arteries and determine the O_2 flux to the brain not only by regulating respiratory reflexes but also by changing brain blood flow. All drugs that affect the carotid bodies will severely hamper these important functions. Hence, it is important to be informed on the effect of commonly (and uncommonly) used anaesthetics and opioids on the chemo sensors of the carotid bodies and their afferent pathways to the respiratory centres in the brain stem.

In cats, Berkenbosch *et al.* studied the peripheral ventilatory response dynamics to hypoxic stimulation while the arterial PO_2 of the medulla oblongata was kept constant using the technique of artificial brainstem perfusion.[12] Mathematically, the responses were best described by two components: a fast component with a time constant of −2 s and a slow component with a time constant of −73 s. While the fast component was considered to originate at the carotid bodies, it was argued that the slow component was due to central modulation of the carotid body response (*i.e.*, central neuronal dynamics of the respiratory network). Interestingly, in the same animal preparation the response of the peripheral chemoreflex pathway to changes in end-tidal PCO_2 does not show a slow component.[13] This indicates that while peripheral hypoxic stimulation activates central neuronal dynamics, peripheral hypercapnic stimulation does not. Also in humans, the hyperventilatory response to hypoxia is well described by a fast and a slow component, with a fast time constant of 3 s and a slower time constant of 100 s (see Figure 4). Propofol has no effect on the gain of the fast component but reduces the gain of the slow component significantly by more than 50% (Table 1).[3]

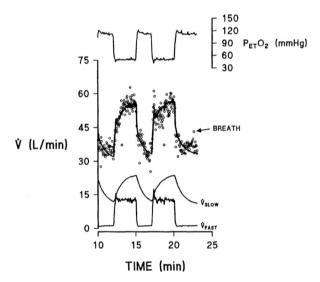

Figure 4. The ventilatory response to hypoxic pulses in an awake subject during mild hypercapnia. Top panel: the hypoxic input function. Bottom panel: each circle represents one breath. The response is separated into a fast component with a time constant of 3 s (V_{FAST}) and a slower component with a time constant of 100 s (V_{SLOW}), using a mathematical model (see reference 12). In this subject the gain of the two components was of similar magnitude. The thick line is the model fit ($V_{TOT} = V_{FAST} + V_{SLOW} + V_0$ + trend term).

These findings contrast with those of the inhalational anaesthetic sevoflurane which as a depressant effect on both components of the acute hypoxic response (Table 1).[14] These data indicate that while sevoflurane affects the carotid bodies (*i.e.*, as observed by the depression of the fast component) as well as central neuronal dynamics (*i.e.*, as observed by depression of the slow component), propofol has a large effect on central neuronal dynamics only, and leaves the carotid bodies unaffected. These observations are in agreement with our findings on the effect of propofol and inhalational anaesthetics on the dynamic ventilatory response to carbon dioxide.[3, 7, 9]

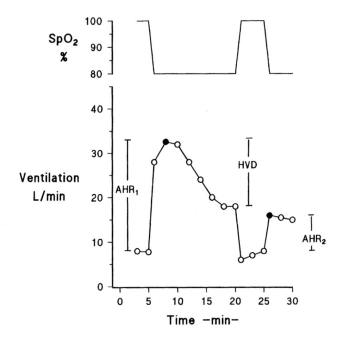

Figure 5. The ventilatory response to sustained isocapnic hypoxia (oxygen saturation 80%). The response is biphasic. An initial hyperventilatory response (initial acute hypoxic response or AHR_1) is followed after about 3-min by a slow ventilatory decline (the hypoxic ventilatory decline or HVD). HVD is due to the central depressant effects of hypoxia and persists beyond the initial hypoxic episode causing a subsequent acute hypoxic response to be severely depressed (AHR_2). The closed data points denote peak ventilation levels. Data adapted from reference 15.

Table 1. The effect of propofol and sevoflurane on the gains of the fast and slow components of the ventilatory response to 3-min hypoxic pulses. The data are from references 3 and 14.

	Fast component	Slow Component
	$G_{DRUG}/G_{CONTROL}$	$G_{DRUG}/G_{CONTROL}$
PROPOFOL 600 ng/ml	0.95 ± 0.35	0.45 ± 0.30 *
SEVOFLURANE 0.25% ET	0.73 ± 0.23 *	0.41 ± 0.32 *

* Significantly different from 1. Values are mean $\pm$ SD. Number of subjects is 12.

6. THE VENTILATORY RESPONSE TO SUSTAINED HYPOXIA

When hypoxia persists for periods > 5 min, the initial hyperventilatory response is not sustained. A slow decline in ventilation develops (time constant about 3 to 4 min); a new steady-state ventilation is reached within 15 to 20 min, still about 25 to 50% above pre-hypoxic baseline values (Figure 5). Interestingly, the depressant effect of sustained hypoxia is not limited to the initial hypoxic period but continues beyond the hypoxic exposure. For example, a second acute hypoxic response, occurring just after a sustained hypoxic episode is severely depressed (Figure 5).[15]

The mechanism of the hypoxic ventilatory decline (HVD) remains unknown. The mechanism(s) and site(s) of generation of HVD in awake humans remain poorly understood. There are several possibilities:

- Mild hypoxia (S_PO_2 > 90%) induced increase in brain blood flow causing the washout of acid metabolites (CO_2 and/or H^+) from the brain compartment and consequently a reduction of CO_2 drive of the central chemoreceptors;
- The central accumulation of inhibitory neuromodulators/transmitters such as adenosine, lactic acid, endorphins, dopamine, (-amino butyric acid (GABA) or dopamine, during central moderate hypoxia (50% > S_PO_2 > 90%) causes a net inhibitory effect on the respiratory neuronal pool in the brainstem. The relatively slow turnover of these substances after the relief of hypoxia may explain the persistent reduction of hypoxic ventilatory responses after 20-min hypoxic exposures;
- During deep hypoxia (S_PO_2 < 50%), the acute lack of oxygen due to an impaired oxygen flux (at mild and moderate hypoxia the oxygen flux is often maintained or only modestly affected) causes direct neuronal dysfunction or the intracellular accumulation of acid metabolites and consequently hypoventilation.

In awake subjects, the ratio of the magnitudes of HVD and the acute hypoxic response (AHR) is fairly constant among and within subjects (HVD/AHR 0.35). Propofol increases the value of HVD/AHR to 0.55 and also increases depression of subsequent hypoxic responses (AHR_2) after 20 min of hypoxia (ratio AHR_2/AHR_1 decreases from 0.7 to 0.5).[2] This indicates that propofol amplifies the relative magnitude of hypoxic ventilatory decline and hence enhances the development of HVD. It is well known that propofol augments GABA-ergic transmission. It is therefore possible that the relative increase in HVD by propofol is related to propofol=s action at the $GABA_A$ receptor complex. Other $GABA_A$ receptor agonists, such as midazolam, produce similar results on the ratio HVD/AHR.[16]

7. PROPOFOL-REMIFENTANIL INTERACTION

Although clinically relevant, the interaction of propofol and opioids on ventilatory control remains understudied. Pavlin and co-workers observed that propofol added to alfentanil increased the level of sedation and analgesia but had only minimal effect on ventilatory parameters such as end-tidal PCO_2 and slope of the hypercapnic ventilatory response (assessed by Read=s rebreathing method).[17] The absence of large effects of the combination of alfentanil and propofol may be explained by the reduction of metabolic rate (VCO$_2$) after the drug combination (which prevented any further rise in end-tidal PCO$_2$), the relatively low doses of propofol tested (max dose 800 ng/ml; at these low doses some excitatory effects are possible, see above), the stimulation of the subjects during experimentation, and well known problems with the specific methodology used to test the effect of these drugs on ventilatory responses (see references 18 and 19 for a further explanation). In a recent set of experiments we tested the combination of propofol (dose range 0 - 2000 ng/ml C$_P$) and remifentanil (dose range 0 – 3.5 ng/ml C$_P$) on resting ventilation, ventilation at a fixed P$_{ET}$CO$_2$ of 55 mmHg, resting P$_{ET}$CO$_2$ and the slope of the hypercapnic ventilatory response,[4] using response surface modelling (RSM) based on a simple pharmacodynamic model (*i.e.*, the 'Richards model'):[20,21]

$$f(x) = \alpha / [\, 1 + \delta \cong x^\gamma\,]^{1/\delta} \tag{3}$$

By fixing δ to –1 we get:

$$f(x) = \alpha\,[\, 1 - x^\gamma\,] \tag{4}$$

To model interactions between two drugs we use the following extension to the model:

$$E(C_1, C_2) = E_0\,[1 - \{(U_1 \cong (\lambda_1)^{1/\gamma} + U_2 \cong (\lambda_1)^{1/\gamma})^\gamma\} \cong I(Q)\,] \tag{5}$$

where U$_1$ = C$_1$/C$_{\lambda 1}$, U$_2$ = C$_2$/C$_{\lambda 2}$, C$_1$ and C$_2$ are the concentrations of remifentanil and propofol (or any other drug), respectively, and C$_{\lambda 1}$ and C$_{\lambda 2}$ the concentrations halfway the range in the study design (in our study 1 ng/ml for remifentanil and 1 μg/ml for propofol). The use of λ's instead of using C$_{50}$'s was done since C$_{50}$'s cannot be well estimated as they typically lie above the applied concentration ranges. A value for λ$_1$ of 50 denotes a 50% depression of the parameter/variable at a concentration of 1 ng/ml remifentanil. Similarly a λ$_2$ of 50 denotes a 50% depression of the parameter/variable at a concentration of 1 μg/ml propofol. γ is a non-linearity parameter and I(Q) is a smooth function (spline) of Q, where[20]

$$Q = U_1 / [U_1 + U_2\,] \tag{6}$$

Q ranges from 0 (drug 2 only) to 1 (drug 1 only). The smooth function has 2 parameters I$_{MAX}$ and Q$_{MAX}$. I$_{MAX}$ is the maximum value of the interaction term, and Q$_{MAX}$ is the value of Q (*i.e.*, concentration ratio) for which I attains I$_{MAX}$. An I$_{MAX}$ of less than 1 denotes antagonism; an I$_{MAX}$ of 1 denotes no interaction, and an I$_{MAX}$ of more than 1 synergy. The choice of the specific pharmacodynamic model, an adaptation of the Richards model (see ref. 21; by setting δ equal to –1) was made for three reasons:

- At certain drug concentrations, the model allows a zero effect to occur as may happen in complex non-linear systems such as ventilatory control (*i.e.*, abrupt central apnoea during drug infusion);[20]
- At high concentrations negative responses (*i.e.*, E(C$_x$) < 0) are possible which may be described by our model (for example, in response to a hypoxic challenge ventilation decreases);[20]
- Linear responses are possible when γ = 1, as may occur when only a limited dose range is tested.[7-9, 20]

The results observed in one subject are shown in figure 6. It depicts the synergistic interaction between propofol and remifentanil on the slope of the hypercapnic ventilatory response. The population analysis (performed using NONMEM, see Table 2 and Figure 7), yielded a synergistic effect on resting ventilation, ventilation at a fixed $P_{ET}CO_2$ of 55 mmHg and resting $P_{ET}CO_2$.

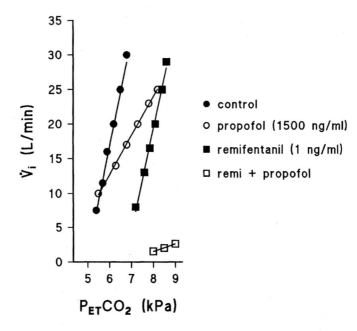

Figure 6. Influence of propofol, remifentanil and their combination on the ventilatory response to carbon dioxide. Values of the slopes are for control 15.5 L/min per kPa, remifentanil 15.0 L/min per kPa, propofol 6.5 L/min per kPa and for the combination 1.1 L/min per kPa, exemplifying the synergistic nature of the drug combination. Data are from one subject. Data from reference 4.

Table 2. Response surface modelling of the interaction of propofol-remifentanil on respiration: population pharmacodynamic model parameters ($n = 22$ healthy male volunteers). Data from ref. 4.

	Resting ventilation (L/min)	Ventilation at fixed $P_{ET}CO_2$ of 55 mmHg (L/min)	Resting $P_{ET}CO_2$ (mmHg)
Baseline value	9.4 ± 0.3	31.4 ± 1.5	41.2 ± 0.1
λ **remifentanil** [ℵ]	28 ± 4.0	58.0 ± 3.5	15.4 ± 1.2
λ **propofol** [ℶ]	13.0 ± 3.3	44.9 ± 3.9	4.2 ± 0.9
$I_{MAX}(Q)$ [ℷ]	1.9 ± 0.2	1.2 ± 0.1	1.3 ± 0.2
γ [ℸ]	0.5 ± 0.1	0.4 ± 0.1	0.7 ± 0.1
C_{50} **remifentanil** [ℸ]	3.3	0.7	5.6
C_{50} **propofol** [ℶ]	16	1.4	36.9

ℵ: % depression at 1 ng/ml.   ℸ: $\gamma \neq 1$ denotes nonlinearity.
ℶ: % depression at1 μg/ml.   ℸ: in ng/ml (extrapolated C_{50}).
ℷ: > 1 denotes synergy.   ℶ: in μg/ml (extrapolated C_{50}).

The differences in synergy strength (resting ventilation > resting $P_{ET}CO_2$ > ventilation at a fixed $P_{ET}CO_2$) is remarkable and may be related to the fact that resting ventilation is dependant on behavioural and chemical control of breathing while stimulated breathing is most dependent on chemical control of breathing.[22] Furthermore, resting ventilation was measured under closed loop conditions (apart from an effect of the drug(s) on respiratory neurons in the CNS, there is an indirect effect of these same drug(s) on ventilation *via* the accumulation of CO_2 in the body) which may be an other cause for the observed synergistic effect, while stimulated breathing was measured under open loop conditions.

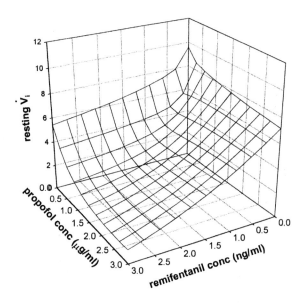

Figure 7. Population response surface model of the interaction of propofol and remifentanil on resting ventilation (number of subjects = 22; number of data points = 94, see also table 2). For both propofol and remifentanil $\gamma \neq 1$, indicating the non-linear relationship between drug and effect. The interaction is synergistic since I(Q) of > 1. (see text for parameter values). Resting ventilation in L/min. Data from reference 4.

8. CONCLUDING REMARKS

Our studies summarized in this paper shed important light on the effect of propofol on ventilatory control in healthy young volunteers. They show the sometimes-impressive respiratory depressant properties of this popular intravenous anaesthetic and increase our insight in its mechanisms and sites of action. Our results show further that the ventilatory control systems may be used as experimental model of anaesthetic effect and outcome.

Although propofol is used in clinical practice in spontaneously breathing patients on a daily basis, knowledge on its effect on ventilatory control in patients is limited. Especially the specific dose range and infusion rate allowing optimal sedation with limited respiratory effect (in the absence and presence of an opioid and/or pain/stress) is not known. Further studies focussing on these latter items are required in order to optimised propofol=s use in spontaneously breathing patients undergoing procedures in which the anaesthetic regimens range from conscious sedation to monitored anaesthesia care.

9. ACKNOWLEDGMENTS

Grant MW 902-19-144 from the Netherlands Organization for Pure Research (Zorgonderzoek Nederland Medische Wetenschappen-NWO), The Hague (Den Haag), The Netherlands, to Dr. Dahan made this paper possible.

10. REFERENCES

1. C. Yang, H. Luk, S. Chen, C. Wu and C. Chai, Propofol inhibits medullary pressor mechanisms in cats, *Can. J. Anaesth.* **44**, 775–781 (1997).
2. D. Nieuwenhuijs, E. Sarton, L. Teppema and A. Dahan, Propofol for monitored anesthesia care: Implications on hypoxic control of cardiorespiratory responses, *Anesthesiology*, **92**, 46–54 (2000).
3. D. Nieuwenhuijs, E. Sarton, L. Teppema, E. Kruyt, I. Olievier, J. van Kleef and A. Dahan, Respiratory sites of action of propofol: Absence of depression of peripheral chemoreflex loop by low-dose propofol, *Anesthesiology*, **95**, 889–895 (2001).
4. D. Nieuwenhuijs, E. Sarton, R. Romberg, E. Olofsen, D. Ward, J. Vuyk, F. Engbers, L. Teppema and A. Dahan, Response surface model of remifentanil-propofol interaction on cardiorespiratory control and bispectral index, Manuscript in preparation.
5. A. Dahan, J. DeGoede, A. Berkenbosch, I. Olievier, The influence of oxygen on the ventilatory response to carbon dioxide in man, *J. Physiol. (Lond.)* **428**, 485B–499 (1990).
6. A. Dahan. The ventilatory response to carbon dioxide and oxygen in man: methods and implications, PhD thesis, Leiden University (1990).
7. A. Dahan, M. van den Elsen, A. Berkenbosch, J. DeGoede, I. Olievier, J. van Kleef and J. Bovill, Effects of subanesthetic halothane on the ventilatory responses to hypercapnia and acute hypoxia in healthy volunteers, *Anesthesiology* **80**, 727–38 (1994).
8. A. Dahan, M. van den Elsen, A. Berkenbosch, J. DeGoede, I. Olievier, A. Burm and J. van Kleef, Influences of a subanesthetic concentration of halothane on the ventilatory response to step changes into and out of sustained isocapnic hypoxia in healthy volunteers, *Anesthesiology* **81**, 850–59 (1994).
9. M. van den Elsen, A. Dahan, J. DeGoede, A. Berkenbosch and J. van Kleef, Influences of subanesthetic isoflurane on ventilatory control in humans, *Anesthesiology* **83**, 478–90 (1995).
10. E. Sarton, A. Dahan, L. Teppema, M. van den Elsen, E. Olofsen, A. Berkenbosch and J. van Kleef, Acute pain and central nervous system arousal do not restore impaired hypoxic ventilatory response during sevoflurane sedation, *Anesthesiology* **85**, 295–03 (1996).
11. K. Buckler, B. Williams and E. Honore, An oxygen-, acid- and anaesthetic-sensitive TASK-like background channel in rat arterial chemoreceptor cells, *J. Physiol. (Lond.)* **525**, 135–42 (2000).
12. A. Berkenbosch, J. DeGoede, D. Ward, C. Olievier and J vanHartevelt, Dynamic response of peripheral chemoreflex loop to changes in end-tidal O_2, *J. Appl. Physiol.* **71**, 1123–1128 (1991).
13. A. Berkenbosch, J. DeGoede, D. Ward, C. Olievier and J vanHartevelt, Dynamic response of peripheral chemoreflex loop to changes in end-tidal CO_2, *J. Appl. Physiol.* **64**, 1779–1785 (1988).
14. E. Sarton, M. van der Wal, D. Nieuwenhuijs, L. Teppema, J.L. Robotham and A. Dahan, Sevoflurane-induced reduction of hypoxic drive is sex-independent, *Anesthesiology*, **90**, 1288–1293 (1999).
15. A. Dahan, D. Ward, M. van den Elsen, J. Temp and A. Berkenbosch, Influence of reduced carotid body drive during sustained hypoxia on hypoxic depression of ventilation in humans, *J. Appl. Physiol.* **81**, 565–572 (1996).
16. A. Dahan and D. Ward, Effect of i.v. midazolam on the ventilatory response to sustained hypoxia in man, *Br. J. Anaesth.* **66**, 454–457 (1991).

17. D. Pavlin, B. Coda, D. Shen, J. Tschanz, Q. Nguyen, R. Schaffer, G. Donaldson, R. Jacobson and C. Chapman, Effects of combining propofol and alfentanil on ventilation, analgesia, sedation and emesis in human volunteers, *Anesthesiology*, **84,** 23–37 (1996).

18. A. Berkenbosch, J.G. Bovill, A. Dahan, J. DeGoede and I.C.W. Olievier, The ventilatory CO_2 sensitivities from Read=s rebreathing method and the steady-state method are not equal in man, *J .Physiol. (Lond.)* **411,** 367–377 (1989).

19. A. Dahan, A. Berkenbosch, J. DeGoede, I.C.W. Olievier and J.G. Bovill, On a pseudo-rebreathing technique to assess the ventilatory sensitivity to carbin dioxide in man, *J. Physiol. (Lond.)* **423,** 615–629 (1990).

20. A. Dahan, D. Nieuwenhuijs, E. Olofsen, E. Sarton, R. Romberg and L. Teppema, Response surface model of alfentanil-sevoflurane interaction on cardiorespiratory control and bispectral index, *Anesthesiology*, **94,** 982–991 (2001).

21. F.J. Richards, A flexible growth function for empirical use, *J. Exp. Botany* **10,** 290–300 (1959).

22. E. Sarton, A. Dahan, L. Teppema, M. van den Elsen, E. Olofsen, A. Berkenbosch and J.W. van Kleef, Acute pain and central nervous system arousal do not restore impaired hypoxic ventilatory response during sevoflurane sedation, *Anesthesiology* **85,** 295-303 (1996).

SECTION 2

MONITORING AND CLINICAL APPLICATION OF INTRAVENOUS ANAESTHESIA

BISPECTRAL INDEX SCALE (BIS) MONITORING AND INTRAVENOUS ANAESTHESIA

Jaap Vuyk and Martijn Mertens[*]

1. INTRODUCTION

Since the first application of an anaesthetic, anaesthesia providers have been looking for a parameter that reliably predicts the depth of anaesthesia. Over the past decades the mechanisms of action of the various groups of anaesthetic agents have been elucidated. The notion that different anaesthetic agents propagate the anaesthetic state through different mechanisms and receptor systems has lead to the believe that no such thing as a single anaesthetic state exists but that anaesthesia may embody different levels of sedation/unconsciousness, analgesia, autonomic nervous system stability and muscle relaxation. Consequently, it may be unrealistic to search for a single parameter that reliably reflects the depth of anaesthesia. Nevertheless, over the past decades the search for such a parameter has been intense. Since 5 years now the bispectral index scale (BIS) monitor is the one and only clinical available device that has culminated from this search and became available for clinical practice. This manuscript describes the current state of knowledge on the bispectral index scale monitor and its present place in clinical practice.

2. ELECTRO-ENCEPHALOGRAPHIC MONITORING

Already in 1875 Richard Caton[1] described the electro-encephalogram (EEG) as a way of determining cerebral electrical activity on the cortical surface of the skull of animals. Then, in 1937, Gibbs and colleagues discovered that the EEG activity was affected by the administration of anaesthetic agents.[2] Since then, technical advances in EEG monitoring have run parallel with the search for a parameter derived from the EEG

[*] Jaap Vuyk and Martijn Mertens, Department of Anaesthesiology P5-38, Leiden University Medical Center, 2300 RC Leiden, The Netherlands. Email: j.vuyk@lumc.nl

Advances in Modelling and Clinical Application of Intravenous Anaesthesia
Edited by Vuyk and Schraag, Kluwer Academic/Plenum Publishers, 2003

that consistently correlates with anaesthetic agent concentration and the level of anaesthetic depth.[3]

Because the raw EEG is hardly interpretable online this quest for a parameter derived from the EEG has great importance. Initially, the search focused on the analysis of the time domain of the EEG. Time domain derived parameters are e.g. the change in total power or median frequency in time, the occurrence of activity in time in certain EEG frequency bands, or the frequency of occurrence of burst suppression. The effect of various anaesthetic agents on time domain derived EEG parameters have been described and claimed to be clinical useful.[4, 5] However, apart from various publications in this field, time domain EEG parameters have never been exploited on a large scale in clinical practice. Next to the analysis of time domain derived EEG parameters the frequency domain has been the subject of numerous studies in the search for a clinically related meaningful EEG parameter. The most frequently used frequency domain type analytical method of the EEG is by means of Fast Fourier Transformation (FFT). During FFT the EEG signal is spliced into small époques of a few seconds. The FFT analysis then results in the projection of the power spectrum versus the EEG frequency in e.g. the 0-30 Hz range. For every time epoch the power spectrum versus frequency is determined and displayed with the result of the most recent analysed epoch projected over the previous one thus resulting in a landscape like figure of the power versus frequency analysis in time, the so called compressed spectral array.

The FFT in its turn then gives rise to the derivation of clinically useful parameters. Two of the most often studied FFT derived EEG parameters are the spectral edge and the median frequency. The spectral edge (SE_{95}) is the FFT derived frequency below which 95% of the power in the spectrum is found; the median frequency (SE_{50}) is defined as the frequency below which 50% of the power in the FFT spectrum is found. Numerous studies describe the effects of various related agents on the SE_{95} and SE_{50} and their relation with the depth of anaesthesia. In general, both SE_{95} and SE_{50} decrease with increasing depth of anaesthesia and increasing blood and central nervous system concentrations of anaesthetic agents. Opioid concentration correlates very well with FFT derived parameters.[6, 7] With increasing opioid concentration the EEG changes from a low amplitude high frequency signal to a high amplitude low frequency signal. This results in the FFT as an increase in power at lower frequencies (0-5 Hz) with a reduction of power at higher frequencies (10-30 Hz) and results in a decrease of the SE_{95} and SE_{50}. Also, intravenous hypnotic agents like propofol, etomidate and methohexitone correlate well with frequency domain derived EEG parameters. With propofol the EEG amplitude shows a characteristic biphasic response to increasing blood propofol concentrations in all frequency bands.[8] Patients lose responsiveness when EEG amplitudes in the high frequency bands are decreasing after having reached a maximum. EEG changes also appear to be different during infusion and emergence. Also etomidate, methohexital and thiopental[9-12] cause a significant slowing of the EEG finally resulting in burst suppression.[13] With variable results frequency domain derived EEG parameters have been used in closed loop settings to control the depth of anaesthesia. Similarly to the clinical application of time domain derived parameters, although sometimes adequately functioning in experimental settings, these parameters have never been used on a broader scale in clinical anaesthesia to help the anaesthesiologist to control the depth of anaesthesia. However, the derivation of EEG parameters and the determination of relationships of these parameters with anaesthetic drug concentrations has led to the consistent and easy to replicate definition of the potency of the various agents on the basis of their EEG slowing capability (EC_{50}) and to the determination of the effect site equilibration half-life on the basis of the delay between the peak blood drug concentrations and maximum EEG depression.[6, 7]

3. BISPECTRAL INDEX ANALYSIS

The bispectral index monitor has been ongoing developed since 1992 with the premarket approval by the FDA in 1996 (Aspect Medical Systems, Inc., Natick, MA). The bispectral analysis is a further computation of time domain and frequency domain parameters. In general, Fourier analysis determines the phase of the various wave components starting at the beginning of the epoch, whereas the bispectral analysis determines the correlation between the phases of the various wave components of which the raw EEG is built. Recently, Ira Rampil published a thorough description of electroencephalographic analysis in general and of the BIS in particular.[3] The bispectral analysis considers the relationship between the sinusoids at two frequencies $f1$ and $f2$ and a modulation of these two $f1+ f2$. For this set of three frequency components the bispectrum can be calculated on the basis of the phase information or bicoherence (BIC $f1,f2$) and the sum of the magnitude of the 3 members known as the real triplet product (RTP $f1,f2$). Finally, the bispectral index then is composed of time domain, frequency domain and higher order spectral parameters. In this way the BIS is a computation of the burst suppression ratio (BSR) and QUAZI, 2 time domain derived parameters, the beta ratio, a frequency domain parameter defining the power in the 30-47 Hz band relative to the 11-20 Hz band, and lastly the SyncFastSlow parameter determined from the bispectrum as the ratio of bispectrum peaks in the 0.5-47 Hz band relative to the 40-47 Hz frequency band. An important feature in the calculation of the bispectral index is that the weight of any of these 4 subparameters (BSR, QUAZI, β-ratio and SyncFastSlow) changes with the level of sedation. The β-ratio weighs heavier in the final computation of BIS at levels of light sedation, the SyncFastSlow parameter dominates at excitation and surgical levels of hypnosis and the BSR and QUAZI are more important in the BIS calculation at the most deep levels of EEG depression. The specific weight of the various subparameters of BIS at various clinical states has been determined, during the development of the BIS by Aspect Medical Systems, on the basis of a body of data gathered from a group of patients that received various anaesthetics while EEG and behavioural data were collected. In the end the BIS is determined as a running average of 15-30 seconds of EEG signal collection and visualized as a dimensionless non-linear parameter between 0-100. With 0 equalling no electrical activity and with 100 defining the awake state (see Figure 1). In general, the Bispectral Index Scale (BIS) reflects the awake state at values exceeding 95, a state of sedation at BIS values of 65-85, an arousal state depression suited for general anaesthesia at BIS values of 40-65 and burst suppression patterns become evident at BIS levels below 40.[14] The Aspect BIS monitor provides on screen the raw EEG, indicators of the quality of signal detection and the electrode resistance and numerical data regarding the incidence of burst suppression displayed as SR; the suppression ratio. A tape is provided with the monitor that includes 3 EEG electrodes that should be fixed with strength to the forehead and temples of the patient to assure optimal signal detection.

Alkire describes in a study on the effects of propofol and isoflurane a relationship between BIS and metabolic rate. He found a linear relationship between the cerebral metabolic reduction caused by propofol and isoflurane anaesthesia and BIS. These data suggest that a physiologic link exists between the EEG and cerebral metabolism during anaesthesia that is mathematically quantifiable using BIS.[15, 16]

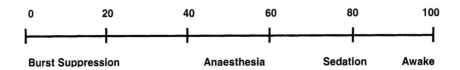

Figure 1. The Bispectral Index Scale (BIS) reflects the awake state at values exceeding 95, a state of sedation at BIS values of 65-85, an arousal state depression suited for general anaesthesia at BIS values of 40-65 and burst suppression patterns become evident at BIS levels below 40.[14]

4. INFLUENCE OF ANAESTHETICS ON BIS

The effect of various anaesthetic agents on the bispectral index scale appears to be agent specific. In general, hypnotic agents like propofol, midazolam or thiopental have a strong depressant effect on BIS, inhalational anaesthetic agents propagate an intermediate depressant effect on BIS whereas the opioids have little or no influence on the BIS at clinically relevant concentrations. This may be interpreted as BIS relating well to sedation and hypnosis but not properly reflecting the level of analgesia or depth of anaesthesia. Blood propofol concentrations of 2 µg/ml decrease the BIS to 60-80, with anaesthetic propofol concentrations of 3-6 µg/ml (see Figure 2) the BIS becomes 40-50 and with blood propofol concentrations exceeding 10 µg/ml burst suppression patterns become apparent and the BIS gets close to 0.[17] Thiopental induced BIS changes closely correspond to those of propofol.[18] Midazolam similarly depresses EEG activity and BIS but at clinical concentrations does not seem to be able to invoke burst suppression like propofol does. Thiopental and propofol appear to be able to induce deep levels of central nervous system depression thus allowing them to be used as monoanaesthetic agents.[19] Benzodiazepines may not be capable of this same level of CNS depression. Sedation with midazolam occurs at plasma midazolam concentrations of 100-200 ng/ml at BIS levels of 60-70. Plasma midazolam concentrations of 600 ng/ml still do not depress the BIS any further than 50.[17]

Also inhalational anaesthetic agents depress the BIS with increasing concentrations. An expired isoflurane concentration of 0.5% reduces the BIS to 50-60 and 1.2% to 30. Similarly, sevoflurane depresses BIS.[20] Increasing age reduced sevoflurane requirements to suppress responses to a verbal command but did not change bispectral index and 95% spectral edge frequency associated with this end point. In a population with a wide age range, bispectral index could predict depth of sedation better than end-tidal sevoflurane concentration.[20] In contrast, clinically relevant opioid concentrations hardly affect the BIS. Plasma alfentanil concentrations of up to 300 ng/ml only reduce BIS values to 80-90. This, while in the presence of nitrous oxide these plasma alfentanil concentrations are capable of assuring adequate anaesthesia for abdominal surgery in the majority of patients.[21] In another study the other synthetic opioids fentanyl, sufentanil or remifentanil were not capable of influencing the BIS during propofol induction of anaesthesia.[22] In contrast, members of the latest branch of the pharmacological anaesthesia tree, the α_2-agonists that have sedative properties, do depress the EEG and the BIS.[23]

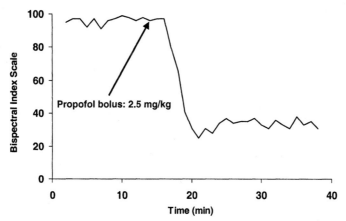

Figure 2. The Bispectral Index Scale (BIS) versus time during induction of anaesthesia with propofol 2.5 mg/kg i.v. in an ASA 1 male patient aged 28 years, followed by a propofol infusion of 10 mg.kg^{-1}.h^{-1}.

Lastly, nitrous oxide and ketamine appear to have paradoxical effects on the BIS. In two studies ketamine was found to counteract the BIS depression inflicted by propofol or midazolam. Ketamine did reduce propofol requirements for loss of consciousness but reversed the decrement in BIS value compared to when propofol was given as single agent.[24] Ketamine-induced dissociative anaesthesia produced persistently an elevated BIS index, which is different from thiamylal and those reported with other conventional anaesthetic agents. The established range of the BIS index appears not to be applicable in patients under ketamine anaesthesia. Monitoring the depth of ketamine anaesthesia remains to be a challenging problem.[25] Along a similar line nitrous oxide appears to induce conflicting BIS changes as well. Nitrous oxide 70% induces loss of consciousness but causes no change in BIS. BIS may indicate a sufficient hypnotic depth to prevent awareness during surgery, but the study by Barr et al. demonstrated that pharmacological unconsciousness-hypnosis may also be reached by mechanisms to which BIS is not sensitive. These authors conclude that BIS is a sufficient but not a necessary criterion for adequate depth of anaesthesia or prevention of awareness with nitrous oxide.[26]

Pharmacodynamic interactions between agents combined during anaesthesia also affect BIS values. Only very few data describe the effect of combinations of agents on BIS. Opioids reduce propofol requirements for induction of anaesthesia. Parallel to this observation loss of consciousness with propofol occurs at higher BIS values when opioids are preadministered than when propofol is given as sole agent.[22] In contrast, the addition and removal of nitrous oxide administration during isoflurane anaesthesia causes paradoxical changes in the EEG. Addition of nitrous oxide causes the BIS to rise whereas discontinuation of nitrous oxide administration during isoflurane anaesthesia resulted in a decrease in BIS.[27]

5. CLINICAL APPLICATION OF BISPECTRAL INDEX MONITORING

Bispectral index monitoring is applicable in patients of all ages. The BIS correlates with depth of sedation independently of age. Sevoflurane concentration for a BIS_{50} is 1.55% in infants (< 1 yr) and 1.25% in children. The concentration-response difference between infants and children was consistent with data showing that minimum alveolar concentration is higher in children less than 1 yr of age.[28] Age-related EEG differences exist in the normal population but they do not affect the BIS. Senile dementia may be associated with significantly lower BIS values. Increasing age reduces sevoflurane requirements to suppress responses to a verbal command but does not change bispectral index associated with this end point. Therefore also in the very old BIS performs just as good as in adults and children.[29]

The most promising application of the bispectral index monitor may be as a monitor of consciousness-sedation-unconsciousness levels. In the absence of central nervous system monitoring hypnotic agents are often administered on the basis of prescribed dosing regimens (12-10-8 mg/kg/h step-down propofol infusion scheme) that may be adjusted to the response of the individual patient. The prescribed dosing regimens do not take into account the pharmacokinetic variability of ± 70% or the pharmacodynamic variability of ± 300-400% in between patients. This huge interindividual PK/PD variability next to the sometimes-poor predictability of the surrogate measures of sedation and anaesthesia (haemodynamic parameters, movement responses etc.) are the cause of the frequent over- and under dosing of individual patients during sedation and general anaesthesia.

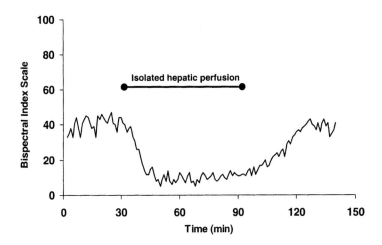

Figure 3. The Bispectral Index Scale (BIS) versus time during continuous infusion with propofol using a TCI system with a constant target concentration of 4 µg/ml in a patient undergoing isolated hepatic perfusion with melfalan for liver metastases of a colon carcinoma. The drop in BIS probably is the result of a rise in the blood propofol concentration resulting from a decrease in propofol clearance due to the temporary absence of hepatic perfusion and thus hepatic enzyme activity. With restoration of hepatic blood flow the BIS increases again.

Figure 3 shows an example of the intraindividual variability in the pharmacokinetics of propofol due to a temporary reduced hepatic clearance of propofol during isolated hepatic perfusion with melfalan. In this and consecutive patients for hepatic perfusions, the BIS could be used to implement a significant decrease in the propofol infusion regimen during isolated hepatic perfusion. The monitoring of the bispectral index scale thus allows for an almost instant focusing out of the huge inter- and intraindividual PK/PD variability to the specific needs of the individual patient at any time. In this context one should keep in mind that different agents affect the BIS differently, that different combinations of agents have a different effect on the BIS and that the BIS may be affected by the intensity of nociception. The BIS therefore probably is most easily interpreted and may relate best to the actual level of sedation during sedation with a single agent in the absence of painful stimuli. In contrast, when two agents are combined, e.g. propofol and an opioid, loss of consciousness occurs at higher BIS values than when propofol is given alone. However, in the presence of clinically relevant opioid concentrations (e.g. plasma alfentanil concentration of 100 ng/ml) the change in BIS_{50} only is 10-15% due to the addition of alfentanil. This, in contrast to the huge interpatient variability in pharmacokinetics of 70% and pharmacodynamics of 300-400%. The BIS-sedation relationship thus is influenced only little by additional agents, painful stimuli and various other matters like e.g. hypothermia, when compared to the huge PK/PD variability in the general pharmacological response. As a result, although no single BIS value exists that assures an adequate hypnotic level in every patient in the presence of any possible anaesthetic agent combination or type of stimulation, the BIS has proven acceptably reliable as a measure of hypnosis during sedation and general anaesthesia with most anaesthetic agents. Clinically, the optimised focusing of drug administration to the specific needs of the patient with BIS monitoring may result in a reduced agent administration and increased speed of return of consciousness and recovery.[30]

A last important question on the intraoperative use of bispectral analysis then is whether the BIS can be used to prevent or detect awareness. Because the BIS very closely correlates with the level of (un)consciousness it is very tentative to state that the use of bispectral index analysis will reduce or prevent the occurrence of awareness. However, because the incidence of awareness is relatively low and because awareness has been reported in the presence of BIS monitoring, showing that the efficiency of awareness prevention by the BIS is not 100%,[31] to get absolute prove that BIS monitoring would reduce the risk of awareness it would take great numbers of patients.[32] Barr et al. even suggest that because of the huge interindividual variability, the real-time BIS-index for the individual subject cannot reliably discriminate wakefulness from unconsciousness during propofol infusion.[33] On the other hand, the long-term effects of intraoperative awareness can be so detrimental, any monitoring device that reduces the risk to this event may be of significant help. Recent case reports regarding awareness detection during anaesthetic agents interruption induced awareness, stress a possible beneficial effect of BIS monitoring in this respect.[37] The probability of awareness and recall appear not be related to the absolute BIS level alone but also to the duration of an increased BIS level. In conclusion, BIS monitoring on itself will not prevent intraoperative awareness. Its ability to track states of (un)consciousness, however, will provide backup to other clinical observations used to evaluate the level of (un)consciousness and may thereby be a significant tool in the prevention of awareness.

Can the BIS also be used as a measure of anaesthetic depth or analgesia? Various studies have tried to determine whether BIS could predict movement to various noxious stimuli. The general picture that arises from early studies is that BIS may be able to predict movement to nociception but only during low opioid - high hypnotic type anaesthetics. However, more recently, using recent versions of the BIS monitor some studies point out that BIS may be as reliable as haemodynamic parameters in predicting movement to noxious stimulation also in the presence of opioids. In the absence of reliable haemodynamic parameters BIS then may be used as an additional parameter of depth of anaesthesia.

Can the BIS be used as a measure of depth of sedation on the ICU? Only few studies have been done in the ICU and the results so far only indicate that the application of BIS may be promising but that more studies need to be done to determine quantitive measures to which the sedation in the ICU may be guided.[34]

6. OTHER APPLICATIONS OF BISPECTRAL INDEX SCALE MONITORING

Next to for clinical applications, the BIS has been used for research purposes in studies on implicit and explicit memory showing that implicit memory formation still occurs at BIS levels between 40-60.[35] Again stressing that the level of consciousness suppression that generally is applied during general anaesthesia does not prohibit the formation of implicit memory. Furthermore, BIS has been used as a parameter to quantify the blood-brain equilibration delay of various agents. In this way it showed its value, similarly to the previously used EEG parameters spectral edge or medium frequency, in the determination of the pharmacology of anaesthetic agents.[9]

Lastly, bispectral index monitoring may be used in the near future as the controlled variable during closed loop control of hypnotic agents. In a study by Struys et al. a BIS controlling adaptive model-based control system was very capable of assuring hypnosis with propofol. Compared to standard practice in this study the closed loop system provided a stable anaesthetic and a more rapid recovery.[36] Similarly, BIS proved to provide an adequate level of anaesthesia with propofol closed loop administration in patients under combined general and regional anaesthesia.[38]

7. LIMITATIONS OF BISPECTRAL INDEX SCALE MONITORING

During the development of the bispectral index monitor agent versus behavioural data have been used to optimise the BIS algorithm. Consequently, when new anaesthetic agents arise new data have to be entered and probably the BIS monitor adjusted to enable use with the new agent. As already mentioned some agents like nitrous oxide and ketamine induce their effects by mechanisms that the BIS monitor apparently is unable to track. Adding ketamine or nitrous oxide deepens the anaesthetic level but increases the BIS. In the presence of these agents the BIS monitor therefore should not be used.

Electrocautery will make the BIS disappear or increase; pacemakers have been described to increase the BIS as well. EMG activity has been claimed to increase the BIS, but later versions like the recent XP version may be less susceptible to this. Lastly, hypothermia decreases the BIS by 1.12 units per degree Celsius decline in body temperature.

8. CONCLUSION

Bispectral index monitoring is useful for the intraoperative tracking of the level of unconsciousness especially during high hypnotic-low opioid anaesthesia. It allows for an improved titration of hypnotic agent requirement and may lead to a reduced agent use and improved recovery. No data yet provide sufficient prove that BIS may predict anaesthetic depth or may be used to predict patient responses to noxious stimulation. BIS monitoring may be useful for guidance of sedation e.g. in the ICU but more data are required to judge its value in this setting. Lastly, no data yet provide sufficient proof that bispectral index monitoring reduces the incidence of awareness.

9. REFERENCES

1. R. Caton, The electrical currents of the brain., *British Medical Journal* **2**, 278 (1875).
2. F. Gibbs, E.Gibbs, and W.Lennox, Effect on the electroencephalogram of certain drugs which influence nervous activity., *Archives of Internal Medicine* **60**, 154-66 (1937).
3. I.J. Rampil, A primer for EEG signal processing in anesthesia, *Anesthesiology* **89**, 980-1002 (1998).
4. L.T. Breimer, A.G.Burm, M.Danhof, P.J.Hennis, A.A.Vletter, J.W.de Voogt, J.Spierdijk, and J.G.Bovill, Pharmacokinetic-pharmacodynamic modelling of the interaction between flumazenil and midazolam in volunteers by aperiodic EEG analysis, *Clin.Pharmacokinet.* **20**, 497-508 (1991).
5. L.T. Breimer, P.J.Hennis, A.G.Burm, M.Danhof, J.G.Bovill, J.Spierdijk, and A.A.Vletter, Quantification of the EEG effect of midazolam by aperiodic analysis in volunteers. Pharmacokinetic/ pharmacodynamic modelling, *Clin.Pharmacokinet.* **18**, 245-53 (1990).
6. J.C. Scott, J.E.Cooke, and D.R.Stanski, Electroencephalographic quantitation of opioid effect: comparative pharmacodynamics of fentanyl and sufentanil, *Anesthesiology* **74**, 34-42 (1991).
7. J.C. Scott, K.V.Ponganis, and D.R.Stanski, EEG quantitation of narcotic effect: the comparative pharmacodynamics of fentanyl and alfentanil, *Anesthesiology* **62**, 234-41 (1985).
8. K. Kuizenga, C.J.Kalkman, and P.J.Hennis, Quantitative electroencephalographic analysis of the biphasic concentration-effect relationship of propofol in surgical patients during extradural analgesia, *Br.J.Anaesth.* **80**, 725-32 (1998).
9. V. Billard, P.L.Gambus, N.Chamoun, D.R.Stanski, and S.L.Shafer, A comparison of spectral edge, delta power, and bispectral index as EEG measures of alfentanil, propofol, and midazolam drug effect, *Clin.Pharmacol.Ther.* **61**, 45-58 (1997).
10. M. Buhrer, P.O.Maitre, O.R.Hung, W.F.Ebling, S.L.Shafer, and D.R.Stanski, Thiopental pharmacodynamics. I. Defining the pseudo-steady-state serum concentration-EEG effect relationship, *Anesthesiology* **77**, 226-36 (1992).
11. D.R. Stanski, Pharmacodynamic modeling of anesthetic EEG drug effects, *Annu.Rev.Pharmacol:Toxicol.* **32**, 423-47 (1992).
12. M. Buhrer, P.O.Maitre, C.Crevoisier, and D.R.Stanski, Electroencephalographic effects of benzodiazepines. II. Pharmacodynamic modeling of the electroencephalographic effects of midazolam and diazepam, *Clin.Pharmacol.Ther.* **48**, 555-67 (1990).
13. H. Schwilden, J.Schuttler, and H.Stoeckel, Quantitation of the EEG and pharmacodynamic modelling of hypnotic drugs: etomidate as an example, *Eur.J.Anaesthesiol.* **2**, 121-31 (1985).
14. J.W. Johansen and P.S.Sebel, Development and clinical application of electroencephalographic bispectrum monitoring, *Anesthesiology* **93**, 1336-44 (2000).
15. M.T. Alkire, C.J.Pomfrett, R.J.Haier, M.V.Gianzero, C.M.Chan, B.P.Jacobsen, and J.H.Fallon, Functional brain imaging during anesthesia in humans: effects of halothane on global and regional cerebral glucose metabolism, *Anesthesiology* **90**, 701-9 (1999).
16. M.T. Alkire, Quantitative EEG correlations with brain glucose metabolic rate during anesthesia in volunteers, *Anesthesiology* **89**, 323-33 (1998).
17. P.S. Glass, M.Bloom, L.Kearse, C.Rosow, P.Sebel, and P.Manberg, Bispectral analysis measures sedation and memory effects of propofol, midazolam, isoflurane, and alfentanil in healthy volunteers, *Anesthesiology* **86**, 836-47 (1997).
18. R. Flaishon, A.Windsor, J.Sigl, and P.S.Sebel, Recovery of consciousness after thiopental or propofol. Bispectral index and isolated forearm technique, *Anesthesiology* **86**, 613-9 (1997).

19. J. Vuyk, T.Lim, F.H.Engbers, A.G.Burm, A.A.Vletter, and J.G.Bovill, The pharmacodynamic interaction of propofol and alfentanil during lower abdominal surgery in women, *Anesthesiology* **83**, 8-22 (1995).

20. T. Katoh, H.Bito, and S.Sato, Influence of age on hypnotic requirement, bispectral index, and 95% spectral edge frequency associated with sedation induced by sevoflurane, *Anesthesiology* **92**, 55-61 (2000).

21. M.E. Ausems, J.Vuyk, C.C.Hug, Jr., and D.R.Stanski, Comparison of a computer-assisted infusion versus intermittent bolus administration of alfentanil as a supplement to nitrous oxide for lower abdominal surgery, *Anesthesiology* **68**, 851-61 (1988).

22. C. Lysakowski, L.Dumont, M.Pellegrini, F.Clergue, and E.Tassnyi, Effects of fentanyl, alfentanil, remifentanil and sufentanil on loss of consciousness and bispectral index during propofol induction of anaesthesia., *Br.J.Anaesth.* **86**, 523-7 (2001).

23. H.M. El Kerdawy, E.E.Zalingen, and J.G.Bovill, The influence of the alpha2-adrenoceptor agonist, clonidine, on the EEG and on the MAC of isoflurane, *Eur.J.Anaesthesiol.* **17**, 105-10 (2000).

24. T. Sakai, H.Singh, W.D.Mi, T.Kudo, and A.Matsuki, The effect of ketamine on clinical endpoints of hypnosis and EEG variables during propofol infusion, *Acta Anaesthesiol.Scand.* **43**, 212-6 (1999).

25. C.C. Wu, M.S.Mok, C.S.Lin, and S.R.Han, EEG-bispectral index changes with ketamine versus thiamylal induction of anesthesia, *Acta Anaesthesiol.Sin.* **39**, 11-5 (2001).

26. G. Barr, J.G.Jakobsson, A.Owall, and R.E.Anderson, Nitrous oxide does not alter bispectral index: study with nitrous oxide as sole agent and as an adjunct to i.v. anaesthesia, *Br.J.Anaesth.* **82**, 827-30 (1999).

27. G.D. Puri, Paradoxical changesin bispectral index during nitrous oxide administration., *Br.J.Anaesth.* **86**, 141-2 (2001).

28. W.T. Denman, E.L.Swanson, D.Rosow, K.Ezbicki, P.D.Connors, and C.E.Rosow, Pediatric evaluation of the bispectral index (BIS) monitor and correlation of BIS with end-tidal sevoflurane concentration in infants and children, *Anesth.Analg.* **90**, 872-30 (2000).

29. M. Renna and R.Venturi, Bispectral index and anaesthesia in the elderly, *Minerva Anestesiol.* **66**, 398-402 (2000).

30. T.J. Gan, P.S.Glass, A.Windsor, F.Payne, C.Rosow, P.Sebel, and P.Manberg, Bispectral index monitoring allows faster emergence and improved recovery from propofol, alfentanil, and nitrous oxide anesthesia. BIS Utility Study Group, *Anesthesiology* **87**, 808-15 (1997).

31. K. Kurehara, T.Horiuch, M.Takahash, K.Kitaguchi, and H.Furuya, [A case of awareness during propofol anesthesia using bispectral index as an indicator of hypnotic effect], *Masui* **50**, 886-9 (2001).

32. M.F. O'Connor, S.M.Daves, A.Tung, R.I.Cook, R.Thisted, and J.Apfelbaum, BIS monitoring to prevent awareness during general anesthesia, *Anesthesiology* **94**, 520-2 (2001).

33. G. Barr, R.E.Anderson, A.Owall, and J.G.Jakobsson, Being awake intermittently during propofol-induced hypnosis: A study of BIS, explicit and implicit memory, *Acta Anaesthesiol.Scand.* **45**, 834-8 (2001).

34. C. De Deyne, M.Struys, J.Decruyenaere, J.Creupelandt, E.Hoste, and F.Colardyn, Use of continuous bispectral EEG monitoring to assess depth of sedation in ICU patients, *Intensive Care Med.* **24**, 1294-8 (1998).

35. G.H. Lubke, C.Kerssens, H.Phaf, and P.S.Sebel, Dependence of explicit and implicit memory on hypnotic state in trauma patients, *Anesthesiology* **90**, 670-80 (1999).

36. M.M. Struys, T.De Smet, L.F.Versichelen, D.Van, V, B.R.Van den, and E.P.Mortier, Comparison of closed-loop controlled administration of propofol using Bispectral Index as the controlled variable versus "standard practice" controlled administration, *Anesthesiology* **95**, 6-17 (2001).

37. M. Luginbühl, T.W.Schnider, Detection of awareness with the bispectral index: two case reports, *Anesthesiology* **96**, 241-3 (2002).

38. A.R. Absalom, N.Sutcliffe, G.N. Kenny, Closed-loop control of anesthesia using bispectral index, *Anesthesiology* **96**, 67-73 (2002).

AUDITORY EVOKED POTENTIALS

A clinical or a research tool?

Stefan Schraag and Gavin NC Kenny[*]

1. INTRODUCTION

Since one of the earliest systematic observations of the physiologic effects of anaesthetic agents of John Snow in 1847 our interest of measures of the level of anaesthesia has persisted and a variety of approaches and technologies have meanwhile been introduced and utilized. Today, the practice of anaesthesia remains one of the safest and most effective in medicine. So why monitor the central nervous system (CNS)? Like all new technologies, CNS monitoring devices will certainly add something to the cost of delivering anaesthesia. On the other hand, there is no doubt that significant unpredictability and uncertainty still exists in the delivery of anaesthetic drugs. This is reflected in the variety of suggested dosing regimens, especially in intravenous anaesthesia. Some patients still suffer intra-operative awareness and may consecutively develop posttraumatic stress disorder,[1] whereas others still have prolonged recovery due to relative overdosing even with otherwise short-acting drugs.

Auditory evoked potentials (AEP) derived from the electroencephalogram (EEG) have been identified to be a promising candidate to characterize depth of anaesthesia. The rationale for using auditory evoked response (AER) monitoring in anaesthesia is to create a window to the brain for assessment and adjustment of drug effect, titration and control of transition to and from anaesthesia and to adapt the level of anaesthesia. Therefore, the primary reason for using AEP monitoring designed to reflect the anaesthetic state must be to improve patient care. This chapter will give an overview of current methodology using the auditory evoked response, its impact on both research and clinical anaesthesia, and contemporary debates about AEP in the literature.

[*] Stefan Schraag , Department of Anaesthesiology University of Ulm , 89075 Ulm, Germany and Gavin NC Kenny, Department of Anaesthesia, University of Glasgow, Royal Infirmary, Glasgow G31 2ER, UK.

Advances in Modelling and Clinical Application of Intravenous Anaesthesia   105
Edited by Vuyk and Schraag, Kluwer Academic/Plenum Publishers, 2003

2. ELECTROPHYSIOLOGIC BASIS OF EVOKED RESPONSES

Evoked potentials are the non-random components of the electroencephalogram that follow a brief sensory stimulus. These evoked responses reflect the functional integrity of specific peripheral and central nervous system regions.

Signal averaging of the electroencephalogram recorded from a mastoid-vertex electrode montage after repeated click stimulation of the ear yields a highly reproducible sequence of waveforms. These waveforms arise, in sequence, from the brain stem, the auditory radiation, the auditory cortex, and association areas of the cortex (Figure 1). The brainstem response has a well-documented anatomical relationship with the auditory neuraxis, whereas later responses have origins that are less easy to define.

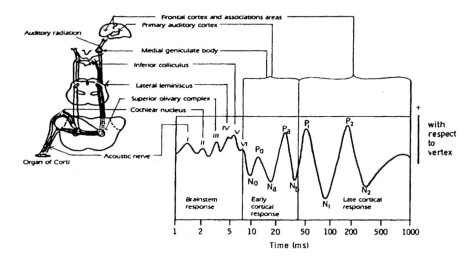

Figure 1. Schematic representation of the auditory evoked response. This diagram describes the nomenclature of the response and shows its anatomical relationship with the auditory neuraxis. Reproduced with permission from Thornton and Sharpe [2].

Of particular interest in the monitoring of the anaesthetic effect are the early cortical responses to auditory stimuli (mid-latency auditory evoked responses), which have been shown to be extremely consistent in terms of different anaesthetics and increasing drug concentrations of these drugs, with only some exceptions.[2] Processing of AEP biosignals usually consist of

- Signal acquisition
- Signal transformation
- Signal classification

In this context a couple of approaches have been successfully studied to describe an index or parameter based on the auditory evoked response, such as the auditory evoked potential index (AEPex),[3] the autoregressive adaptive modelling (ARX),[4] Forty-hertz midlatency auditory evoked potential activity[5] or wavelet analysis of middle latency auditory evoked responses.[6] One of the problems of using evoked potentials for monitoring is the small size of the bioelectric signal, necessitating a prolonged period of averaging between measurements. However, the key issue in AEP monitoring remains the quality of the primary signal presented to subsequent processing and analysis.

2.1. Signal acquisition.

The auditory evoked response is recorded as an electrical potential from bipolar surface electrodes in response to repeated auditory clicks of 1 ms duration, which are presented about 70dB above normal hearing threshold. One electrode is placed on the centre of the top of the head (reference or inactive electrode) and is subtracted from that recorded from an electrode placed over the temporal lobe, on the mastoid process (active) (Figure 2). It is important to ensure impedance levels below 3 kΩ, ideally below 1 kΩ, which can be obtained using modern silver-silver chloride self-attaching electrodes. Impedance checking is one important feature of successful AEP recording.

2.2 Signal transformation.

As with all low-voltage bioelectrical signals (0.1-0.5μV), a sufficient number of stimuli is necessary to generate a reliable signal and to eliminate the background noise. The stimulus presentation rate is clinically important, as increasing this rate can reduce the time to calculate a full signal update. A compromise has to be reached between the clarity of the response and the time taken to obtain it. Usually 256-1024 sweeps are averaged, representing 0.5-2 minutes of data collection at a stimulus rate of about 6 Hz.

2.3. Signal classification and parameter selection.

Every collected series of AEP should be subjected to proper filtering to allow a standardized comparison of waveforms across different populations and to eliminate interferences from ECG. Digital filtering is preferable to analogue filtering as the latter can change latency and distort the signal. The latencies of the peaks and troughs (in ms) along the horizontal axis and their amplitude (in μV) along the vertical axis may be analysed by visual inspection. However, further processing of the original signal may be advantageous to better quantify its changes over time. Dutton and colleagues demonstrated that the 40-Hz power of the frequency spectrum predicts wakefulness better than all latency or amplitude indices.[5] Power spectral analysis (based on fast Fourier transformations) of the evoked response has been applied by Schwender and colleagues.[7] Coherent frequency analysis may also be applied to the steady state evoked response.[8] Thornton and Newton have described an index based on the average second differential of the waveform for a time window which includes the early cortical response,[9] whereas Mantzaridis and Kenny prefer the sum of the square root of the absolute difference between every two successive segments of the AEP waveform to calculate an AEP index (AEPex).[3]

A similar processing of the AEP waveforms was introduced by Jensen and colleagues.[4] They additionally introduced an "autoregressive" (ARX) modelling technique (autoregressive modelling with exogenous input) to overcome the theoretical disadvantage of time consuming signal averaging used in the conventional analysis, for example a full update of 256 sweeps of 144 ms duration takes 36.9 s. The essence of the ARX technique is that filtering parameters are modified on an ongoing basis (Figure 2).

After acquisition of the baseline signal, filtering parameters are adjusted to create what functions as a "keyhole" that will admit only the signal of interest. That allows rapid verification of the continuing presence of that signal. As the signal varies, it cannot pass the keyhole and it is possible therefore to make rapid notification of change. However, the clinical advantage of this modelling over the AEPex or manual methods of AEP analysis has not yet been demonstrated.[10]

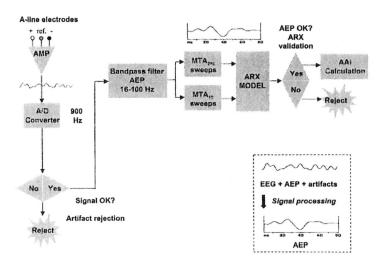

Figure 2. Autoregressive modelling with exogenous input (ARX algorithm) implemented in the A-line® AEP monitor (Alaris Medical). Recently, an automated signal check has been implemented (v. 1.5). With permission of Alaris Medical.

A novel approach has been made by Kochs and colleagues[6] to derive numerical indices from evoked responses using the technique of wavelet transformation. The AEP waveform is decomposed into constituent waveforms using one specific function among a number of known wavelet transformation functions. This approach differs from fast Fourier transformation, which is based on sine and cosine functions only. This sophisticated method of analysis has the advantage that it is objective and can be automated, but it does not necessarily provide additional or better information than the manual methods.

3. INFLUENCE OF ANAESTHETICS ON THE AER

Whereas the brain stem auditory evoked response (BAER) is resistant to the effects of general anaesthetic agents, the wave forms that follow the BAER are increasingly sensitive to anaesthetics with the characteristic pattern of change being increases in latency and decreases in amplitude in response to increasing drug concentrations.[2] The early cortical responses (also called midlatency auditory evoked potentials, MLAEP), notably Pa and Nb, vary in a dose-dependent and consistent manner in response to the administration of both inhaled and intravenous anesthetics.[11-13] This homogenous pattern has been identified as an important characteristic of auditory evoked potentials to quantify anaesthetic action (Figure 3).

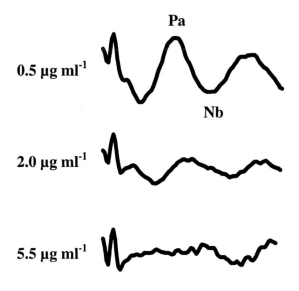

Figure 3. Gradual changes in auditory evoked potentials. Latency increases and amplitude decreases with increasing concentrations of propofol.

A couple of drugs used for general anaesthesia are not adequately reflected in the response of the AER to changes in concentrations. In a clinical study with alfentanil, fentanyl and morphine, Schwender and colleagues demonstrated that there were no dose-dependent effects of opioids on MLAEP.[14] Midazolam has less pronounced effects[15] and, in general, the amplitudes of the Pa and Nab waves are preserved during sedation with benzodiazepines.[16] As the generators of the early cortical AEP are located in the primary auditory cortex and temporal lobe, this suggests that benzodiazepines do not completely suppress cortical processing of auditory stimuli. Ketamine has no effect on the AER.[17]

4. CLINICAL APPLICATION OF AEP MONITORING AND DEPTH OF ANAESTHESIA

Adequate oblivion is a requirement and expectation of patients undergoing general anaesthesia. The main target of drugs used in general anaesthesia is the central nervous system and therefore a reliable signal produced in the CNS is required, which reflects the balance of increasing concentrations of general anaesthetics on one hand and the level of nociceptive stimulation response produced by surgery on the other. In this context AEP monitoring has to be assessed for its utility to distinguish adequate from inadequate anaesthesia.

Several studies suggest that MLAEP have substantial potential to be an effective discriminator between the anaesthetized and conscious states.[18-24] In a study of cardiac surgery patients during near normothermia in the prebypass period, Schwender and colleagues[18] studied the occurrence of implicit memory during the administration of different anaesthetic agents. They observed that implicit memory occurred only in patients in whom the latency increase in Pa was less than 12 ms. That threshold had a sensitivity of 100% for the detection of patients capable of forming implicit memory and a specificity of 77%, i.e., 23% of patients with Pa less than 12 ms did not form implicit memory. Thornton and colleagues[19] found that an Nb latency of 44.5 ms provided 100% sensitivity that patients lost their ability to respond to command in the presence of nitrous oxide after thiopental induction. Newton and colleagues[20] studied the effect of the ability of volunteers to form explicit memory during inhalation of sub-minimum alveolar concentrations (MAC) of isoflurane. An Nb latency of 47 ms separated, with 100% sensitivity and specificity, those who could and could not form explicit memory for words presented during inhalation. Using the isolated forearm technique (IFT), Loveman and co-workers[25] also demonstrated that Nb latency may represent an indicator of awareness in individual patients but also found a wide inter-patient variability.

In addition, three recent comparisons of MLAEP derivatives confirm the high level of sensitivity and specificity in the prediction of consciousness. It is suggested that the distinction between the anaesthetized and awake state is sharper, with less overlap in the ranges of conscious and unconscious values, with MLAEP derivatives, than is the case with the BIS.[21-23] There is still an ongoing evaluation of which derivative of the AEP waveform is optimal,[26] and the performance of either index in a broad range of patients and anaesthetic condition remains to be explored. Although there is reason to believe that AEP may be useful in identifying situations with a risk of awareness, data are equivocal of how effective AEP is in predicting movement in response to surgical stimulation.[27-29] Another area of uncertainty is the question how combined drug effects, especially the combination of opioids with general anaesthetics, may influence the performance of AEP, especially during surgery or other nociceptive stimulations, where clinical signs of consciousness may be masked by opioid analgesia.[30] Whereas Crabb and co-workers[31] report a dose-dependent reduction of auditory evoked responses by remifentanil during isoflurane anaesthesia, a later report by McGregor[32] from the same group could not demonstrate any significant changes to AEP during intubation in patients receiving remifentanil as part of either an inhaled anaesthetic technique using isoflurane or as part of a total i.v. technique using propofol.

6. AEP AS A RESEARCH TOOL

The evolution of quantitative monitors of "hypnosis" tempts one to consider automated control of anaesthetic administration. Closed-loop control of anaesthesia has awaited the development of a sufficiently robust monitor. New designs for automated anaesthetic administration have been successfully evaluated using mid-latency auditory evoked potentials as the input signal utilizing both proportional-integral control algorithms [33] and neural networks and fuzzy logic.[34] These systems are able to provide an unbiased control method of anaesthesia effect when used in pharmacodynamic studies.[35]

Furthermore, results of interaction studies in which AEP is used have revealed more insight into the quantitative contribution of opioids to general anaesthesia and hypnosis [30]. It is now highly evident that the degree of AEP suppression reflects increasing levels of unconsciousness and amnesia produced by hypnotic anaesthetics, whereas other states of unresponsiveness, such as the effect of higher opioid concentrations is less well represented by changes in AEP.[26]

There is still a debate whether the increasing concentrations of hypnotic drugs that produce sedation simultaneously impair memory formation and if so, how these effects relate to each other. Veselis and colleagues recently found electrophysiological evidence that midazolam and propofol affect memory differently from their sedative effects.[36] In their study they identified specific components of the auditory event-related potential, which is recorded in amplitudes and latencies of 80-700 ms (P1, N1, P2, N2, and P3 , N3) corresponding to the late cortical response. These components are associated with specific, but not necessarily unique, neuroanatomic structures. The authors conclude, that these drugs act by additional mechanisms beyond general central nervous system depression to produce the effects of sedation and memory impairment.

8. CONCLUSION

In summary, recent developments in AEP monitoring have contributed to an increasing predictability and safety of titrating general anaesthetics. The AEP signal is one of most robust and universally applicable measure to quantify concentration-effect responses of anaesthetic drugs and is therefore suitable to act as an unbiased calibration tool in pharmacodynamic research. Although predominantly used in experimental settings yet, a first commercially available AEP device is now undergoing clinical validation studies.[10] Whereas AEP monitoring will definitely contribute to an improved patient care, its potential to detect and subsequently avoid intraoperative memory formation and recall remains to be demonstrated.

9. REFERENCES

1. R. Sandin, G. Ennlund, P. Samuelsson, C. Lennmarken, Awareness during anaesthesia: a prospective case study, *Lancet* **355**, 707-711 (2000).
2. C. Thornton, R.M. Sharpe, Evoked responses in anaesthesia, *Br.J.Anaesth.* **81**, 771-781 (1998).
3. H. Mantzaridis, G.N.C. Kenny, Auditory evoked potential index: A quantitative measure of changes in auditory evoked potentials during general anaesthesia, *Anaesthesia* **52**, 1030-1036 (1997).
4. E.W. Jensen, P. Lindholm, S.W. Henneberg, Autoregressive modeling with exogenous input of auditory evoked potentials to produce an online depth of anaesthesia index, *Methods Inform. Med.* **35**, 256-260 (1996).
5. R.C. Dutton, W.D. Smith, I.J. Rampil, B.S. Chortkoff, and E.I. Eger, Forty-hertz midlatency auditory evoked potential activity predicts wakeful response during desflurane and propofol anesthesia in volunteers, *Anesthesiology* **91**, 1209-1220 (1999).
6. E. Kochs, G. Stockmanns, C. Thornton, W. Nahm, and C.J. Kalkman, Wavelet analysis of middle latency auditory evoked responses, *Anesthesiology* **95**, 1141-1150 (2001).
7. D. Schwender, I. Keller, S. Klasing, and C. Madler, Akustisch evozierte Potentiale mittlerer Latenz (AEPML) unter hochdosierter Opioidanalgesie, *Anaesthesist* **39**, 299-305 (1990).
8. R. Munglani, J. Andrade, D.J. Sapsford, A. Baddeley, J.G. Jones, A measure of consciousness and memory during isoflurane administration: the coherent frequency, *Br. J. Anaesth.* **71**, 633-641 (1993).

9. C. Thornton and D.E.F. Newton, The auditory evoked response: a measure of depth of anaesthesia, *Balliere's Clinical Anaesthesiology* **3**, 559-585 (1989).

10. H. Litvan, E.W. Jensen, M. Revuelta, S.W. Henneberg, P. Paniagua, J.M. Campos, P. Martinez, P. Caminal and J.M.V. Landeira, Comparison of auditory evoked potentials and the A-line ARX index for monitoring the hypnotic level during sevoflurane and propofol induction, *Acta Anaesthesiol. Scand.* **46**, 245-251 (2002).

11. C. Thornton, C.P. Heneghan, M.F.M. James and J.G. Jones, Effects of halothane or enflurane with controlled ventilation on auditory evoked potentials, *Br. J. Anaesth.* **56**, 315-323 (1984).

12. C. Thornton, C.P. Heneghan, M. Navaratnarajah, P.E. Bateman and J.G. Jones, Effect of etomidate on the auditory evoked response in man, *Br. J. Anaesth.* **57**, 554-561 (1985).

13. F.W. Davies, H. Mantzaridis, G.N.C. Kenny and A.C. Fisher, Middle latency auditory evoked potentials during repeated transitions from consciousness to unconsciousness, *Anaesthesia* **51**, 107-113 (1996).

14. D. Schwender, T. Rimkus, R. Haesler, S. Klasing, E. Pöppel and K. Peter, Effects of increasing doses of alfentanil, fentanyl and morphine on mid-latency auditory evoked potentials, *Br. J. Anaesth.* **71**, 622-628 (1993).

15. D. Schwender, M. Daunderer, N. Schnatmann, S. Klasing, S. Finsterer and K. Peter, Midlatency auditory evoked potentials and motor signs of wakefulness during anaesthesia with midazolam, *Br. J. Anaesth.* **79**, 53-58 (1997).

16. D. Schwender, S. Klasing, C. Madler, E. Pöppel and K. Peter, Effects of benzodiazepins on mid-latency auditory evoked potentials, *Can. J. Anaesth.* **40**, 1148-1154 (1993).

17. D. Schwender, S. Klasing, C. Madler, E. Pöppel and K. Peter, Mid-latency auditory evoked potentials during ketamine anaesthesia in humans, *Br. J. Anaesth.* **71**, 629-632 (1993).

18. D. Schwender, A. Kaiser, S. Klasing, K. Peter and E. Pöppel, Midlatency auditory evoked potentials and explicit and implicit memory in patients undergoing cardiac surgery, *Anesthesiology* **80**, 493-501 (1994).

19. C. Thornton, M.P. Barrowcliffe, K.M. Konieczko, P. Ventham, C.J. Doré, D.E. Newton and J.G. Jones, The auditory evoked response as an indicator of awareness, *Br. J. Anaesth.* **63**, 113-115 (1989).

20. D.E. Newton, C. Thornton, K.M. Konieczko, C. Jordan, N.R. Webster, N.P. Luff, C.D. Frith and C.J. Doré, Auditory evoked response and awareness: A study in volunteers at sub-MAC concentrations of isoflurane, *Br. J. Anaesth.* **69**, 122-129 (1992).

21. R.J. Gajraj, M. Doi, H. Mantzaridis and G.N.C. Kenny, Analysis of the EEG bispectrum, auditory evoked potentials and the EEG power spectrum during repeated transitions from consciousness to unconsciousness, *Br. J. Anaesth.* **80**, 46-52 (1998).

22. R.J. Gajraj, M. Doi, H. Mantzaridis and G.N.C. Kenny, Comparison of the bispectral EEG analysis and auditory evoked potentials for monitoring depth of anaesthesia during propofol anaesthesia, *Br. J. Anaesth.* **82**, 672-678 (1999).

23. S. Schraag, U. Bothner, R.J. Gajraj, G.N.C. Kenny and M. Georgieff, The performance of the electraoencephalogram bispectral index and auditory evoked potential index to predict loss of consciousness during propofol infusion, *Anesth. Analg.* **89**, 1311-1315 (1999).

24. V. Bonhomme, G. Plourde, P. Meuret, P. Fiset and S. Backman, Auditory steady-state response and bispectral index for assessing level of consciousness during propofol sedation and hypnosis, *Anesth. Analg.* **91**, 1398-1403 (2000).

25. E. Loveman, J.C. Van Hooff and D.C. Smith, The auditory evoked response as an awareness monitor during anaesthesia, *Br. J. Anaesth.* **86**, 513-518 (2001).

26. J.C. Drummond, Monitoring depth of anesthesia. With emphasis on the application of the bispectral index and the middle latency auditory evoked response to the prevention of recall, *Anesthesiology* **93**, 876-882 (2000).

27. E. Kochs, C.J. Kalkman, C. Thornton, D.E. Newton, P. Bischoff, H. Kuppe, J. Abke, E. Konecny, W. Nahm and G. Stockmanns, Middle latency auditory evoked responses and electroencephalographic derived variables do not predict movement to noxious stimulation during 1 minimum alveolar anesthetic concentration isoflurane/nitrous oxide anesthesia, *Anesth. Analg.* **88**, 1412-1417 (1999).

28. T. Kurita, M. Doi, T. Katoh, H. Sano, S. Sato, H. Mantzaridis and G.N.C. Kenny, Auditory evoked potential index predicts the depth of sedation and movement in response to skin incision during sevoflurane anesthesia, *Anesthesiology* **95**, 364-370 (2001).

29. M. Doi, R.J. Gajraj, H. Mantzaridis and G.N.C. Kenny, Prediction of movement at laryngeal mask insertion: comparison of auditory evoked potential index, bispectral index, spectral edge frequency and median frequency. *Br. J. Anaesth.* **82**, 203-207 (1999).

30. I.A. Iselin-Chaves, H.E. El Moalem, T.J. Gan, B. Ginsberg and P.S.A. Glass, Changes in the auditory evoked potentials and the bispectral index following propofol or propofol and alfentanil, *Anesthesiology* **92**, 1300-1310 (2000).

31. I Crabb, C. Thornton, K.M. Konieczko, A. Chan, R. Aquilina, N. Frazer, C.J. Doré and D.E. Newton, Remifentanil reduces auditory and somatosensory evoked responses during isoflurane anaesthesia in a dose-dependent manner, *Br. J. Anaesth.* **76**, 795-801 (1996).
32. R.R. McGregor, L.G. Allan, R.M. Sharpe, C. Thornton and D.E. Newton, Effect of remifentanil on the auditory evoked response and haemodynamic changes after intubation and surgical incision, *Br. J. Anaesth.* **81**, 785-786 (1998).
33. G.N.C. Kenny and H. Mantzaridis, Closed loop control of anaesthesia, *Br. J. Anaesth.* **83**, 223-228 (1999).
34. R. Allen and D. Smith, Neuro-fuzzy closed-loop control of depth of anaesthesia, *Art Intell Med* **21**, 185-191 (2001).
35. U. Bothner, S. Milne, G.N.C. Kenny, M. Georgieff and S. Schraag, Bayesian probabilistic network modeling of remifentanil and propofol interaction on wakeup time after closed-loop controlled anesthesia, *Int. J. Clin. Monit.* **17**, 31-36 (2002).
36. R.A. Veselis, R.A. Reinsel and V.A. Feshchenko, Drug-induced amnesia is a separate phenomenon from sedation. Electrophysiologic evidence, *Anesthesiology* **95**, 896-907 (2001).

FUNCTIONAL BRAIN IMAGING AND PROPOFOL MECHANISMS OF ACTION

Pierre Fiset[*]

1. INTRODUCTION

Positron Emission Tomography (PET) and functional Magnetic Resonance Imaging (fMRI) allow researchers to study brain function in vivo. These techniques are used to refine our understanding of the nature of anaesthetic effects as well as of the influence of anaesthetic drugs on sensory and pain transmission.

2. HOW THE VARIOUS TECHNIQUES WORK

2.1. Positron emission tomography

Positron emission tomography uses a combination of scintigraphic and computerized tomography techniques. A biological compound labelled with a radioactive tracer (^{11}C, ^{13}N, ^{15}O, ^{18}F) is injected into a subject so that its distribution in the target tissue can be determined. Depending on the information desired, a variety of compounds can be labelled. For functional brain studies, ^{15}O labelled water is often used for determination of regional Cerebral Blood Flow (rCBF) based on the assumption that changes in rCBF are coupled with those of neuronal activity.[1-3] Cerebral metabolic rate studies are performed with labelled glucose or oxygen. It is also possible to study neurotransmission by looking at the displacement of a labelled ligand from its binding sites.[4] For example, ^{11}C benztropine, an M_1 and M_2 non-specific antagonist, is used by our group to study cholinergic muscarinic transmission under anaesthesia.

---

[*] Pierre Fiset, Department of Anaesthesia, McGill University, Montréal, Québec, Canada

Advances in Modelling and Clinical Application of Intravenous Anaesthesia
Edited by Vuyk and Schraag, Kluwer Academic/Plenum Publishers, 2003

Positron emission tomography has been used for more than a decade in man for localization of the neural substrate of cognitive operations.[5] The basis of PET studies is to submit a group of individuals to a series of different conditions and to statistically compare the images to determine the physiologic changes induced by a given condition. Examples of conditions are: increasingly painful stimuli, increasing levels of drug sedation or a more complex pattern mixing painful stimuli at increasing levels of sedation.

2.2 Functional magnetic resonance imaging (fMRI)

Functional magnetic resonance imaging (fMRI) uses a different principle. Again, the basis of the studies is to compare changes in brain activation associated with various conditions in a strictly controlled experimental environment. However, there is no need for administration of radioactive tracers, and the temporal and spatial resolutions are much better than with PET.

During an fMRI scan, the magnetic fields from hydrogen nuclei of water molecules orient themselves along the strong magnetic field of the scanner. Radio frequency pulses are sent to disturb this orientation. The resulting realignment causes the emission of a radio frequency signal that can be detected by a receiver coil.[6]

In brain regions activated during neuronal stimulation, the signal is increased by a change in the ratio of deoxyhaemoglobin. During neuronal activity, local metabolism increases and local blood flow increases more than in proportion for the demand, inducing a paradoxical decrease in the ratio of deoxyhaemoglobin. It is the resulting "blood oxygen level dependent" (BOLD) signal that constitutes the basis of fMRI.[7]

3. BRAIN IMAGING AND PROPOFOL ACTION

Brain imaging offers unique possibilities for improving our knowledge of anaesthetic effects. Anaesthesia induces a host of dose-specific and controllable changes in central nervous system function. Our knowledge of propofol pharmacology and the availability of powerful tools to achieve and maintain stable drug concentrations allow us to use propofol as a prototypical anaesthetic drug that modulates the level consciousness. Stable plasma levels, or conditions in the brain imaging vocabulary, can be obtained that correspond to specific levels of sedation. Dose specific changes in brain activity can be measured, and the neurophysiological correlates of the regional changes can be explored. Brain imaging allows us to have a systems approach to the investigation of mechanisms of anaesthesia based on the premise that propofol, and by extension other anaesthetic drugs, possibly has a dose-dependant effect on specific neural systems.

4. PET STUDIES ON REGIONAL CEREBRAL EFFECTS

Michael Alkire and his group (U.C. Irvine) have done a series of propofol studies in human volunteers using [18]fluorodeoxyglucose (FDG) to measure the changes in the central nervous system glucose metabolic rate produced by anesthesia[8] and showed that it was not uniform. Cortical metabolism was depressed more than sub-cortical and marked differences in regional cortical changes were seen. In another study, these authors correlated EEG changes with the cerebral metabolic reduction caused by propofol and isoflurane and proposed that a physiologic link exists between those variables.[9]

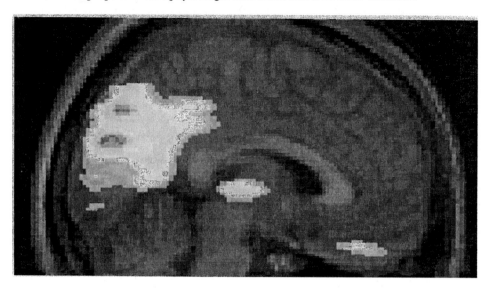

Figure 1. The thalamus, pre-cuneus, cuneus and posterior cingulated cortex are preferentially affected by propofol. Additionally, a large area of the parieto-occipital sulcus (not shown here) shows a decrease in regional cerebral blood flow. The shades of gray indicate the intensity of the effect (propofol concentration versus cerebral blood flow)[10].

Our group has studied the effects of propofol on the central nervous system using PET. In a first study, we determined the effect of different levels of propofol sedation, from light sedation to unconsciousness, on rCBF using $^{15}H_2O$. We found a significant decrease in rCBF in the thalamus, the orbito-frontal cortices, and a large area of the medial parieto-occipital cortex extending bilaterally to the parieto-occipital sulcus area.[10] These anatomical sites are involved in the control of consciousness and in various integrative and associative tasks. In particular, given the importance of thalamic function in conscious processes, this study as well as others[11] show that "the level of functional thalamic activity occurring in a brain during anaesthesia is likely to be related in some manner to a person's level of consciousness[12] These results also support the hypothesis that propofol has regional effects and that certain brain structures may demonstrate particular sensitivity to anaesthetic drugs. If these results are confirmed, the notion that precise neural networks are selectively affected by anaesthetics should help guide research on the cellular and molecular mechanisms of anaesthesia (see below).

The neural pathways for conducting and perceiving pain and vibro-tactile stimulation are well known and their activation can be accurately shown using PET.[13,14] Anaesthesia alters the perception of external stimuli thus allowing patients to undergo painful procedures. Very little is known on the exact mechanism by which such a disruption of neural conduction occurs. Is the transmission of sensory information blocked at the level of the dorsal horn, the thalamus, or at the primary or secondary sensory cortex? Is the modulation of the associative and affective functions related to pain perception? Do these areas of the central nervous system show a dose-dependant sensitivity to anaesthetics?

As a first step to answering these questions, we studied the influence of the level of propofol sedation on vibro-tactile stimulation.[15] Volunteers were administered increasing target concentrations of propofol while presented with standardized vibratory stimuli. We found a significant decrease in activation of the primary sensory cortex at very low sedative doses of propofol (0.5 $\mu g \cdot ml^{-1}$). A more profound effect was seen at higher levels of sedation, with almost complete abolition of activation in the thalamus when pharmacological unconsciousness was produced. This suggests that even when a patient is only mildly sedated, there may be a significant diminution of cortical activation, which accounts for the relative indifference to certain external tactile stimuli.

We then proceeded to investigate the effect of propofol on pain perception.[16] At light levels of sedation, pain perception (intensity and unpleasantness) increased with a concomitant increase in anterior cingulate cortex (ACC) activation. After loss of consciousness, some nociceptive information reached cortical and sub cortical structures (e.g. the insular cortex), but the transfer of information to the thalamus and anterior cingulate cortex was greatly reduced. These results support the notion that concentration specific effects of propofol can be linked to specific regional central nervous system effects.

5. PET STUDIES ON NEUROTRANSMISSION

Although most of the brain imaging research in anaesthesia has been done with blood flow and metabolic markers, some groups have used positron emission tomography with ligand displacement techniques to investigate changes in neurotransmission during anaesthesia.[17,18]

We have used ^{11}C-Benztropine[19], a non-specific M1 and M2 antagonist, to study muscarinic receptor occupancy during propofol-induced unconsciousness. There are reports in the literature of reversal of anaesthetic effects with physostigmine, an anticholinesterase drug that crosses the blood-brain barrier.[20-25] In fact Antilirium® has been used for years to "speed up awakening". Scopolamine, on the other hand, an antimuscarinic drug which also crosses the blood-brain barrier, induces sedation and potentiates the anaesthetic effect.

These facts, coupled with the extensive knowledge of the modulatory effect of the central cholinergic system on sleep-wake states,[26,27] suggest that anaesthetics may produce changes in the level of consciousness by altering central muscarinic transmission.[23,27,28] Our preliminary results (unpublished) show that propofol produces a decrease in benztropine binding (reflecting a decrease in central acetyl choline (ACh) binding) under anaesthesia in central nervous system areas rich in M1 receptors. This would support the hypothesis that propofol affects ACh-binding in one of two ways. First, it is possible that propofol causes a change in receptor configuration or affinity so that it becomes less available for binding. Alternatively, it is possible that propofol binds directly with the M1 receptor and prevents binding with ACh (or benztropine).

The availability of ligands related to the serotonin, dopamine, benzodiazepine and other receptors would provide powerful tools for further refining our understanding of anaesthetic effects on neurotransmission.

6. UNDERSTANDING ANAESTHETIC EFFECTS

Brain imaging helps to refine our understanding of anaesthetic effect and is providing novel information that result in the formulation of hypotheses. In the studies reported here as well as in many others in which various anaesthetics were used, a constant finding is that the drugs that we use seem to exert their action on specific sites within the central nervous system. This is true for a wide variety of drugs like midazolam,[11] inhalational anaesthetics[29,30] and opioids.[31] Although brain imaging can't give precise information on the neurophysiological mechanisms or the anatomical connectivity that underlie anaesthetic effects, it provides an anatomical target for the localization of anaesthetic sensitive neurotransmitters and a framework for the determination of the functional network affected by anaesthetic drugs.

Functional imaging of anaesthetic effects has contributed to the emergence or the reinforcement of some interesting hypothesis on mechanisms of anaesthesia. The thalamus has consistently shown marked deactivation coincident with the anaesthesia-induced loss of consciousness, appearing to be a very important target of anaesthetic effect. This is consistent with findings from other researchers interested in single cell physiology. At the cellular level, anaesthetics have been shown to cause hyper polarization and increased conductance of thalamic ventrobasal relay neurons.[32] This would cause an inhibition of thalamic tonic firing of action potential which, considering the central role of the thalamus in the relay of afferent information and maintenance of consciousness could be well in line with the production of anaesthesia.[32]

Study of the mechanisms of anaesthesia may also reveal the neural substrates of changes in the level of consciousness we experience daily. The use of anaesthetic drugs can be seen as a powerful tool for investigating conscious phenomena. Anaesthetics can be very precisely given to achieve precise states of altered consciousness. Once these conditions are reached, one can look at the functional neural network responsible for that state, gathering information on processes responsible for conscious behaviour. That approach has been elegantly exposed recently by Raichle et al.[33] They suggest that brain imaging of altered conscious states, whether caused by anaesthesia, sleep or coma, is instrumental in the characterization of the baseline state of the resting human brain. By looking at which areas are deactivated when a person is taken from a baseline level of cerebral activity (resting quietly, awake, with eyes closed and no task) to a pharmacologically altered state of consciousness (anywhere from mild sedation to unconsciousness), one can determine which brain networks are involved in the maintenance of the awake state. Such a conceptual approach to the investigation of consciousness offers a golden opportunity for anaesthesia research to bring significant contributions to the wider field of neuroscience.

7. CONCLUSION

Brain imaging is a window on the working brain. It offers tremendous possibilities for understanding the neural processes involved in all aspects of consciousness. Data from research in this field suggest that anaesthetics, and propofol in particular are not simply general depressant of brain activity, but rather act on specific structures of the central nervous system in a dose-dependant fashion.

8. REFERENCES

1. M. Raichle, W. Martin, Herscovitch P, Mintun M, Markham J, Brain blood flow measured with intravenous H$_2$O^{15} II. Implementation and validation, *Jf Nucl Med* **24**, 790-8, (1983).
2. M. Kato, Ueno T, Black P, Regional cerebral blood flow of the main visual pathways during photic stimulation of the retina in intact and split-brain monkeys, *Exp Neurol* **42**, 65-77 (1974).
3. A. Villringer, Understanding functional neuroimaging methods based on neurovascular coupling, *Adv Exp Med Biol* **413**, 177-93 (1997).
4. G.B. Saha, MacIntyre WJ, Go RT, Radiopharmaceuticals for brain imaging, *Semin Nucl Med* **24**, 324-49 (1994).
5. M.I. Posner, Petersen SE, Fox PT, Raichle ME, Localization of cognitive operations in the human brain, *Science* **240**, 1627-31 (1988).
6. D. Le Bihan, Jezzard P, Haxby J, Sadato N, Rueckert L, Mattay V, Fuctional magnetic resonance imaging of the brain, *Annals of Internal Medicine* **122**, 296-303 (1995).
7. S. Ogawa, Tank DW, Menon R, Ellermann JM, Kim S-G, Merkle H, Ugurbil K, Intrinsic signal changes accompanying sensory stimulation: functional brain mapping with magnetic resonance imaging, *Proc Natl Acad Sci* **89**, 5951-5 (1992).
8. M.T. Alkire, Haier RJ, Barker SJ, Shah NK, Wu JC, Kao J, Cerebral metabolism during propofol anesthesia in humans studied with positron emission tomography, *Anesthesiology* **82**, 393-403 (1995).
9. M.T. Alkire, Quantitative EEG correlations with brain glucose metabolic rate during anesthesia volunteers, *Anesthesiology* **89**, 323-33 (2001).
10. P. Fiset P, Paus T, Daloze T, Plourde G, Meuret P, Bonhomme V, Hajj-Ali N, Backman SB, Evans AC, Brain mechanisms of propofol-induced loss of consciousness in humans: a Positron Emission Tomography study, *J Neurosci* **19**, 5506-13 (1999).
11. R.A. Veselis, Reinsel RA, Beattie BJ, Mawlawi OR, Feshchenko VA, DiResta GR, Larson SM, Blasberg RG, Midazolam changes cerebral blood flow in discrete brain regions, *Anesthesiology* **87**, 1106-17 (1997).
12. M.T. Alkire, Haier RJ, Fallon JH, Toward a unified theory of narcosis: brain imaging evidence for a thalamocortical switch as the neurrophysiologic basis of anesthetic-induced unconsciousness, *Consciousness and Cognition* **9**, 370-86 (2000).
13. R.C. Coghill, Talbot JD, Evans AC, Meyer E, Gjedde A, Bushnell MC, Duncan GH, Distributed processing of pain and vibration by the human brain, *J Neurosci* **14**, 4095-108 (1994).
14. J.D. Talbot, Marret S, Evans AC, Meyer E, Bushnell MC, Duncan GH, Multiple representations of pain in human cerebral cortex, *Science* **251**, 1355-7 (1991).
15. V. Bonhomme, Fiset P, Meuret P, Backman S, Plourde G, Paus T, Bushnell C, Evans A, Effect of propofol-induced general anesthesia on changes in regional cerebral blood flow elicited by vibrotactile stimulation: a positron emission tomography study, *J Neurophysiol* **85**, 1299-308 (2001).
16. R.K. Hofbauer, Fiset P, Plourde G, Backman SB, Bushnell MC, Cortical correlates of the conscious experience of pain, *J Neurosci*, Submitted (2002).
17. F. Gyulai, L. Firestone, J. Price, P. Winter, In vivo imaging of volatile anesthetic action at the 5HT$_{2A}$-receptor (5HT$_{2A}$-R) in humans: a quantitative positron emission tomography (PET) study, *Society for Neuroscience* **23**, 59.18 (1997).
18. F.E. Gyulai, Mintum MA, Firestone LL, Dose-dependent enhancement of in vivo GABA$_A$-benzodiazepine receptor binding by isoflurane, *Anesthesiology* **95**, 585-93 (2001).
19. S.L. Dewey, Brodie JD, Fowler JS, MacGregor RR, Schyler DJ, King PT, Alexoff DL, Volkow ND, Shiue C-L, Wolf AP, Bendriem B, Positron Emission Tomography (PET) studies of dopaminergic/cholinergic interactions in the baboon brain, *Synapse* **6**, 321-7 (1990).
20. U. Ebert, Oertel R, Kirch W: Physostigmine reversal of midazolam-induced electroencephalographic changes in healthy subjects, *Clin Pharmacol Ther* **67**, 538-48 (2001).
21. A.A. Artru, Hui GS, Physostigmine reversal of general anesthesia for intraoperative neurological testing: Associated EEG changes, *Anesth Analg* **65**, 1059-62, (1986).
22. P. Hartvig, Lindström B, Petterson E, Wiklund L, Reversal of postoperative somnolence using a two-rate infusion of physostigmine, *Acta Anaesthesiol Scand* **33**, 681-5 (1986).
23. P. Meuret, Backman SB, Bonhomme V, Plourde G, Fiset P, Physostigmine reverses propofol-induced unconsciousness and attenuation of the auditory steady state response and bispectral index in human volunteers, *Anesthesiology* **93**, 708-17 (2000).
24. A. Toro-Matos, Rendon-Platas AM, Avila-Valdez E, Villarreal-Guzman RA, Physostigmine antagonizes ketamine, *Anesth Analg* **59**, 764-7 (1980).

25. M. Talbot, G. Plourde, S.B. Backman, D. Chartrand, P. Fiset, Effect of physostigmine on the loss of consciousness and analgesia produced by remifentanil, *Anesthesiology* **93**, A389 (2000).
26. R. Lydic R, Biebuyck JF, Sleep neurobiology: relevance for mechanistic studies of anaesthesia, *Br J Anaesth* **72**, 506-8 (1994).
27. R. Lydic, Baghdoyan HA, Cholinergic contribution to the control of consciousness, Anesthesia: Biologic Foundations. Edited by Yaksh TLeal. Philadelphia, Lippincott-Raven, 1997, pp 433-50
28. J.C. Keifer, Baghdoyan HA, Becker L, Lydic R, Halothane decreases pontine acethylcholine release and increases EEG spindles, *Neuroreport* **5**, 577-80 (1995).
29. M.T. Alkire, Haler RJ, Shah NK, Anderson CT, Positron emission tomography study of regional cerebral metabolism in humans during isoflurane anesthesia, *Anesthesiology* **86**, 549-57 (1997).
30. M.T. Alkire, Pomfrett CJ, Haier RJ, Gianzero MV, Chan CM, Jacobsen BP, Functional brain imaging during anesthesia in humans: effects of halothane on global and regional cerebral glucose metabolism, *Anesthesiology* **90**, 701-9 (1999).
31. L.J. Adler, Gyulai FE, Diehl DJ, Mintum MA, Winter PM, Firestone LL, Regional brain activity changes associated with fentanyl analgesia elucidated by positron emission tomography, *Anesth Analg* **84**, 120-6 (1997).
32. C.R. Ries, Puil E, Mechanism of anesthesia revealed by shunting actions of isoflurane on thalamocortical neurons, *J Neurophysiol* **81**, 1795-801 (1999).
33. D.A. Gusnard, Raichle ME, Raichle ME, Searching for a baseline: functional imaging and the resting human brain, *Nature Reviews Neuroscience* **2**, 685-94, (2001).

THE DEVELOPMENT AND FUTURE OF
TARGET CONTROLLED INFUSION

John B Glen[*]

1. INTRODUCTION

Fortunately, the simplicity of the clinical application of target controlled infusion (TCI) is far removed from the complexity of the mathematical basis of the concept, as originally proposed by Kruger –Theimer[1] and Schwilden.[2] A small group of pioneers with an understanding of mathematics, pharmacokinetics, computers and anaesthesiology has translated the complex equations described into the reality of a simple method to achieve and maintain a pseudo steady-state blood or brain concentration of various iv therapies. The 'Diprifusor'TCI system (AstraZeneca) for the administration of propofol was the first commercial system to be approved by regulatory authorities. Users of this system do not require a detailed knowledge of the basic sciences on which this device has been built. As a clinical tool, a TCI system simplifies the administration of iv agents, and provides the anaesthetist with greater precision in the control of depth of anaesthesia or sedation, as the target drug concentration can be titrated upwards and downwards in a predictable and reproducible manner. In this way, control is similar to that achieved by adjustment of the inspired concentration of an inhalational agent and a TCI system can be seen as the iv. equivalent of a vaporizer. This article summarizes briefly the evolution of TCI systems and looks at recent enhancements and possible future developments

2. THE CONCEPT OF TCI

Target Controlled Infusion (TCI) is an alternative mode of infusion for iv agents whereby the user, instead of setting an infusion rate in ml/h or μg/kg/min, sets a desired (target) blood concentration in μg/ml or ng/ml. With conventional infusion, drug

* John (Iain) B. Glen, Glen Pharma Limited, 35A Bexton Road, Knutsford, Cheshire, WA16 0DZ, UK

Advances in Modelling and Clinical Application of Intravenous Anaesthesia   123
Edited by Vuyk and Schraag, Kluwer Academic/Plenum Publishers, 2003

concentration increases gradually over time and the rate at which steady state is approached depends on the pharmacokinetics of the agent. With TCI systems, pharmacokinetic parameters are incorporated in infusion control software. Infusion rate control algorithms in an external computer, or in a microprocessor incorporated within a pump, control the amount of drug delivered to ensure that the target concentration is attained rapidly and the infusion rate is automatically reduced over time to maintain a constant blood concentration:

- Conventional infusion: Infusion rate constant
                            Blood concentration increases over time

- TCI: Blood concentration constant
                            Infusion rate decreases over time

If the target concentration setting is changed by the user, the control algorithms ensure that a new steady state blood concentration is attained rapidly.

3. EARLY DEVELOPMENTS AND NOMENCLATURE

In 1968, Kruger-Theimer[1] derived equations specifying the intravenous infusion rate profile required to achieve and maintain a constant specified plasma concentration of a drug whose pharmacokinetics could be described by a linear multicompartment model. In 1981, Schwilden[2] suggested and demonstrated the use of computer controlled infusion pumps to implement exponentially declining infusion schemes based on the concept proposed by Kruger-Theimer. The first drugs administered in this way were etomidate and alfentanil.[3] The infusion profile delivered by these pumps was described as a BET (bolus, elimination, transfer) scheme. This scheme provided a loading dose (bolus) to fill the initial volume of distribution of the drug, a final infusion rate equal to the clearance (elimination) of the drug and an interim infusion scheme to match the redistribution (transfer) of drug from the central volume of distribution to more peripheral sites. Later infusion schemes were modified and infusion rate control algorithms developed to allow the anaesthesiologist to vary the target plasma drug concentration as clinically indicated.[4-6] The use of a prototype TCI system for the administration of propofol was first described in 1988.[7] This was followed by a system developed by the University of Glasgow based on an external computer connected to a volumetric infusion pump.[8] The control software in this system later formed the basis of the 'Diprifusor' TCI module which was developed by ICI (now AstraZeneca) and was approved in Europe in 1996.

Early research systems were described as CATIA (computer assisted total intravenous anaesthesia)[3], TIAC (titration of intravenous agents by computer),[9] CACI (computer-assisted continuous infusion)[4] and CCIP (computer-controlled infusion pump).[10] In an attempt to simplify terminology and achieve a degree of standardization, TCI has been proposed as a descriptive term for all of these systems and the following abbreviations have been suggested;[11] Cp_T = target plasma concentration, Ce_T = target effect site concentration, Cp_M = measured plasma concentration, Cp_{CALC} = calculated plasma concentration, Ce_{CALC} = calculated effect site concentration. TCI systems display both the Cp_T, the target set by the user, and Cp_{CALC}, the plasma concentration calculated by the TCI system.

When a given target setting is being maintained, these two figures will be the same. However, when a lower Cp_T is set, Cp_{CALC} will lag behind Cp_T as the rate of decline in the blood concentration is dependent on the distribution and elimination of drug from the body, as calculated by the pharmacokinetic model in the system. In evaluating the predictive performance of TCI systems, indices based on the difference between Cp_M and Cp_{CALC} are calculated.[12]

4. THE DEVELOPMENT OF DIPRIFUSOR TCI

The development of the Diprifusor TCI system, including pharmacokinetic concepts[13] and associated technology[14] has been described in detail elsewhere[15], but a brief summary of key aspects is included here to illustrate principles which will be important in the development of commercial systems for other molecules. Despite lengthy academic experience, TCI was a new concept for drug and device regulatory agencies and a regulatory process had to be defined in discussions with these authorities. There was also a need for clear delineation of the responsibilities of the drug company, in selecting the pharmacokinetic (PK) model and providing guidance on target concentration settings in the drug labelling, from those of the infusion pump manufacturer. This was achieved by the supply of a Diprifusor TCI module by AstraZeneca to pump companies. This module contains infusion control algorithms developed by one of the research groups[8] and the PK model described by Marsh et al.[16] This model was selected for clinical trials in 1992, following discussion with academic groups, as the most accurate available at that time. This was confirmed in a later prospective study by Coetzee et al.[17] Incorporation of the Diprifusor module in pumps from different manufacturers ensures that the output of all pumps will be the same with any particular target profile input. In addition, while many different PK models for propofol have been used successfully, guidance on target concentration settings is relevant only to the output achieved with standardized systems incorporating the Diprifusor module with the Marsh PK model. The pump manufacturer, having incorporated the module in a pump, has no need to repeat clinical studies but must demonstrate, with a laboratory study, that the delivery performance profile of their integrated pump meets a specification derived by the drug company with devices used in clinical trials. This laboratory study provides a link for the regulators between the drug and device components of the regulatory submission. Amended labelling for propofol required approval as a variation to the marketing authorisation for propofol. The Diprifusor TCI module and pumps incorporating this module were evaluated by Notified Bodies before approval for marketing in Europe with the grant of a CE mark of conformity.

5. FURTHER DEVELOPMENT OF DIPRIFUSOR

The use of Diprifusor TCI for the delivery of propofol was first approved for induction and maintenance of anaesthesia in adults. Recently, additional submissions have been made requesting the extension of Diprifusor TCI use to conscious sedation for procedures conducted under regional anaesthesia and to intensive care sedation of adult ventilated patients. Research modifications of Diprifusor have been used with encouraging results for patient maintained sedation,[18] and for paediatric anaesthesia,[19] but formal clinical validation of these modifications has not yet been completed. Two enhancements, not available in the original user interface, have been added to Diprifusor TCI systems.

The time required to reach a lower concentration, if the infusion were to be stopped, is indicated as the 'decrement time'. If the lower concentration input by the user is the propofol blood concentration at which waking is anticipated, an estimated waking time can be provided by the system. However, it is important to understand that the propofol blood concentration at waking will depend on the amount of concomitant analgesia given (i.e. waking will occur at a higher calculated blood propofol concentration if minimal analgesic supplementation has been given) and that the model predicts a decline in propofol concentration for an average patient without accounting for pharmacokinetic variability. With an understanding of these limitations, information on decrement time may help to promote the use of appropriate analgesic supplementation to avoid the delay in recovery which could be anticipated if high propofol target settings are still in use at the end of anaesthesia.

A second addition involved the provision of information on Ce_{CALC} in the pump display. The value of k_{e0} incorporated in Diprifusor systems is 0.26/min[20] and again it must be appreciated that this is an average value and, as discussed later, debate continues on the most appropriate k_{e0} for propofol. Nevertheless, information on the calculated effect-site concentration of propofol has provided a number of benefits. The extent of the delay in equilibration between blood and brain propofol concentrations is illustrated and this allows more rational adjustment of the target blood concentration setting to achieve a desired brain concentration more quickly. Computer simulations predict that if a given effect-site concentration of propofol is desired, this can be achieved more rapidly, and without overshoot, by doubling this target setting as a blood propofol concentration for 2 minutes, then decreasing to the desired target. Such an approach would not be appropriate for elderly or haemodynamically unstable patients. In these patients, it is desirable to increase the target blood concentration gradually until a desired effect is achieved. In this situation, the effect site concentration may lag well behind the blood concentration suggesting that it would be appropriate to reduce the target blood concentration setting towards the calculated effect site concentration when the desired effect has been achieved, to prevent an unnecessary overshoot in the effect site concentration.

Population pharmacokinetic models have now been described for propofol[21,22] and modified parameters for elderly patients have been proposed.[23] These models, that include covariates for various patient characteristics such as age or gender, should allow improved individualization of drug dosage for research studies, but were not available at the time of clinical validation of the Diprifusor system. The PK model in a TCI system can be seen as analogous to the gearbox in a car that converts a given throttle setting into a speed. The PK model in a TCI system converts a target setting into an exponentially decreasing infusion rate profile and changing the PK model in Diprifusor would potentially alter the performance of an established system whose 12,000 users have become familiar with the current 'gearbox'. Apart from this practical problem, a change in the PK model would require further regulatory validation studies. As can be seen in Figure 1, the amount of drug delivered in plasma concentration control mode (Cp_T) with the Schnider model is much less than with the Marsh PK model.

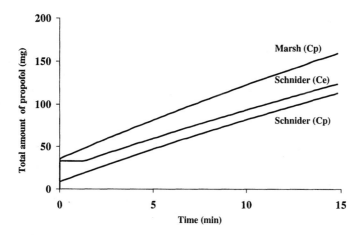

Figure 1. Computer simulation of the cumulative amounts (mg) of propofol delivered in a 53 year male patient, body weight 77 kg, height 177 cm, to achieve a target propofol concentration of 2.0 µg/ml. Cp = plasma concentration target control, Ce = effect-site concentration target control. Marsh[16] and Schnider[21] PK models.

Thus different target settings would be required to achieve the same effect, particularly during the first 15 minutes of a procedure where the simulation shows that the Schnider model delivers only 37% and 71 % of the amount provided with the Marsh model at 1 and 15 minutes respectively. This difference is primarily dependent on the much smaller V_1 of the Schnider model; 4.27 L versus 17.6 L for the Marsh model for the patient illustrated. Even with effect-site control (Ce_T) with the Schnider model, the amount of drug delivered at 1 and 15 minutes is 72% and 85% respectively of that provided by the Marsh model. Thus, at a given target setting, onset of effect can be predicted to be more rapid with Diprifusor TCI than with a TCI system incorporating the Schnider PK model, even if the latter system were to be operated in effect-site control mode. In view of both practical and regulatory considerations, it is unlikely that the PK model in Diprifusor TCI systems will now be amended. However, in future, when it is hoped that commercial TCI systems become available for other drugs, it is likely that the more sophisticated models, which have been developed for drugs such as remifentanil,[24] will be employed.

6. FURTHER DEVELOPMENT OF TCI

Two topics will be considered here. Firstly, as the effect of anaesthetic drugs does not occur in the blood but in the brain, there is increasing interest in TCI systems that control the concentration at the effect-site. Secondly, as the benefits of the TCI mode of administration become more widely recognised, consideration will be given to the possible development of commercial TCI systems for drugs other than propofol.

6.1. Effect-Site TCI Control

Algorithms to achieve and maintain stable drug concentrations at the site of drug effect have been described[25,26] and a number of research TCI systems have incorporated this facility. All of these algorithms require a value for k_{e0}, a rate constant which influences the rate of equilibration of the concentration of drug at the effect-site in the brain with the concentration in blood; and all create an overshoot in the plasma concentration to drive drug to the effect site more quickly. Different PK models for a given drug may deliver drug in a significantly different manner as shown in Figure 1, such that the same k_{e0} value may not be appropriate for all PK models. For propofol, Schnider et al. [27] have proposed a value for k_{e0} of 0.456/min for use in conjunction with the population PK model described by this same group.[21] Other studies have reported k_{e0} values for propofol ranging from 0.2[28] to 1.21/min. The latter value was proposed by Struys et al.[29] for use in conjunction with the Marsh PK model for propofol to achieve a time to peak effect of 1.6 min as observed by Schnider et al.[27] A k_{e0} value of 0.26/min is currently incorporated in Diprifusor TCI systems to allow the display of Ce_{CALC} but effect site control is not currently available with this system. This value was derived from a study of the pharmacodynamics of propofol as determined by auditory evoked potentials.[20]

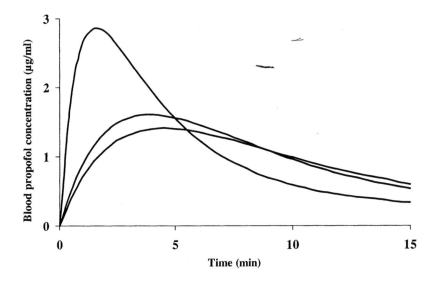

Figure 2. Computer simulation of the influence of k_{e0} on calculated effect-site concentrations of propofol following a bolus of 1mg/kg over 5 s. Values of k_{e0} = 1.21 (highest peak), 0.26 and 0.2/min (lowest peak).

With plasma concentration control, the k_{e0} value incorporated in a TCI system has no influence on the amount of drug delivered and does not influence the rate of onset of effect. The k_{e0} value does however affect the estimated value of the effect site concentration (Ce_{CALC}) displayed by a TCI pump and thus the displayed rate of equilibration between blood and brain concentrations. Computer simulation of the effect of different k_{e0} values for propofol on the time to peak effect after a bolus dose is of limited value in confirming an optimum value for k_{e0}, as the peak concentration achieved with a given amount of drug is influenced by the k_{e0} value used, and only small differences in the time to peak effect can be expected (Figure 2). On the other hand, with the spectrum of k_{e0} values reported in the literature and simulations based on plasma concentration control by TCI, a wide spread of times to peak effect is predicted (Figure 3).

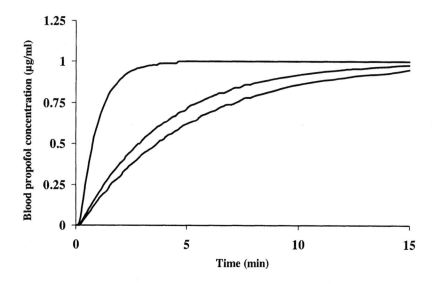

Figure 3. Computer simulation of calculated effect-site concentrations of propofol with k_{e0} values of 1.21 (steepest curve), 0.26 and 0.2/min (lowest curve) with Cp_T of 1 µg/ml and the Marsh[16] PK model.

With this approach the maximum effect eventually obtained is independent of the k_{e0} value. Most studies have used surrogate indices of effect, usually based on processed EEG parameters to determine a k_{e0} value. Before the commercial development of effect-site control systems for propofol can be envisaged, it is considered that a consensus needs to be reached on the most appropriate k_{e0} value for use with the Marsh PK parameters. With the separation in time to predicted peak effect with different k_{e0} values illustrated in Figure 2 (80% of peak effect at 1.4 min with k_{e0} of 1.21/min versus 8 min with k_{e0} of 0.20/min) it should be possible, if a subanaesthetic propofol concentration is targeted, to use some form of simple psychometric testing to obtain an objective assessment of the actual time to peak effect to compare with the values determined from more complex EEG studies. The k_{e0} value of 0.3 /min obtained in the detailed study by Kazama et al.[30] (t½ k_{e0} 2.3 min) in a study using BIS monitoring may prove to be close to ideal.

The other problem in validation of an effect-site control system is that concentrations at this site cannot be directly measured. Their assessment may require evaluation of the influence of "overpressure" of the plasma concentration on haemodynamics and characterisation of the delivery performance of the system. Figure 4 illustrates that with the Marsh PK model, effect site control with a k_{e0} of 1.21/min leads to only a moderate increase in the amount of drug delivered over the first 2 min but a k_{e0} value of 0.2/min leads to a greatly increased delivery of propofol over the first 5 min. Hence the importance of confirming the correct k_{e0} for this model.

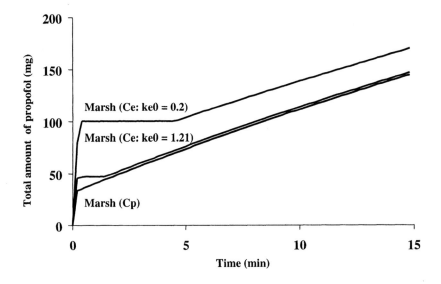

Figure 4. Computer simulation of the cumulative amounts of propofol (mg) delivered in a 70 kg adult to achieve a propofol concentration of 2 µg/ml with the Marsh[16] PK model. Cp = plasma concentration control. Ce = effect site control with k_{e0} values of 0.2 or 1.21/min.

7. COMMERCIAL TCI SYSTEMS FOR OTHER DRUGS

The TCI mode of administration of drugs provides a number of practical advantages to the user as follows:

- Improved control and predictability of the pharmacodynamic effect achieved.
- Therapeutic concentration achieved rapidly and maintained constant.
- Control over onset time by slow upward titration of target if desired in elderly.
- Proportional changes in blood concentration rapidly achieved.
- Improved titratability.
- Avoidance of peak blood concentrations and possible risk of associated toxicity
- No need for calculation of infusion rate.
- Automatic adjustment for differences in body weight, lean body mass, age or gender if complex model available.
- Displayed effect-site concentration facilitates titration of the blood concentration.
- Estimation of the time required to reach a lower plasma concentration.
- Target concentration regained automatically after a syringe change.
- A more logical and modern approach.

In comparative studies where user preference has been elicited, the majority of users has preferred the TCI mode of administration and found it easier to use than conventional manually controlled infusion.[31] The benefits of TCI as summarized above have encouraged the development of a number of experimental TCI systems which have been used to administer a large range of anaesthetic and ancillary drugs.

Software programs such as RUGLOOP (Michel Struys, Ghent, Belgium), STANPUMP (Steven Shafer, Stanford, USA) and STELPUMP (Johan Coetzee, Stellenbosch, South Africa) can be loaded into a laptop computer and used to control a computer compatible infusion pump. These programs, when used in this way, are considered to be medical devices and hence fall within the scope of medical device legislation. The originators of these programs clearly indicate that these are experimental programs and responsibility for their use lies with the individual user or their institution. As they are not approved systems (i.e. not CE marked in Europe) they should only be used in clinical investigations following local ethics committee approval. With the increasing awareness of the benefits of TCI there is now activity among infusion pump manufacturers to produce validated TCI systems, independent of the Diprifusor approach. Once validated, these systems could be advocated for the delivery of other drugs by TCI, but a prerequisite will be the willingness of pharmaceutical companies to ensure the standardization of such systems by identifying a particular PK model and delivery performance specification for their drug, and adding guidance in drug labelling on target concentration settings. Any intravenous drug that is administered over a moderate duration by infusion could potentially benefit from the TCI mode of administration. Of these, remifentanil, sufentanil, alfentanil, fentanyl, etomidate, midazolam and dexmedetomidine have all been given by TCI with experimental systems and other candidates could be found among iv antibacterials, antiarrhythmics, chemotherapeutic agents and inotropes. In the near future one can envisage iv anaesthesia work stations with the facility to deliver a range of drugs by TCI, together with associated monitoring and ventilation capabilities, and commercial developments in this direction are already underway.

8. PHARMACOKINETIC/PHARMACODYNAMIC MODELLING

The ability to achieve and maintain steady drug concentrations with TCI has facilitated research investigations into the interaction between hypnotic and analgesic agents[32]. A simple benefit of TCI systems is that measures of relative potency can be based on blood or effect site concentrations, obviating the need for consideration of the differences in pharmacokinetics between agents leading to differences in onset time and duration of effect. As a research tool, experimental TCI systems have been developed for the administration of thiopentone in rats[33] and for propofol in dogs[34]

TCI systems have also been used as the control actuator in feedback control systems to achieve a given depth of sedation[35] or anaesthesia[36] with a controlled variable derived from the EEG. Further development of these systems can be anticipated in the future. Research studies and understanding of the pharmacokinetic behaviour of drugs and PK/PD interactions have been greatly facilitated by the availability of computer simulation programs (see chapter by Billard).

9. CONCLUSIONS

Over a period of 20 years, TCI systems have developed from an early research prototype to simple to use integrated systems in commercially available syringe pumps. As the benefits of the TCI mode of administration become more widely appreciated, both for research studies and general clinical use, it is likely that commercial systems for drugs other than propofol will be developed. The principal benefit of TCI, the precise control of effect obtained by titration of the target concentration setting, would be attractive for a range of iv drugs used in anaesthesia and critical care.

10. REFERENCES

1. E.Kruger-Thiemer, Continuous intravenous infusion and multicompartment accumulation, *Eur. J. Pharmacol.* **4**, 317-24 (1968).
2. H. Schwilden, A general method for calculating the dosage scheme in linear pharmacokinetics, *Eur. J. Clin. Pharmacol.* **20**, 379-86 (1981). (1937).
3. J.Schuttler, H. Schwilden and H Stoeckel, Pharmacokinetics as applied to intravenous anaesthesia: practical applications, *Anaesthesia* **38** (Supp), 53-56 (1983).
4. J.M. Alvis, J.G.Reves, A.V.Govier, P.G. Menkhaus, C.E. Henling, J.A. Spain and E. Bradley, Computer assisted continuous infusion of fentanyl during cardiac anesthesia: comparison with manual method, *Anesthesiology* **63**, 41-49 (1985).
5. J Jacobs, Algorithm for optimal linear model-based control with application to pharmacokinetic model-driven drug delivery, IEEE Trans. *Biomed. Eng.***37**, 107-109 (1990).
6. J.M Bailey and S.L.Shafer, A simple analytical solution to the three-compartment pharmacokinetic model suitable for computer-controlled infusion pumps, *IEEE Trans. Biomed. Eng.* **38**, 522-25 (1997).
7. J. Schuttler, S.Kloos, H.Schwilden and H. Stoeckel, Total intravenous anaesthesia with propofol and alfentanil by computer assisted infusion, *Anaesthesia* **43**, Supp, 2-7 (1988).
8. M. White and G.N.C. Kenny, Intravenous propofol anaesthesia using a computerised infusion system, *Anaesthesia* **45,** 204-09 (1990).
9. M.E.Ausems, D.R.Stanski and C.C. Hug, An evaluation of the accuracy of pharmacokinetic data for the computer assisted infusion of alfentanil, *Br J. Anaesth.* **57**, 1217-25 (1985).
10. S.L. Shafer, J.R. Varvel, N. Aziz and J.C. Scott, Pharmacokinetics of fentanyl administered by computer controlled infusion pump, *Anesthesiology* **73**, 1091- 1102 (1998).
11. P.S.A. Glass, J.B. Glen, G.N.C. Kenny, J. Schuttler and S.L. Shafer, Nomenclature for computer-assisted infusion devices, *Anesthesiology* **86**, 1430-31 (1997).
12. J.R. Varvel, D.L. Donoho and S.L. Shafer, Measuring the predictive performance of computer-controlled infusion pumps, *J. Pharmacokin. Biopharm.* **20**, 63-93 (1992).
13. E. Gepts, Pharmacokinetic concepts for TCI anaesthesia, *Anaesthesia* **53**, Supp. 1: 4-12 (1998).
14. J.M.Gray and G.N.C. Kenny, Development of the technology for 'Diprifusor' TCI systems, *Anaesthesia* **53**, Supp.1: 22-27 (1998).
15. J.B. Glen, The development of 'Diprifusor': a TCI system for propofol, *Anaesthesia* **53**, Supp.1:13-21 (1998).
16. B. Marsh, M. White, N. Morton and G.N.C. Kenny, Pharmacokinetic model driven infusion of propofol in children, *Br. J.* Anaesth. **67**, 41-48 (1991).
17. J.F. Coetzee, J.B. Glen, C.A. Wium and L. Boshoff, Pharmacokinetic model selection for target controlled infusions of propofol, *Anesthesiology* **82**, 1328-1345 (1995).
18. J.A.C. Murdoch, S.A. Grant and G.N.C. Kenny, Safety of patient-maintained propofol sedation using a target-controlled system in healthy volunteers, *Br J. Anaesth.* **85**, 299-301 (2000).
19. E.Doyle, W. McFadzean and N.S. Morton, I.V. anaesthesia with propofol using a target controlled infusion system: comparison with inhalation anaesthesia for general surgical procedures in children, *Br. J. Anaesth.* **70**, 542-545 (1993).
20. M.White, F.H.M. Engbers, M.J.Schenkels, A.G.L. Burm and J.G.Bovill, The pharmacodynamics of propofol determined by auditory evoked potentials, *Proc. 11th WCA*, 14-20th April, Sydney: P610 (1996).
21. T.W. Schnider, C.F. Minto, P.L.Gambus, C. Andresen, D.B. Goodale, S.L. Shafer and E. Youngs, The influence of method of administration and covariates on the pharmacokinetics of propofol in adult volunteers, *Anesthesiology* **88**, 1170-82 (1998).

22. J. Schuttler and H.Ihmsen, Population pharmacokinetics of propofol, *Anesthesiology* **92**, 727-738 (2000).

23. J. Vuyk, C.J. Oostwouder, A.A. Vletter, AG.L. Burm and J.G.Bovill, *Br J. Anaesth.* **86**, 183-88 (2001).

24. C.F. Minto, T.W.Schnider, T.D.Egan, E.Youngs, H.J.M.Lemmens, P.L.Gambus, V.Billard, J.F.Hoke, K.H.P.Moore, D.J.Hermann, K.T.Muir, J.W.Mandema and S.L.Shafer, Influence of age and gender on the pharmacokinetics and pharmacodynamics of remifentanil, *Anesthesiology* **86**, 10-23 (1997).

25. S.L. Shafer and K.M. Gregg, Algorithms to rapidly achieve and maintain stable drug concentrations at the site of drug effect, *J. Pharmacokin. Biopharm.* **20**, 147-69 (1992).

26. J.R. Jacobs and E.A. Williams, Algorithm to control "Effect Compartment" drug concentrations in pharmacokinetic model-driven drug delivery, *IEEE Trans. Biomed. Eng.* **40**, 993-99 (1993).

27. T.W. Schnider, C.F.Minto, S.L.Shafer, P.L.Gambus, C. Andresen, D.B.Goodale and E.J.Youngs, The influence of age on propofol pharmacodynamics, *Anesthesiology* **90**, 1502-16 (1999).

28. V. Billard, PL Gambus, N.Chamoun, D.R. Stanski, S.L. Shafer, A comparison of spectral edge, delta power, and bispectral index as EEG measures of alfentanil, propofol and midazolam drug effects, *Clin. Pharmacol. Ther.* **61**, 45-58 (1997).

29. M.M.R.F. Struys, T. De Smet, B. Depoorter, L.F.M. Versichelen, E.P. Mortier, F.J.E. Dumortier, S.L. Shafer and G. Rolly, Comparison of plasma compartment versus two methods for effect compartment-controlled target controlled infusion of propofol, *Anesthesiology* **92**, 399-406 (2000).

30. T. Kazama, K. Ikeda, K. Morita, M. Kikura, M. Doi, T. Ikeda, T. Kurita and Y.Nakajima, Comparison of the effect-site ke0s of propofol for blood pressure and EEG bispectral index in elderly and younger patients, *Anesthesiology* **90**, 1517-27 (1999).

31. D Russell, Intravenous anaesthesia: manual infusion schemes versus TCI systems, *Anaesthesia* **53**, Supp 1: 42-45 (1998).

32. J.Vuyk, T.Lim, F.H.M. Engbers, A.G.L.Burm, A.A.Vletter and Bovill JG. Thepharmacodynamic interaction of propofol and alfentanil during lower abdominal surgery in women, *Anesthesiology* **83**, 8-22 (1995).

33. L.L.Gustafsson, W.F.Ebling, E.Osaki, S Harapat, D.R.Stanski and S.L.Shafer, Plasma concentration clamping in the rat using a computer-controlled infusion pump, *Pharmaceutical Res.* **9**, 800-07 (1992).

34. T.Beths, J.B.Glen, J.Reid, A.M. Monteiro and A.M.Nolan, Evaluation and optimisation of a target-controlled infusion system for administering propofol to dogs as part of a total intravenous anaesthetic technique during dental surgery, *Veterinary Record* **148**, 198-203 (2001).

35. S.Albrecht, C.Frenkel, H.Ihmsen and J.Schuttler, A rational approach to the control of sedation in intensive care unit patients based on closed-loop control, *Europ. J. Anaesthesiol.* **16**, 678-87 (1999).

36. A.R.Absalom, N.Sutcliffe and G.N.Kenny, Closed-loop control of anaesthesia using bispectral index, *Anesthesiology* **96**, 67-73 (2002).

AWARENESS 1960 – 2002, EXPLICIT RECALL OF EVENTS DURING GENERAL ANAESTHESIA

Rolf H. Sandin[*]

1. INTRODUCTION

In 1960 Ruth Hutchinson[1] published the first study on the incidence of awareness during general anaesthesia (GA). She found that 1.2% among 656 surgical patients remembered having been aware. The year after, in 1961, Meyer and Blacher[2] illustrated the mental consequences after awareness. Patients who had awakened paralysed during cardiac surgery tended to suffer from repetitive nightmares, anxiety, irritability and preoccupation with death. This was before the posttraumatic stress disorder (PTSD) had been identified as a syndrome.[3,4]

Four decades have elapsed since the pioneering papers by Hutchinson, and Meyer and Blacher were published. We have witnessed the potent inhaled agents and the MAC-concept being introduced. Focus was shifted from vaporizer setting to a measure more relevant for the brain when continuous measurement of end-tidal anaesthetic gas concentrations (ET_{AGC}) became possible. Non-depolarising neuromuscular blocking agents with moderate duration of action, and the possibility to monitor a limited degree of neuromuscular blockade are other leaps forward. Total intravenous anaesthesia (TIVA) became a real possibility with the introduction of propofol, although some feared that this technique would be associated with an increased incidence of awareness. Spinal anaesthesia has reduced the number of general anaesthetics for Caesarean section – a procedure with increased risk for awareness. The laryngeal mask airway made relaxation for intubation unnecessary in a large number of procedures. The knowledge about pharmacokinetics and pharmacodynamics has increased tremendously leading to new concepts as "context-sensitive half time" and "$t_{1/2}ke0$", while leaving old parameters like $t_{1/2}\beta$ out in the cold. Cognitive function during anaesthesia is not only addressed in terms of explicit memory, much interest is currently devoted to implicit memory.

---

[*] Rolf H. Sandin, The Karolinska Institute, 141 86 Stockholm, Sweden

Advances in Modelling and Clinical Application of Intravenous Anaesthesia
Edited by Vuyk and Schraag, Kluwer Academic/Plenum Publishers, 2003

135

However, to what extent has progress in anaesthesia actually affected the risk for wakening in the middle of surgery since 1960, and if this should happen, what do we know about the general severity of this complication?

2. INCIDENCE OF AWARENESS

Five prospective incidence studies based on reasonable numbers of patients, representing various types of surgery have been published since 1991.[5-9] These studies indicate an incidence of awareness of 0.2% (0.1%-0.4%).[5-9] Studies in which a structured interview was used suggest that the present incidence of awareness with explicit recall has been reduced to approximately 20% as compared with older data, albeit the specific reason for this remains unknown (see[6] for older references).

However, detailed data concerning under what conditions the result was obtained are lacking in most available incidence studies, and some factors that may affect the incidence of awareness will therefore be discussed.

2.1. Delayed memory for explicit recall

Most studies on awareness have been limited to a single postoperative interview soon after anaesthesia, usually within the first 24h after surgery. However, retrieval of material learned under subhypnotic concentrations of anaesthetics may be temporarily impaired. Memory for words learned soon after anaesthesia was less well preserved when tested after 2h, but had improved 1week later.[10] A patient given TIVA had no explicit recall when she left the PACU. She remembered a dream the day after, and recalled details from her surgery on day 8.[6] In a subsequent study, 11,785 patients were questioned on 3 occasions after anaesthesia. The last structured interview took place during the second week after surgery. Memory for intraoperative wakefulness was delayed by several days in 50% of ultimately identified awareness cases, and no relation was found between when memory for explicit recall first occurred and the severity of the patients experiences.[9] Thus, previous studies may have significantly underestimated the true incidence of awareness.

2.2. Neuro-Muscular Blockade

Although no randomized controlled trial (RCT) has been conducted to demonstrate an increased incidence of awareness when muscle relaxants are used, this is probably the case, and muscle relaxants should be used only when necessary. Despite the fact that severe suffering due to awareness has only been described in relaxant anaesthesia, it may occur in non-relaxant anaesthesia as well. Four patients among 4032 non-relaxed cases (0.1%) recalled intraoperative events, but had not experienced any major mental distress.[9] Two of those patients denied any attempt to move despite that they realized their situation during wakefulness. The extremely low number of reported cases of awareness during non-relaxant anaesthesia, and the apparent tendency not even to remember wakefulness during non-relaxant anaesthesia unless memory is "jogged" by repeated interviews,[9] it seems that awareness without paralysis is of limited significance to the patient.

2.3. Total Intravenous Anaesthesia

No RCT has compared the incidence of awareness in TIVA with other types of GA. One prospective case study using a structured interview was confined to intravenous anaesthesia with muscle relaxation.[6] In this study the incidence of explicit recall was 0.2%, thus similar to other types of anaesthesia.[5,7-9] However, lack of recall is not necessarily a guarantee for absence of high-level cognitive function during anaesthesia. Twenty female patients were deliberately awakened from propofol anaesthesia.[11] While intermittently conscious, these patients were able to respond to verbal command and asked to verbally acknowledge a visual stimulus before they again were anaesthetised, and the surgical procedure was completed. Sixty-five percent of these patients were unable to remember having been awakened or any of the cognitive tasks performed during wakefulness when they were questioned on the following day. A similar finding has recently been published by other authors.[12] Using the isolated forearm technique (IFT), Flashion obtained response to command in 40 paralysed patients when the hypnotic effect of bolus induction doses of propofol or thiopental wore off, but no patient had recall.[13] Thus, amnesia for intermittent wakefulness during propofol anaesthesia seems quite possible, even if the possibility of delayed explicit memory emerging after several days, not investigated in these studies, should be remembered.[9] This issue was further explored by Russell and Wang also using the IFT.[14] Seven among 45 patients anaesthetised with propofol and alfentanil responded to command on a total of 12 occasions, but no patient had explicit recall. The authors emphasized the discrepancy between the incidence of wakefulness with amnesia demonstrated by IFT, 16%, and the 0.2% incidence of explicit recall found by Nordström,[6] also using TIVA based on propofol, alfentanil and muscle relaxation. However, there were considerable differences concerning protocol and drug doses between the two studies[15,16] that precludes a direct comparison. Thus, several studies[11-14] have demonstrated the discrepancy between amnesia and anaesthesia when propofol is used as the principal anaesthetic, but no RCT has so far shown that TIVA is associated with an increased incidence of awareness, with or without explicit recall, as compared with any other type of relaxant anaesthesia.

2.4. Nitrous oxide (N₂O)

In a frequently cited meta-analysis[17] it was concluded that: "The clinically important risk of intraoperative awareness with a N_2O-free anaesthetic reduces the usefulness of this method of preventing postoperative vomiting." A closer look at the data[18-24] in this meta-analysis casts doubt on the validity of the conclusion that the omission of N_2O *per se* is associated with an increased incidence of awareness. Seven of the eight awareness cases in the meta-analysis came from the same study,[18] 6 patients without, and 1 patient who was given N_2O. The 6 patients with explicit recall after N_2O-free anaesthesia had received, on average, an ET_{AGC} of 0.70±0.35% of isoflurane in O_2, and in 4 of the cases, the average end-tidal alveolar gas concentration (ET_{AGC}) was only 0.52±0.29%, which is close to MAC_{awake} for isoflurane. This insufficient concentration of isoflurane to reliably prevent consciousness obviously accounts for the 4.4% incidence of awareness in this study group, and this should not be misinterpreted as being due to omission of N_2O *per se*. It should also be noted that in this meta-analysis,[17] N_2O-free anaesthesia is not equal to TIVA. No patient in this meta-analysis anaesthetised with propofol reported awareness.[17]

There is currently no evidence that omission of N_2O is associated with an increased incidence of awareness provided that a reasonable concentration of another anaesthetic is used.

2.5. End-Tidal Anaesthetic Gas Concentration

No RCT has evaluated the effectiveness of ET_{AGC} in order to prevent awareness. The only available cohort study differentiating between relaxant anaesthesia with and without ET_{AGC} found a similar incidence of awareness - 0.2% - whether ET_{AGC} was used or not.[9] In that study, at least 5 of the 14 awareness episodes in relaxant anaesthesia occurred during laryngoscopy or intubation, before any inhaled agent had been administered. Even if generally accepted guidelines for "safe" ET_{AGC}[25] seem to work well in clinical practice, it should be noted that those recommendations are based on very limited numbers of experimental cases as compared to the inverted prevalence of awareness. A 76 years old lady was aware during combined epidural and general anaesthesia at a lowest ET_{AGC} sevoflurane of 1% in N_2O-O_2[26], and two of the cases in [9] were aware despite a lowest recorded ET_{AGC} of 1.2%, and 1.5% sevoflurane in 66% N_2O, respectively. These ET_{AGC} correspond to 1.3, 1.3, and 1.5 $MAC_{skin\ incision}$, respectively (3.0, 3.2, and 3.4 times MAC_{awake}), when corrected according to Eger[27] for age, but not for temperature or the slight antagonistic effect between sevoflurane and N_2O demonstrated by Katoh.[28] Thus, outliers concerning anaesthetic gas requirements for unconsciousness may exist. Furthermore, in some cases it may not be considered possible to maintain the desired ET_{AGC} due to circulatory compromise. In those cases, when the inspired fraction of anaesthetic gas is rapidly and frequently altered, and cardiac output changes considerably over a short time, the ET_{AGC} does not reliably mirror the cerebral concentration of anaesthetic. Thus, while being a very useful device in anaesthetic practice, monitoring of ET_{AGC} can for several reasons not be expected to eliminate awareness.

2.6. Procedures with increased risk for awareness

Caesarean section, trauma-, and cardiac surgery have been considered to be associated with increased risk for awareness. Today, most cases of Caesarean section are performed under regional anaesthesia. In case of general anaesthesia, it seems likely that the risk for awareness has been reduced by more reasonable induction doses of thiopental, and by rational handling of the halogenated anaesthetics in this situation. An incidence of awareness of 0.4% was reported by Lyons and McDonald[29] as early as 1991. Despite the fact that difficult intubation - a definite risk for awareness[9] - is more likely to be encountered in pregnant women, the current incidence of awareness during Caesarean section should not be significantly higher than in any other procedure although no recent study has been conducted.

Awareness during cardiac anaesthesia has for a long period been considered to occur in 1.1%[30] to 23%[31] of patients.[32] It seems that both the choice of drugs and other aspects of anaesthetic regimen are of importance. Ranta[33] demonstrated that feedback to the anaesthesiologists about outcome led to a change of practice and a reduced incidence of aware-ness from 4% to 1.5%. In a recent, prospective study in 617 "fast-track" cardiac cases given inhaled or intravenous anaesthetics continuously, Dowd[34] found an incidence of awareness of 0.3% when the patients were questioned after 24h. Thus, it seems possible to reduce the incidence of awareness also in cardiac anaesthesia to a level not far from that in any other type of surgery.

Trauma surgery has been associated with explicit recall in up to 43% of cases.[32,35] In a more recent study no case of explicit recall was found among 96 cases of trauma surgery (although evidence of implicit memory was found).[36] Even if more studies would be needed to illuminate the current situation, this clearly means that most trauma cases need not be aware during surgery.

3. SUFFERING DURING AND AFTER AWARENESS

Suffering due to awareness can be immediate in terms of pain, mental distress or both. Despite sufficient cognitive capacity to experience pain and anxiety, victims of awareness may not always be able to understand what is going on. In addition to immediate suffering, neurotic symptoms may follow.[4]

Much information about suffering due to awareness is published as case reports. However, all patients do not suffer during wakefulness, and it seems less likely that a case of awareness will be reported if the patient did not find any reason to tell anyone about intraoperative experiences and did not care about it.[9,37] Thus, selection bias makes it impossible to assess the average severity of suffering due to awareness from case reports.

Myles and colleagues[8] investigated reasons for postoperative dissatisfaction among 10,811 anaesthetised patients. Within 24 hours after anaesthesia they identified 12 cases with explicit recall (0.1%). The adjusted odds ratio (OR) for patient dissatisfaction in case of awareness was 54.9, an OR several times higher than that for moderate/severe pain (OR 6.95), severe nausea and vomiting (OR 4.09), or multiple complications (OR 6.25). However, patients may anticipate pain and nausea after surgery, but they may not expect to consciously attend their own surgery, and the result obtained by Myles et al. does not necessarily reflect the degree of suffering due to awareness.

It is very laborious to collect a sufficiently large prospective cohort to draw any conclusions about the general severity of suffering among awareness cases. A significant number of non-consecutive cases have been enrolled in 4 peer-reviewed studies by the use of other methods, i.e. by advertising,[38] referral from colleagues of historical cases,[39] and both these methods[40,41] (Table 1). Another way to provide data from non-consecutive awareness cases, analysis of "closed-claims", was used in a recent publication[42] (Table 1). However, all these methods carry a risk for biased sampling of "complainers", patients seeking economic compensation or patients with more severe suffering.[39,42] Avoidance, one of the symptoms of PTSD,[4] may also constitute a possible source of selection bias. While some patients with PTSD due to violent crime or accidents avoid situations that remind them of the corresponding eliciting event, victims of awareness may avoid health care providers and, thus, be reluctant to participate in an investigation about previous wakefulness during anaesthesia. Data on immediate suffering, pain, and delayed mental symptoms in the retrospective studies[38-42] are given in Table 1.

In addition to retrospective data, there is one reasonably large prospectively identified cohort of awareness cases giving details about late mental symptoms[9] (Table 1). In that study, 4 of 19 patients with awareness (n=18) or inadvertent paralysis (n=1) experienced neurotic symptoms, but all these patients claimed to have recovered within 3 weeks. However, this was found to be a false impression of the true severity of the late mental symptoms. A more disappointing view was obtained when it was attempted to locate all the previously identified 18 awareness cases after approximately 2 years.[43] Two patients could not be located, another patient had died, and 6 patients declined to participate. Four of the 9 interviewed patients were found to still suffer from PTSD after 2 years. Two of the patients with persisting PTSD had contact with a psychiatrist.

These patients admitted that they had falsely claimed to have recovered mentally within a few weeks after anaesthesia in order to avoid being reminded of their awareness episodes. Another 3 patients had experienced some, but not all symptoms required for a diagnosis of PTSD. These 3 patients now reported diminishing, and no longer unbearable symptoms. Thus, depending on how the fact that only 9 of the 18 awareness cases (50%) in the previously prospectively identified cohort were eligible for evaluation should be interpreted, the incidence of long term mental problems after awareness was 39-78%, and the incidence of PTSD was 22-44% (Table 1).

In addition, the person who located the patients was entirely confident that at least 2 of the 6 patients who declined to participate did so because they wanted to avoid everything that reminded them of their previous, unsuccessful anaesthetic. Thus, data[43] from a prospectively identified cohort of awareness cases[9] support the findings on long term consequences in the previous retrospective studies.[38-42]

Taken together, more than 80% of prospectively identified cases with explicit recall after relaxant anaesthesia suffered from pain, panic or immediate psychological problems,[9] and this complication carry a significant risk for long-term mental problems. It is not known if early professional therapy can reduce the likelihood of mental consequences and the duration of symptoms after awareness. Furthermore, delayed memory for explicit recall may reduce the possibility to identify these patients. Thus, further attempts to prevent this complication are justified.

Table 1. Studies on immediate suffering and late mental symptoms after awareness with explicit recall.

Author and year	n	Method[a]	Mental distress	Pain	Late symptoms
Evans 1987[38]	27	RET, ADV	78%	41%	-
Moerman 1993[39]	26	RET, REF	92%	39%	69%
Schwender 1998[40]	45	RET, REF+ADV	49%[b]	24%	49%
Osterman 2001[41]	18	RET, REF+ADV			56%[c]
Domino 1999[42]	79	RET, CCA	11%	21%	84%[d]
Sandin 2000[9]	19	PRO	47%	37%	21%[e]
Lennmarken 2002[43]	9	PRO			39-78%[f]

[a] RET=retrospective, PRO=prospective, ADV=advertising, REF=referral, CCA=closed claims analysis
[b] 60% described helplessness.
[c] All 56% classified as PTSD.
[d] 10% classified as PTSD.
[e] The incidence of late symptoms according to the patient's statements within 3 weeks after surgery.
[f] The incidence of late symptoms among awareness cases identified in[9] when evaluated after approximately 2 years. The incidence of PTSD was 22-44%.

4. MONITORING AND PREVENTION

A large variety of methods aimed to avoid awareness have been reviewed elsewhere.[44,45] One of those methods is the isolated forearm technique (IFT). Despite the fact that this method is generally regarded as a scientific "Gold-Standard" for detecting cognitive function during relaxant anaesthesia, it has failed to reach widespread clinical use. Some of the arguments for the reluctance to use the IFT have been reviewed and evaluated by Russell.[46]

Currently, no single study has demonstrated a reduced incidence of awareness by the use of any proposed method for prevention or detection. For some measures such as avoiding muscle relaxants when not necessarily needed, and the use of potent, volatile anaesthetics for Caesarean section, this lack of evidence is probably due only to the fact that no relevant study has been conducted, while for other proposals the true benefit remains more obscure.

Much attention is currently drawn to neurophysiologic techniques based on either EEG or middle latency auditory evoked potentials (MLAEP or "AEP")[45]. Ideally, peer-reviewed, controlled, randomised studies should guide our decisions as to whether we should incorporate devices like Aspect 2000™ (BIS), AlarisAEP™, Narcotrend™ or PSA 4000™ in clinical routine, or if limited health care resources in this era of financial constrains are better used in other ways.

However, awareness is a rare complication in terms of statistics, and studies advocating the merits of various prevention techniques have almost invariably aimed at other primary end-points than awareness *per se*. Sufficiently large RCTs will be very difficult to conduct,[9] and the current situation has many similarities to when pulse oximetry became available. Despite the initial inability to advocate the use of pulse oximetry by "evidence based medicine", the wide-spread use eventually created a situation of "medicine based evidence", i.e. the benefit from using pulse oximetry was indicated by apparently reduced numbers of deaths due to respiratory complications (this trend was probably due also to the introduction of end-tidal CO_2 monitoring).[47,48]

In order to interpret the relevance of available data in terms of avoiding awareness by the use of new, sophisticated methods, and possible differences in performance between the various techniques, it is important to realize limiting and confounding facts. The number of publications concerning the BIS is the far largest among the commercially available techniques. A substantial number of publications about non-commercially applications of AEP are available, but there is no consensus about the most appropriate algorithm to interpret the data from the various AEP technologies, and they may not be equivalent. Concerning the so far only commercially available AEP technology, the AlarisAEP™ (previously A-line™), the number of publications is very limited. Furthermore, updating of algorithms, not least concerning suppression of EMG artefacts, have been frequent both for AlarisAEP™ and the BIS, and older, less favourable data, obtained by previous algorithms are not necessarily relevant for currently available versions.

There has also been confusion about what to expect from these monitors. Ability to predict movement in response to noxious stimulation has been investigated, but detecting anaesthetic suppression of spinal reflexes is not relevant for the ability to discriminate between consciousness and unconsciousness.[49,50]

4.1. The Possibility to Prevent Awareness by BIS and AEP - Some Indications

4.1.1. Case reports and manufacturer feedback

Considering the estimated number of cases monitored by the BIS (2.75 million, March 2001),[51] and the general interest in whether this technique is reliable or not, it may be worth noting that only two peer reviewed case reports claiming that awareness has occurred at a low BIS value have been published. One report[52] stated that awareness had been evident during sternotomy at a BIS value of 47. However, the stored data were subsequently downloaded by the manufacturer and analysed. It was found that BIS was 47 two min before the first incision, and thereafter it increased.[53] The BIS value had reached 60 within 5 min after the first incision and continued to between 60-70. A firm conclusion about this case does not seem possible as suggested in a subsequent Letter to the Editor[54] titled "False negative BIS? Maybe, maybe not!". The second case report[55] is published in Japanese. According to personal communication (Paul Manberg, Aspect Medical Systems, MA) the patient declared on discharge from the OR, that she had heard voices and had felt the abdominal surgery. The authors assumed that awareness had occurred during an episode of elevated blood pressure and movement when the BIS had been about 40, although no firm conclusion from the patient to support this assumption could be obtained. Periods of "high BIS values" had been evident also during this case. In addition to these two case reports, another 12 inconclusive cases with explicit recall have been reported to the manufacturer.[51] This makes a total of 14 BIS monitored cases with explicit recall in which the time-point for awareness was not possible to establish. Awareness may in these cases have occurred at BIS values below 60, but it should be noted that episodes with BIS >60 were evident in all these patients. There is currently no case reported to the manufacturer in which awareness unequivocally has occurred at a BIS value below 60.[51] No corresponding estimate has yet been provided for the more recently launched AlarisAEP™ or non-commercial AEP applications. However, this type of argument for effectiveness is weak for several reasons, and is probably best regarded in an opposite way, i.e. that the BIS has not been shown unable to prevent awareness.

4.1.2. Sensitivity and Specificity

A relevant experimental approach has been to evaluate if monitoring technologies identify subhypnotic anaesthetic action in a way that correspond to accepted sedation scores, and, in terms of awareness even more interesting, whether the transition between consciousness and unconsciousness can be predicted. Sigmoid relations between the probability for unresponsiveness and monitor reading have been demonstrated for BIS when isoflurane, midazolam, and propofol were used[56], and for AEP (calculated and displayed as "AEP index" or AEP_i) using sevoflurane.[57] Both BIS (A-1000™, version 3.2) and AEP_i showed high predictive performance for depth of sedation when sevoflurane was used.[57] The relation between BIS value and sedation score, evaluated as P_K (prediction probability),[58] was superior to a non-commercial AEP technique, whereas Pa and Nb latency of the AEP were equal to the BIS in predicting loss of consciousness.[59] However, inter-individual variability in BIS and AEP derived parameters at the different sedation score levels were evident. When the A-1000™ version of the BIS, using software algorithm 3.0 and 60 second "smoothing", and AEP_i were compared, both techniques were considered able to differentiate between consciousness and unconsciousness during propofol-N_2O-opioid anaesthesia,[60] although AEP_i was considered to discriminate somewhat better. A similar conclusion was reached when these monitors were compared in patients anaesthetised with propofol and a concomitant regional block.[61] In another study using propofol, the A-line[TM] AEP monitor (earlier version of AlarisAEP[TM]) and the Aspect 2000[TM] version 3.3 displayed similar performance with a certain degree of inter-individual overlap during transitions between verbal response and no response.[12]

Thus, BIS and AEP technologies display a relation to the sedative and hypnotic anaesthetic action when ordinary anaesthetic drugs are used, but there is a certain degree of inter-individual variability. However, while less than optimal sensitivity and specificity may limit some scientific applications, this does not necessarily imply inability to reduce the incidence of awareness. In order to prevent awareness, the primary end point is a very high sensitivity (virtually no false negatives). As illustrated by the studies above, high sensitivity will be associated with a less impressive specificity (several patients will be given more anaesthetics than actually needed). Thus, the question is if potentially negative consequences from overdosing in some cases can be an acceptable price for high sensitivity or not. There are at least 6 peer-reviewed studies[62-67] in which the use of anaesthetics was reduced by between 13% and 40% when BIS was used to guide the administration. One study reported no significant difference.[68] There is no published trial in which the use of BIS has been associated with an increased consumption of anaesthetics. BIS-guided reduction of anaesthetic consumption have also been reported in 4 recent abstracts.[69-72] It seems that routine anaesthetic techniques generally result in more excessive drug doses than if the recommended BIS criteria favouring sensitivity at the expense of specificity are applied. Thus, the less than optimal specificity of BIS need not be a major drawback in the current context. If adherence to the recommended threshold for sensitivity when the AlarisAEP[TM] is used also leads to less consumption of anaesthetics as compared to standard practice has not yet been investigated.

Although "running close to the edge" (recommended monitored value) may improve various aspects of outcome and save money, this is not a primary goal in terms of avoiding awareness. It should be remembered that the recommended thresholds for sensitivity, different for the various technologies, are empirically derived, and remain to some extent arbitrary until otherwise proven in sufficiently large cohorts of patients undergoing surgery. This has to be demonstrated individually for each of the available technologies.

4.1.3. Time for Updating

Intuitively, rapid update of the displayed value would seem advantageous. The required time for updating is different for the AlarisAEP[TM] (after initially analysing 256 sweeps which requires 37s, complete updating is done every 2-6s, depending on signal quality), the Aspect 2000[TM] (updating every 2s as a moving average with a 15s or 30s "window"), and ordinary non-commercials applications of AEP (256 sweeps; 37s, or more frequently updating as a moving average). However, the benefit from these differences concerning updating remains to be evaluated in terms of preventing awareness.

4.1.4. Human response to monitored data

Even if a perfect monitor for awareness were available, it's effectiveness for preventing awareness would still be dependent on the vigilance, knowledge, and actions taken by the anaesthesiologist. Abnormal values displayed by any monitoring technique may cause uncertainty as to whether this is due to malfunctioning technology or physiology. This applies also to neurophysiological monitoring. In a recent report, two cases of awareness during BIS monitoring are described.[73] In one of the cases, it was not noticed that the infusions of propofol and remifentanil were obstructed. In the second case, no desflurane was delivered due to an incorrectly turned valve, and it was initially assumed that the absence of desflurane, as indicated by ET_{AGC} measurement, was due to monitor failure. In these two cases the BIS values increased to 90, and to between 60 and 70, respectively. These cases are interesting, not only to demonstrate that BIS, in clinical routine, actually indicated possible awareness. As pointed out by the authors, this report also illustrates the importance of definite strategies how to act in case of abnormal physiological parameters.

5. CONCLUSIONS

Explicit recall of intraoperative experiences during relaxant anaesthesia is a potentially serious complication with a significant risk for long-term mental problems. There are not sufficient data to assess the role for improving "conservative" measures, such as better education, new strategies for the use of ET_{AGC}, or reliance on "amnesic drugs" to reduce the incidence of this potential mare. Muscle relaxants are probably too frequently used, while the IFT continues to be used by few anaesthesiologists despite the fact that this may constitute under-utilization of a cheap, and at least in some hands, simple method.

Indirect data of relevance for the possibility to avoid awareness by the use of neurophysiological technologies are beginning to accumulate, while a RCT may not ever be conducted due to the enormous number of patients that must be included. Since decisions still have to be made, we have to search also the second-best protocols for information. Studies including large numbers of patients are needed since the apparent utility in small series created by expert hands under study conditions may deviate - in both directions - from the true benefit in broad, clinical practice. Awareness occurring when neurophysiological monitoring was used should be reported in peer-reviewed papers and to the manufacturers, and in order to facilitate the interpretation, neurophysiological monitoring devices should be equipped with a non-volatile memory. Finally, the utility in certain patient groups, and ethical and economical issues, not touched upon in this chapter, have to be considered. Eventually, we will know if cerebral monitoring is the answer.

6. REFERENCES

1. R. Hutchinson, 1960, Awareness during surgery, *Br. J. Anaesth.* **33**, 463-469 (1960).
2. B.C. Meyer, and R.S. Blacher, A traumatic neurotic reaction induced by succinylcholine chloride, *NY State J Med* **61**, 1255-1261 (1961).
3. J.E. Osterman, and B.A. van der Kolk, Awareness during anaesthesia and posttraumatic stress disorder. *Gen Hosp. Psychiatry* **20**, 274-281 (1998).
4. American Psychiatric Association: Diagnostic and statistical manual of mental disorders. 4th edition. (Washington DC, American Psychiatric Association, 1994.)
5. W.H. Liu, T.A. Thorp, S.G. Graham, and A.R. Aitkenhead, Perception and memory during general anaesthesia, *Anaesthesia* **46**, 435-437 (1991).
6. O. Nordström, A.M. Engström, S. Persson, and R. Sandin, Incidence of awareness in total i.v. anaesthesia based on propofol, alfentanil and neuromuscular blockade, *Acta Anaesthesiol. Scand.* **41**, 978-984 (1997).

7. S.O.V. Ranta, R. Laurila, J. Saario, T. Ali-Melkkilä, and M. Hynynen, Awareness with recall during general anesthesia: incidence and risk factors, *Anesth . Analg.* **86**, 1084-1089 (1998).
8. P.S. Myles, D.L. Williams, M. Hendrata, H. Anderson, and A.M. Weeks, Patient satisfaction after anaesthesia and surgery: results of a prospective survey of 10,811 patients, *Br. J. Anaesth.* **84**, 6-10 (2000).
9. R.H. Sandin, G. Enlund, P. Samuelsson, and C. Lennmarken, Awareness during anaesthesia: a prospective case study, *Lancet* **355**, 707-711 (2000).
10. N. Adam, Disruption of memory functions associated with general anaesthetics, in: Functional disorders of memory, Kihlstrom J.F., Evans F.J. eds., Lawrence Erlbaum Associates, Hillsdale, New Jersey, pp. 219-238.
11. O. Nordström, and R. Sandin, Recall during intermittent propofol anaesthesia, *Br. J. Anaesth.* **76**, 699-701 (1996).
12. G. Barr, R.E. Andersson, and J.G. Jakobsson, A study of bispectral analysis and auditory evoked potential indices during propofol-induced hypnosis in volunteers, *Anaesthesia* **56**, 888-893 (2001).
13. R. Flashion, A. Windsor, J. Sigl, and P.S. Sebel, Recovery of consciousness after thiopental or propofol, *Anesthesiology* **86**, 613-619 (1997).
14. I.F. Russell, and M. Wang, Absence of memory for intra-operative information during surgery with total intravenous anaesthesia, *Br. J. Anaesth.* **86**, 196-202 (2001).
15. R. Sandin, Incidence of awareness in total intravenous anaesthesia, *Br. J. Anaesth.* **87**, 320 (2001).
16. I.F. Russell, and M. Wang, In reply, *Br. J. Anaesth.* **87**, 320 (2001).
17. M. Tramèr, A. Moore, and H. McQuay, Omitting nitrous oxide in general anaesthesia: meta-analysis of intraoperative awareness and postoperative emesis in randomized controlled trials, *Br. J. Anaesth.* **76**, 186-193 (1996).
18. E.I. Eger II, G.H. Lampe, L.Z. Wauk, P. Whitendale, M.K. Calahan, and J.H. Donegan, Clinical pharmacology of nitrous oxide: an argument for its continued use, *Anesth. Analg.* **71**, 575-585 (1990).
19. G. Girardi, R. Rossi, M.P. Cellai, E. Pieraccioli, and G.P. Novelli, Anaesthesia with isoflurane in air and with isoflurane and nitrous oxide, *Minerva Anestesiol.* **60**, 321-328 (1994).
20. D.S. Lonie, and N.J. Harper, Nitrous oxide anaesthesia and vomiting. The effect of nitrous oxide anaesthesia on the incidence of vomiting following gynaecological laparoscopy, *Anaesthesia* **41**, 703-707 (1986).
21. G.H. Lampe, L.Z. Wauk, J.H. Donegan, L.H. Pitts, R.K. Jackler, L.L. Litt, I.J. Rampil, and E.I. Eger, Effect on outcome of prolonged exposure of patients to nitrous oxide, *Anesth. Analg.* **71**, 586-590 (1990).
22. M.A. Gregory, T. Gin, G. Yau, R.K. Leung, K. Chan, and T.E. Oh, Propofol infusion anesthesia for caesarean section, *Can. J. Anaesth.* **37**, 514-520 (1990).
23. P. Sengupta, and O.M. Plantevin, Nitrous oxide and day-case laparoscopy: effects on nausea, vomiting and return to normal activity, *Br. J. Anaesth.* **60**, 570-573 (1988).
24. S.R. Wrigley, J.E. Fairfield, R.M. Jones, and A.E. Black, Induction and recovery characteristics of desflurane in day case patients: a comparison with propofol, *Anaesthesia* **46**, 615-622 (1991).
25. C.H. McLeskey, Awareness during anesthesia, *Can. J. Anaesth.* **46**, 80-87 (1999).
26. S. Miura, S. Kashimoto, T. Yamaguchi, and T. Matsukawa, A case of awareness with sevoflurane and epidural anesthesia in ovarian tumorectomy, *J. Clin. Anesth.* **13**, 227-229 (2001).
27. E.I. Eger 2nd, Age, minimum alveolar anesthetic concentration, and minimum alveolar anesthetic concentration-awake, *Anesth. Analg.* **93**, 947-953 (2001).
28. T. Katoh, K. Ikeda, and H. Bito, Does nitrous oxide antagonize sevoflurane-induced hypnosis? *Br. J. Anaesth.* **79**, 465-468 (1997).
29. G. Lyons, and R. McDonald, Awareness during caesarean section, *Anaesthesia* **46**, 62-64 (1991).
30. A.A. Phillips, R.F. McLean, and J.H. Devitt, Recall of intraoperative events during open-heart surgery. *Can. J. Anaesth.* **40**, 922-926 (1993).
31. L. Goldman M.V. Shah, and M.W. Hebden, Memory of cardiac surgery. Anaesthesia **42**: 596-603 (1987).
32. T. Heier, and P.A. Steen, Awareness in anaesthesia: incidence consequences and prevention, *Acta Anaesth. .Scand.* **40**, 1073-1086 (1996).
33. S. Ranta, J. Jussila, and M. Hynynen, Awareness of awareness during cardiac anaesthesia: influence of feedback information to the anaesthesiologist, *Acta Anaesth. Scand.* **40**, 554-560 (1996).
34. N.P. Dowd, D.C.H. Cheng, J.M. Karski, D.T. Wong, J.C. Munro and A.N. Sandler, Intraoperative awareness in fast-track cardiac anesthesia, *Anesthesiology* **89**, 1068-1073 (1998).
35. M.S. Bogetz, and J.A. Katz, Recall of surgery for major trauma, *Anesthesiology* **61**, 6-9 (1984).
36. G.H. Lubke, C. Kerssens, H. Phaf, and P.S. Sebel, Dependence of explicit and implicit memory on hypnotic state in trauma patients, *Anesthesiology* **90**, 670-680 (1999).
37. R. Sandin, and O. Nordström, Awareness during total i.v. anaesthesia, *Br. J. Anaesth.* **71**, 782-787 (1993).
38. J.M. Evans, Patients´experiences of awareness during general anaesthesia, in: Consciousness, awareness and pain in general anaesthesia, Rosen M., Lunn J.N. eds., Butterworths, London, 1997, pp 184-192.

39. N. Moerman, B. Bonke, and J. Oosting, Awareness and recall during general anesthesia, *Anesthesiology* **79**, 454-464 (1993).
40. D. Schwender, H. Kunze-Kronawitter, P. Dietrich, S. Klasing, H. Forst, and C. Madler, Conscious awareness during general anaesthesia: patients perceptions, emotions cognition and reactions, *Br. J. Anaesth.* **80**, 133-139 (1998).
41. J.E. Osterman, J. Hopper, W.J. Heran, T.M. Keane, and B.A. van der Kolk, Awareness under anaesthesia and the development of posttraumatic stress disorder, *Gen. Hosp. Psychiatry* **23**, 198-204 (2001).
42. K.B. Domino, K.L. Posner, R.A. Caplan, and F.W. Cheney, Awareness during anesthesia, *Anesthesiology* **90**, 1053-1061 (1999).
43. C. Lennmarken, K. Bildfors, G. Enlund, P. Samuelsson, and R. Sandin, Victims of awareness, *Acta Anaethesiol. Scand.* **46**, 229-231 (2002).
44. T. Heier, P.A. Steen, Assessment of anaesthesia depth, *Acta Anesthesiol. Scand.* **40**, 1087-1100 (1996).
45. J.C. Drummond, Monitoring depth of anesthesia, *Anesthesiology* **93**, 876-882 (2000).
46. I.F. Russell, Memory when the state of consciousness is known: studies of anaesthesia with the isolated forearm technique, in: Awareness during anaesthesia, Ghoneim M.M. ed., Butterworth-Heinemann, Oxford, 2001, pp129-143.
47. J.H. Tinker, D.L. Dull, R.A. Caplan, R.J. Ward, and F.W. Cheney, Role of monitoring devices in prevention of anesthetic mishaps: a closed claims analysis, *Anesthesiology* **71**, 541-546 (1989).
48. J.H. Eichhorn, Prevention of intraoperative anaesthesia accidents and related severe injury through safety monitoring, *Anesthesiology* **70**, 572-577 (1989).
49. I.J. Rampil, Anesthetic potency is not altered after hypothermic spinal cord transection in rats, *Anesthesiology* **80**, 606-610 (1994).
50. J.F. Antognini, and K. Schwartz, Exaggerated anesthetic requirements in the preferentially anesthetized brain, *Anesthesiology* **79**,1244-1249 (1993).
51. P.J. Manberg, D. Zraket, L. Kovitch, and L. Christman, Awareness during anesthesia with BIS monitoring: 2001 update, *Anesthesiology* **95**, A564 (2001).
52. G. Mychaskiew, M. Horowitz, V. Sachdev, and B.J. Heath, Explicit recall at a bispectral index of 47, *Anesth. Analg.* **92**, 808-809 (2001).
53. G. Mychaskiew, M. Horowitz M., In reply, *Anesth. Analg.* **93**, 798-799 (2001).
54. I. Rampil, False negative BIS? Maybe, maybe not! *Anesth. Analg.* **93**, 798 (2001).
55. K. Kurehara, T. Horiuch, M. Takahash, K. Kitaguchi, and H. Furuya H., A case of awareness during propofol anesthesia using bispectral index as an indicator of hypnotic effect, *Masui.* **50**, 886-889 (2001).
56. P.S. Glass, M. Bloom, L. Kearse, C. Rosow, P. Sebel, and P. Manberg, Bispectral analysis measures sedation and memory effects of propofol, midazolam, isoflurane, and alfentanil in healthy volunteers, *Anesthesiology* **86**, 836-847 (1997).
57. T. Kurita, M. Doi, T. Katoh, H. Sano, S. Sato, H. Mantzaridis, and G.N.C. Kenny, Auditory evoked potential index predicts the depth of sedation and movement in response to skin incision during sevoflurane anesthesia, *Anesthesiology* **95**, 364-370 (2001).
58. W.D. Smith, R.C. Dutton, and T. Smith, Measuring the performance of anesthetic depth indicators, *Anesthesiology* **84**, 38-51 (1996).
59. I.A. Iselin-Chaves, H.E. El Moalem, T.J. Gan, B. Ginsberg, and P.S.A. Glass, Changes in the auditory evoked potentials and the bispectral index following propofol or propofol and alfentanil, *Anesthesiology* **92**, 1300-1310 (2000).
60. R.J. Gajraj, M. Doi, H. Mantzaridis, and G.N.C. Kenny, Comparison of bispectral EEG analysis and auditory evoked potentials for monitoring depth of anaesthesia, *Br. J. Anaesth.* **82**, 672-678 (1999).
61. S. Schraag, U Bothner, R Gajraj, G.N.C. Kenny, and M. Georgieff, The performance of electroencephalogram bispectral index and auditory evoked potential index to predict loss of consciousness during propofol infusion, *Anesth. Analg.* **89**, 1311-1315 (1999).
62. D. Song, G.P. Joshi, and P.F. White, Titration of volatile anaesthetics using bispectral index facilitates recovery after ambulatory anesthesia, *Anesthesiology* **87**, 842-848 (1997).
63. B. Guignard, C. Coste, C. Menigaux, and M. Chauvin, Reduced isoflurane consumption with bispectral index monitoring, *Acta Anaesthesiol. Scand.* **45**, 308-314 (2001).
64. R. Tufano, R. Palomba, G. Lambiase, and L.G. Giurleo, The utility of bispectral index monitoring in general anaesthesia, *Minerva Anestesiol.* **66**, 389-393 (2000).
65. S. Paventi, A. Santevecchi, E. Metta, M.G. Annetta, V. Perilli, L. Sollazzi, and R. Ranieri, Bispectral index monitoring in sevoflurane and remifentanil anaesthesia. Analysis of drugs management and immediate recovery, *Minerva Anestesiol.* **67**, 435-439 (2001).
66. A. Yli-Hankala, A. Vakkuri, P. Annila, and K. Korttila, EEG bispectral index monitoring in sevoflurane or propofol anaesthesia: analysis of direct costs and immediate recovery, *Acta Anaesthesiol. Scand.* **43**, 545-549 (1999).

67. D.J. Pavlin, J.Y. Hong, P.R. Freund, M.E. Koerschgen, J.O. Bower, and T.A. Bowdle, The effect of bispectral index monitoring on end-tidal gas concentration and recovery duration after outpatient anesthesia, *Anesth. Analg.* **93**, 613-619 (2001).

68. M. Struys, L. Versichelen, G. Byttebier, E. Mortier, E. Moerman, and G. Rolly, Clinical usefulness of the bispectral index for titrating propofol target effect-site concentration, *Anaesthesia* **53**, 4-12 (1998).

69. C.F. Bannister, K.K. Brosius, and B.J. Meyer, The effect of BIS monitoring on emergence, PACU discharge and anesthetic utilization in children receiving sevoflurane anesthesia, *Anesthesiology* **93**, A1276 (2000).

70. Z.T. Gabopoulou, P.D. Mavrommati, V.A. Vrettou, M.M. Petsicopoulos, G. Kyraki, and K.G. Velmachou, Bispectral index monitoring in patients undergoing long-lasting microsurgical procedures where muscle-relaxation is not indicated, *Anesthesiology* **93**, A93 (2000).

71. W.F. Madei, and H.P. Klieser, Clinical utility of the bispectral index during S(+)ketamine/propofol anesthesia, *Anesthesiology* **93**, A304 (2000).

72. M. Luginbuhl, S. Wuthrich, S. Petersen-Felix and T.W. Schneider, Utility of BIS monitoring in inhalation and total intravenous anesthesia compared, *Anesthesiology* **95**, A 280 (2001).

73. M. Luginbuhl, and T.W. Schneider, Detection of awareness with the bispectral index: two case reports, *Anesthesiology* **96**, 241-243 (2002).

SEDATION FOR LOCOREGIONAL ANAESTHESIA

Armin Holas [*]

1. INTRODUCTION

Intravenous sedation is a valuable adjunct during surgery under regional anaesthesia, since the availability of more recent sedative agents and more sophisticated application systems were introduced into clinical practice. With this improved background it has been possible to perform an ever-increasing variety of surgical procedures under loco-regional anaesthesia. The advantages of local anaesthetic techniques include the preservation of protective airway reflexes, residual postoperative analgesia, and the avoidance of side-effects associated with general anaesthesia, for example respiratory and cardio-vascular depression, postoperative nausea and vomiting or drowsiness.

Surgical procedures performed under local anaesthesia may be uncomfortable for patients for a variety of reasons. Firstly, the subcutaneous injection of the local anaesthetic is often painful, especially when multiple injections are required. Secondly, traction on "deep" structures and the need for patients to remain immobile for prolonged periods of time on a hard, narrow operating table may also cause significant discomfort.

In many cases, only light sedation is required, with patients remaining in verbal contact with their anaesthesiologists throughout the surgical procedure. Therefore, this kind of sedation is known as "conscious sedation" or "monitored anaesthesia care" (MAC) and is defined as a specific anaesthesia service involving monitoring of vital signs provided during an operation in connection with local anaesthesia[1].

The goal of conscious sedation is to enhance patient comfort, to guarantee his protective airway reflexes, to avoid painful stimuli and to help maintain haemodynamic stability during the surgical procedure.

---

[*] Armin Holas, Department of Anaesthesiology and Intensive Care Medicine, University of Graz, 8045 Graz, Austria

Advances in Modelling and Clinical Application of Intravenous Anaesthesia
Edited by Vuyk and Schraag, Kluwer Academic/Plenum Publishers, 2003

149

2. ASSESSMENT OF SEDATION

Sedative agents are essential in local anaesthesia but both the drugs and an inappropriate level of sedation may have adverse effects. More commonly, accumulation of sedative or analgesic agents may have unwanted side-effects associated with over-sedation which may cause respiratory depression with airway obstruction and also hypotension. On the other side, under-sedation may lead to discomfort and stress for the patients often combined with pain and haemodynamic instability. Therefore, the assessment of sedation is an important tool allowing the doses of sedative drugs to be titrated against the clinical response. With a regular assessment of conscious sedation, adjuvant drugs can be used more safely and also more effectively. Each patient requires an individual balance between anxiolysis, sedation, analgesia or ventilatory control and this balance may change during the surgical procedure. All these factors should be considered separately, treated appropriately and also monitored regularly.

For sedation, in many European countries, the most commonly used scoring system is the scale according to Ramsay[2] (table 1), described for the first time in 1974. This sedation scale defines six points, three levels of wakefulness and three levels of sleep. The desired level of sedation is a score of 2 or 3. Those levels of sedation are very easy to determine in patients and, with some experience, a consistent scoring of the sedative level can be achieved.

Table 1. The Ramsay sedation score

Awake levels	Score
Patient anxious, agitated and restless	1
Patient co-operative, oriented and tranquil	2
Patient responds to commands only	3
Asleep levels	
Brisk response to loud stimulus	4
Slow response to loud stimulus	5
No response to loud or painful stimulus	6

Predominantly, in the United States, a different scoring system is very common for the assessment of sedation. That is the "Observer's Assessment of Alertness and Sedation" (OAA/S) described by Chernik and co-workers[3] in 1990 which also seems to be an objective way of measuring the level of alertness in sedated patients (table 2). This composite sedation score takes several separate variables into account, such as responsiveness, speech, facial expression, and different degrees of ptosis. The desired level of sedation is ideally achieved with an OAA/S score of 3 or 4.

3. CHOICE OF SEDATIVE AGENTS

The centrally active adjuvant drugs available to optimize surgical conditions for both the patient and the surgeon include some benzodiazepines which allow an adequate control of action like midazolam, sedative doses of hypnotic agents like propofol and also short acting opioid analgesics like remifentanil. In addition, a variety of routes of administration (e.g. oral, rectal and intravenous) are available to apply adjuvant drugs to patients receiving regional anaesthesia. However, the oral route is limited by the delayed onset of clinical effects, and thus by the lack of precise control of the resulting level of sedation. Therefore, at the present time, the intravenous route is the most popular approach for conscious sedation.

An understanding of the pharmacokinetic and pharmacodynamic effects of the commonly used anxiolytic, sedative and analgesic agents is essential in order to achieve optimal surgical conditions and acceptable patient outcome when using sedation-based techniques. Since sedative and analgesic medications are more often combined, the possibility of adverse drug interactions must also be considered.

Table 2. The Observer's Assessment of Alertness and Sedation (OAA / S)

Responsiveness	Speech	Eyes	Score level
Response readily to name	Normal	Clear, no ptosis	awake / alert: 5
Lethargic reponse to name	Mild slowing	Glazed or mild ptosis	light sedation: 4
Response after name is called loudly	Slurring	Glazed or marked ptosis	moderate sedation: 3
Response after mild shaking	Few recognizable words		deep sedation: 2
Response only after squeezing the trapezius			unconscious: 1

3.1. Benzodiazepines

All benzodiazepines have the ability to produce anxiolysis, as well as varying degrees of amnesia and sedation. Benzodiazepine-induced central nervous system depression is dose-dependent and can vary from light sedation to deep unconsciousness. Individual responses may vary widely.

3.1.1. Diazepam

Diazepam has quite a long elimination half-life ($t_{1/2}$ ß) of on average 50 hours, which may result in delayed recovery and possible re-sedation after an initial period of recovery due to active metabolites and entero-hepatic re-circulation. This fact is particularly undesirable for ambulatory patients since it may occur following discharge from the hospital.

Furthermore, the effects of diazepam are intensified in older patients, in whom local anaesthetic techniques are frequently used, because of a linear prolonged elimination half-life: The elimination half-life in a 20-year-old patient is about 20 hours and in contrast, in a 80-year-old patient it is approximately 90 hours.

Intravenous diazepam causes modest respiratory depression, with decreases in tidal volume of about 25%. Opioid analgesics or other hypnotics potentiate its respiratory depressant properties, even when administered at low dosages.

Finally, diazepam is insoluble in water, requiring organic solvents like propylene glycol (40%) and ethyl alcohol (10%) to produce a stable intravenous solution. Therefore, intravenous use of diazepam is often associated with a high incidence of local irritation, phlebitis or even venous thrombosis, although these untoward effects may be reduced by using diazepam in a lipid emulsion, like Diazepam Lipuro®.

Recommended doses of diazepam for sedation are 0.1 - 0.2 mg/kg given quite carefully and slowly according to individual needs. During the last 10 years, the use of diazepam as a sedative agent has been reduced because of its poor control of the desired sedative level.

3.1.2. Midazolam

For many years, midazolam has been the most popular intravenous benzodiazepine because it is water soluble and does not cause pain on injection or irritation to veins. It has a potency that is two or three times greater than that of diazepam. It is a more rapid-acting agent than diazepam with a relatively short elimination half-life of about 2-4 hours and no active metabolites. Thus, midazolam allows a more predictable recovery after surgical procedures. However, midazolam requires careful intravenous titration to the desired sedation level and to minimize side-effects resulting from inadvertent overdosage. The effects of aging can increase the patient's sensitivity to midazolam.

In many studies, midazolam has a more rapid onset of clinical effect and also produces more profound anterograde amnesia, anxiolysis and sedation than diazepam. For conscious sedation with midazolam, dosages of 0.05 to 0.1 mg kg^{-1} or 0.03 to 0.2 mg kg^{-1} h^{-1} are recommended and have to be titrated conscientiously to individual response. Individual differences in drug-response appear to be less with midazolam than with diazepam. Although full recovery from sedative effects is more rapid than after diazepam, accumulation can occur after multiple doses or prolonged infusions of midazolam producing postoperative residual sedation and amnesia that can delay recovery after outpatient procedures.[4] In addition, the sedative effects of midazolam are also more prolonged and intensified in the elderly.

3.2. Propofol

Propofol has been commonly used in sub-hypnotic dosages for conscious sedation to accompany local anaesthesia, mainly because it is a very short acting, easily controllable and individually titrable hypnotic and sedative agent.[5] The unique pharmacokinetic properties of propofol result in a quick recovery from the effects of a single bolus dose, as well as following a continuous infusion, because of the early redistribution from the brain and a high metabolic clearance rate.[6] The rapid onset and short duration of action of propofol ensures prompt responsiveness to changes in its infusion rates, with optimal titration achieved by using a variable-rate infusion. Furthermore, propofol has a low incidence of undesirable side-effects when used in sedative dosages.[7] Its use is rarely associated with excitatory phenomena or involuntary movements, and there is a low incidence of postoperative nausea and vomiting (PONV). Following outpatient surgery, postoperative nausea and vomiting is particularly undesirable not only because of the unpleasantness for the patient, but also because it may significantly delay discharge from the hospital.

Of particular importance, low-dose infusions of propofol have little depressant effect on cardiovascular and respiratory variables like tidal volume, minute ventilation or end-expiratory carbon dioxide.[8] Nevertheless, the monitoring of oxygen saturation is recommended and supplemental oxygen should be given throughout surgery, especially when propofol is administered combined with an opioid analgesic.

3.2.1. Manually controlled infusion of propofol for conscious sedation

Propofol has been well investigated as a sedative agent in regional anaesthesia for ophthalmic, orthopaedic or urological surgery. The use of propofol for conscious sedation was initially described by Mackenzie and colleagues in the late eighties.[5] They utilized a variable-rate propofol infusion with a mean dose of 3.8 mg kg^{-1} h^{-1} to provide sedation for patients undergoing lower limb surgery under spinal anaesthesia. With these dosages, patients were all calm but arousable with verbal commands. More important, the maintenance of the desired sedation level was easily achieved by varying the propofol infusion rate. Within 4 minutes of terminating the propofol infusion, patients were completely awake and rapidly became fully orientated. In a following study, the same group[9] compared a similar infusion rate of propofol (mean 3.7 mg kg^{-1} h^{-1}) with that of midazolam (mean 0.27 mg kg^{-1} h^{-1}) used to supplement spinal anaesthesia. However, propofol was associated with a significantly faster recovery. After discontinuing the sedative infusions, patients receiving propofol were fully awake within 2.1 ± 0.3 minutes, compared to 9.2 ± 1.5 minutes after midazolam. Finally, White and Negus found in 1991 that propofol for sedation allowed greater accuracy in titration of the sedative effect compared to midazolam.[10]

Propofol is an appealing sedative agent particularly for use in ophthalmic surgery not only because of its sedative properties but also because of the sustained associated reduction in intra-ocular pressure and low incidence of PONV postoperatively. In the early nineties, Holas and colleagues compared propofol with diazepam for sedation of patients undergoing ophthalmic surgery in retrobulbar blockade.[11] One hundred elderly patients of comparable anaesthetic risk (American Society of Anesthesiologists physical status 2 or 3) undergoing cataract surgery received either propofol (n=50) or diazepam (n=50). Propofol was infused continuously at a rate of 0.8 to 3.0 (mean 1.18) mg kg^{-1} h^{-1} while diazepam was administered as a very slow intravenous bolus of 5 mg before surgery. During the procedure, patients sedated with propofol showed much better results in oxygen saturation with no signs of motor unrest. In contrast, marked respiratory depression and motor agitation during the procedure, as well as postoperative fatigue and slow mobilization were common in patients receiving diazepam.

Similar results are described in many other publications when propofol is compared with benzodiazepines for conscious sedation. Even when the residual effects of midazolam are antagonised by flumazenil at the end of the surgical procedure, recovery was not faster than following propofol infusion.[12]

3.2.2. Target-controlled infusion (TCI) of propofol for conscious sedation

One of the great advantages of propofol's pharmacokinetic profile relates to the ease with which the resulting level of sedation can be altered. Therefore, a target-controlled infusion is a logical approach to the development of improved administration techniques for an intravenous agent. TCI is based on the understanding of the drug's pharmacokinetic properties. A TCI-system for propofol uses an open three-compartment pharmacokinetic model[13] to predict the necessary initial bolus-dose and following infusion rates to achieve and maintain a given predicted blood concentration. Once achieved, this target blood concentration may be similarly altered depending on clinical needs.

Already in 1993, Skipsey and colleagues described their first experience with a target-controlled infusion system for propofol for sedation during surgery under local blockade[14]. They found that alteration of sedation levels is easy to achieve with a TCI-system as changes made to the target concentration to either "deepen" or "lighten" the level of sedation result in patients achieving the desired sedation score only within a few minutes. Therefore, a TCI-system allows a more rapid adjustment of the propofol blood concentration according to individual requirements than a manually controlled infusion. In elderly patients, not surprisingly, the authors found an age-related decrease in the required propofol blood concentrations for adequate levels of sedation. Finally, the median blood concentration of propofol in this study was at 0.9 µg ml^{-1} and 88% of the total infusion time was found at the desired level of sedation without undue over-sedation. Only a few years later, a quite important step forward was taken concerning better control sedation with TCI-systems. In 1996, Kenny, for the first time, described the concept of the "effect-site concentration".[15] As we know, the effect-site for anaesthetic and sedative agents is the brain. Thus, after intravenous infusion, there is a short delay before effect-site concentrations equilibrate with blood concentrations. Taking this equilibration into account, it was possible to calculate and display the theoretical effect-site concentration on a TCI-system. This information may be very useful because it gives a more accurate reflection of the drug effect and the associated degree of sedation than the target blood concentration does. It may also help to prevent overdosing the sedative agent.

A proposed and popular technique for conscious sedation is to select a low target blood concentration initially, and to increase this target concentration once the theoretical effect-site concentration has reached a very similar level. Using this "biophase concentration" as a guide, target blood concentrations can be titrated slowly and gradually until the desired level of sedation is achieved. With such improved TCI devices, it is possible to achieve a smooth control of patient sedation without unwanted over-sedation. Casati and colleagues[16] recently found that propofol at target blood concentrations of 0.4 - 1.0 (1.2) µg/ml are adequate for conscious sedation with a TCI system but also depend on the age of the patient, the surgical procedure and the kind of and magnitude of premedication.

4. OPIOID ANALGESICS AS ADJUNCTS FOR CONSCIOUS SEDATION

While opioid analgesics can be used as the sole supplement to local anaesthesia, they do not produce reliable sedation without considerable respiratory depression. Therefore, opioids may be used in combination with sedative drugs to provide analgesia and patient comfort and to maintain haemodynamic stability during nerve blockade and surgery.[17] Combinations of analgesic and sedative agents can enhance the degree of sedation, improve surgical conditions and can make local anaesthetic-based techniques more acceptable to most ambulatory patients.

But while providing effective pain relief, all opioid analgesics also increase the incidence of untoward side-effects. In particular, opioids increase the incidence of PONV and can also produce respiratory depression during the intraoperative period. Supplemental oxygen, combined with close monitoring of spontaneous respiration, is therefore mandatory throughout the entire surgical procedure when opioids or combinations of opioid and sedative drugs are administered for conscious sedation.

4.1. Remifentanil

Remifentanil is the first representative of a new class of esterase-metabolized opioid drugs, resulting in a short "context-sensitive half-time". Hughes and co-workers[18] introduced the concept of context-sensitive half-time in 1992 to describe recovery from anaesthetic infusions of varying duration. The context-sensitive half-time is defined as the time required for the drug concentration in the central compartment to decrease by 50% following discontinuation of the infusion. In 1993, Egan[19] described a context-sensitive half-time for remifentanil of about 3.5 minutes, independent of the duration of infusion. Due to this unique pharmacokinetic profile, remifentanil allows a more precise intraoperative titration and has a more predictable offset of effect than all traditional opioids with almost no risk of accumulation, even after prolonged infusion.

In 1999, Servin and colleagues published a summary article[20] about the use of remifentanil as an analgesic adjunct in local anaesthesia in which the results of nine clinical studies about the efficacy and adverse events of remifentanil as an adjunct in „Monitored Anaesthesia Care" are reviewed. In this paper, following key-findings are described:

- Remifentanil provides effective analgesia during nerve block placement when given as a continuous infusion at an initial rate of 0.1 μg kg^{-1} min^{-1} beginning five minutes before placement of the block and thereafter decreased to 0.05 μg kg^{-1} min^{-1} for maintenance of analgesia and comfort, with adjustments of 0.025 μg kg^{-1} min^{-1} according to clinical response.
- In one of these studies[21], the 50% effective dose (ED_{50}) for achievement of adequate sedation with remifentanil was found to be 0.043 μg kg^{-1} min^{-1}.
- Respiratory depression is an expected adverse effect of remifentanil administration. It is more frequently observed with infusion rates higher than 0.2 μg kg^{-1} min^{-1}.
- During conscious sedation, bolus doses should not be administered concurrently with a continuous infusion of remifentanil, especially in eldery patients.

Recently, Holas and colleagues performed a prospective, randomized study comparing the efficacy and safety of remifentanil, propofol or a combination of both for conscious sedation during eye surgery under retrobulbar blockade[17]. Forty-five patients scheduled for elective cataract surgery under local anaesthesia were randomly assigned to receive either remifentanil (group R, n=15), propofol (group P, n= 15) or both agents in reduced doses (group RP, n=15). For conscious sedation, all drugs were administered continuously without an initial bolus dose. Infusion was started five minutes before retrobulbar blockade was applied and stopped at the end of the procedure. The goal was a sedation level at which patients were calm and comfortable but obeyed verbal commands during the procedure aiming at a Ramsay sedation score of 2 or 3. In those patients receiving remifentanil only , the infusion was performed exactly as described in the key-findings above. In patients receiving propofol only, the infusion was started at a rate of 2 mg kg^{-1} min^{-1} , reduced to 1 µg kg^{-1} min^{-1} after retrobulbar blockade, increased again at the start of the procedure and then titrated according to clinical response. In patients receiving remifentanil and propofol together, both drugs were administered at half dosages than in those patients receiving either of the agents alone and then titrated according to individual needs.

As a result, in the remifentanil group, ten patients were sedated at Ramsay sedation level 2 and five at level 3. In the propofol group, twelve patients were at sedation level 2 and three at level 3. In contrast, in the group receiving both remifentanil and propfol, all patients were found at sedation level 2. Results in oxygen saturation were significantly higher in patients receiving remifentanil and propofol at low doses compared to those receiving either of the drugs alone. Pain control during retrobulbar blockade was significantly different among the 3 groups. In the propofol group, there was no patient who was absolutely pain free whereas in the remifentanil and in the combined groups 53% and 60% of patients, respectively, had no pain at all. Nausea was reported in four patients (27%) receiving remifentanil alone within the postoperative period and one of these also vomited about one hour after surgery. No case of PONV was seen in the other groups. In conclusion, combined with propofol at lower concentrations, remifentanil provides superior analgesia during the performance of nerve blockade, thereby enhancing patient comfort during the surgical procedure without compromising haemodynamic stability or respiratory depression.

4.1.1. Target-Controlled Infusion with Remifentanil

A manually controlled infusion of remifentanil will still require a considerable time to achieve steady-state blood concentrations. Each manual adjustment of the infusion rate will again result in a somewhat delayed equilibration to the new steady-state condition. Its effect, according to current dosing recommendations, is highly variable and depends on the condition of the individual patient. For example, the same infusion rate applied to an adipose elderly patient will more than double the blood concentration of remifentanil compared to a young lean patient. A target-controlled infusion of remifentanil which compensates for the distribution and elimination by adjusting the infusion rate based on a pharmacokinetic model, makes individual titration of the drug more predictable. The pharmacokinetic model used in TCI-remifentanil also includes parameters such as age, body-weight, height and body surface area as additional co-variates for better titration of the drug to individual needs. Thus, TCI remifentanil would be an attractive addition to the armamentarium of conscious sedation but is still in the clinical investigation process for this indication.

5. PATIENT-CONTROLLED SEDATION (PCS)

An alternative approach to conscious sedation is to allow patients to self-administer sedative drugs during the surgical procedure by pressing a demand-button using a modified patient-controlled analgesia (PCA) device. That technique of administration is called patient-controlled sedation (PCS). With such an device, adjusted with an appropriate infusion rate and lockout time, patients become able to titrate their own infusion to an appropriate level of sedation with almost no risk of over-sedation. The two commonly used sedative agents for PCS are propofol and midazolam, either alone or combined with opioids. Some studies have compared patient-controlled sedation with propofol and patient-controlled sedation with midazolam.[22,23] The results of these studies showed a faster onset, less over-sedation and better recovery in patients receiving propofol. On the other hand, a higher incidence of respiratory depression, expressed as lower oxygen saturation and higher carbon dioxide tension, was documented in patients treated with midazolam. Conclusively, the investigators found patient-controlled sedation with propofol to be a safe technique which provided good intraoperative conditions and a high degree of patient satisfaction.

The limitation of a standard bolus type PCS is that blood and effect-site concentrations will hardly be stable over time. Each new bolus produces a peak concentration with the potential for over-sedation, the blood concentration then decreases with time until a new bolus is initiated when the patient feels uncomfortable. Because of these limitations, target-controlled infusion and patient-controlled sedation have been combined recently.

5.1. Patient-Controlled Sedation and TCI-Systems

In 1997, an investigation about a modified propofol TCI-system for patient-controlled sedation was published that allows the patient to modify the set target concentration of propofol by pressing a demand button.[24] The term "Patient Maintained Sedation" was created to describe this technique. The equipment was used in 36 un-premedicated orthopaedic patients undergoing regional procedures lasting 10 to 280 minutes. The target-controlled infusion of propofol was started at a target blood concentration (C_T) of 1 µg ml^{-1} and patients were able to increase the target blood concentration by 0.2 µg ml^{-1} increments by pressing the demand button. A lockout time of two minutes was implemented to allow some equilibration between blood and effect-site concentration and a maximum target blood concentration of 3 µg/ml was permitted. Finally, if no demands were made for six minutes, the TCI-system reduced the target blood concentration automatically by 0.2 µg ml^{-1}. It was found that there was considerable inter-individual variability in propofol consumption with a mean of 2.35 mg kg^{-1} h^{-1} (range: 0.18 - 7.86 mg kg^{-1} h^{-1}). Optimum sedation was provided at a median target concentration of 0.8 - 0.9 µg ml^{-1}. The investigators found no cardiovascular instability and only little over-sedation. The recovery period was short and there were no delays in discharge combined with a high patient satisfaction rate after operation.

The advantages of a patient-controlled TCI-sedation system in contrast to a standard bolus type patient-controlled sedation include a rapid onset and offset of sedative effects, a rapid titration to the level of sedation based on the degree of anxiety experienced and, finally, an improved patient safety and satisfaction. In the development of a patient-controlled TCI system for sedation, the initial target concentration, the incremental target concentration achieved by patient demand, the lockout interval and the time before the target concentration is decreased, all are important factors to ensure that the system is safe, yet flexible enough to provide adequate sedation when required. But unfortunately, this technique for conscious sedation is still in an experimental stage and such devices are not yet available commercially.

6. CONCLUSION

The use of loco-regional anaesthesia for a variety of surgical procedures has become more and more popular during the last years as it provides not only satisfactory operating conditions and good intra-and postoperative analgesia, but also has some advantages in terms of health economics. In order to improve patient acceptability, comfort and to reduce stress it is common practice to provide conscious sedation during the surgical procedure. It is clear that only sedative and analgesic drugs with appropriate pharmacokinetic properties like propofol and remifentanil are well suited for this special indication and only these agents are able to guarantee a rapid and smooth recovery profile without untoward side-effects.

Besides the well known application of these drugs as a bolus or a manually controlled infusion, some more sophisticated delivery systems like patient-controlled sedation combined with target-controlled infusion or the administration of remifentanil with a TCI-system have been developed during the last years or are currently under evaluation. So we can hope that these new devices with their improved abilities concerning control of sedation will soon be introduced into clinical practice. This would open a new area of research to further optimise the condition of patients undergoing surgical and diagnostic procedures under sedation with an increasing significance in peri-operative medicine.

7. REFERENCES

1. M. H. Stevens, and P. F. White, Monitored anesthesia care, in: R. E. Miller, ed. *Anesthesia 4th edition,* New York: Churchill Livingstone, 1994; pp 1465-1480.
2. M. A. E. Ramsay, T. M. Savege, B. R. Simpson, and M. Goodwin, Controlled sedation with alphaxalone-alphadolone, *Br Med J* **2**, 656-659 (1974).
3. D. A. Chernik, D. Gillings, H. Laine, J. Hendler, J. M. Silver, A. B. Davidson, E. M. Schwam, and J. L. Siegel, Validity and reliability of the Observer's Assessment of Alertness/Sedation Scale: study with intravenous midazolam, *J. Clin. Psychopharmacol.* **10**, 244-251 (1990).
4. M. L. Urquhart, and P. F. White, Comparison of sedative infusions during regional anesthesia – methohexital, etomidate, and midazolam, *Anesth. Analg.* **68**, 249-254 (1989).
5. N. Mackenzie, and I. S. Grant, Propofol for intravenous sedation. *Anaesthesia* **42**, 3-6 (1987).
6. S. L. Shafer, and D. R. Stanski, Improving the clinical utility of anesthetic drug pharmacokinetics, *Anesthesiology* **76**, 327-330 (1992).
7. I. Smith, P. F. White, M. Nathanson, and R. Gouldson, Propofol: an update on its clinical uses, *Anesthesiology* **81**, 1005-1043 (1994).
8. G. Rosa, G. Conti, P. Orsi, F. D´Alessandro, I. La Rosa, G. Di Giugno, and A. Gasparetto, Effects of low-dose propofol on central respiratory drive, gas exchanges and respiratory pattern, *Acta Anaesth. Scand.* **36**, 128-136 (1992).
9. E. Wilson, N. Mackenzie, and I. S. Grant, A comparison of propofol and midazolam by infusion to provide sedation in patients who receive spinal anaesthesia, *Anaesthesia* **43**, 91-94 (1988).
10. P. F. White, and J. B. Negus. Sedative infusions during local and regional anesthesia: a comparison of midazolam and propofol, *J. Clin. Anesth.* **3**, 32-39 (1991).
11. A. Holas, and J. Faulborn, Propofol versus diazepam for sedation of patients undergoing ophthalmic surgery in regional anaesthesia, *Anaesthesist* **42**, 766-772 (1993).
12. A. F. Ghouri, M. A. Ramirez Ruiz, and P. F. White, Effect of flumazenil on recovery after midazolam and propofol sedation, *Anesthesiology* **81**, 333-339 (1994).
13. B. Marsh, M. White, N. Morton, and G. N. C. Kenny, Pharmacokinetic model driven infusion of propofol in children, *Br J Anaesth* **67**, 41-48 (1991).

14. I. G. Skipsey, J. R. Colvin, N. Mackanzie, and G. N. C. Kenny, Sedation with propofol during surgery under local blockade. Assessment of a target controlled infusion system, *Anaesthesia* **48**, 210-213 (1993).
15. G. N. C. Kenny, Patient sedation: technical problems and developments, *Eur. J. Anaesth.* **13**, Suppl 13: 18-21 (1996).
16. A. Casati, G. Fanelli, E. Casaletti, E. Colnaghi, V. Cedrati, and G. Torri, Clinical assessment of target-controlled infusion of propofol during monitored anesthesia care, *Can. J. Anesth.* **46**, 235-239 (1999).
17. A. Holas, P. Krafft, M. Marcovic, and F. Quehenberger, Remifentanil, propofol or both for conscious sedation under regional anaesthesia., *Eur. J. Anaesthesiol.* **16**, 741-748 (1999).
18. M. A. Hughes, P. S. A. Glass, and J. R. Jacobs, Context-sensitive half-time in multicompartment pharmacokinetic models for intravenous anaesthetic drugs, *Anesthesiology* **76**, 334-341 (1992).
19. T. D. Egan, H. J. M. Lemmens, P. Fiset, D. J. Herrmann, K. T. Muir, D. R. Stanski, and S. L. Shafer, The pharmacokinetics of a new short-acting opioid remifentanil in healthy adult male volunteers, *Anesthesiology* **79**, 881-892 (1993).
20. F. Servin, J. M. Desmonts, and W. D. Watkins, Remifentanil as an analgesic adjunct in local/regional anesthesia and in Monitored Anesthesia Care, *Anesth. Analg.* **89**, 28-32 (1999).
21. M. Lauwers, F. Camu, H. Breivik, A. Hagelberg, M. Rosen, R. Sneyd, A. Horn, D. Noronha, and S. Shaikh, The safety and effectiveness of remifentanil as an adjunct sedative for regional anesthesia, *Anesth. Analg.* **88**, 134-140 (1999).
22. G. E. Rudkin, G. A. Osborne, B. P. Finn, D. A. Jarvis, and D. Vickers, Intraoperative patient controlled sedation. Comparison of patient-controlled propofol with patient-controlled midazolam, *Anaesthesia* **47**, 376-381 (1992).
23. C. K. Pac-Soo, S. Deacock, G. Lockwood, and C. Carr, J. G. Whitwam, Patient controlled sedation for cataract surgery using peribulbar block, *Br. J. Anaesth.* **77**, 370-374 (1996).
24. M. G. Irwin, N. Thompson, and G. N. C. Kenny, Patient maintained propofol sedation, *Anaesthesia* **52**, 525-530 (1997).

TARGET-CONTROLLED INFUSION IN CHILDREN

Xavier Viviand, Aurélie Bourgoin[*]

1. INTRODUCTION

Target-controlled infusion (TCI) is a new technique for the administration of intravenous agents based on real-time pharmacokinetic calculations. Its aim is to control and maintain steady therapeutic levels of drugs with a narrow margin of safety. TCI systems are intended to be similar to the vaporizers for halogenated agents. This technique is increasingly used in adults thanks to the recent availability of a marketed system designed to deliver propofol (Diprifusor®). Its utilization is much more limited in children due to theoretical and practical limits (Table 1). This presentation will focus mainly on the applicability of the technique in children and on the available literature. The reader may find a more detailed discussion about TCI administration in two recent reviews.[1, 2]

2. AGENTS AND PHARMACOKINETICS

The performance of a TCI system is directly correlated to the appropriateness of the pharmacokinetic parameter set in a given patient. It is well known that body composition and function greatly vary during childhood and differ from adults. Body water content and fat stores change with age. In full-term newborns, water represents 70 percent of the total body weight. This value decreases with age to reach 50 percent in adults. Other modifications such as mass and maturation of the liver and kidneys, concentration of plasma proteins and cardiac output also have an impact on distribution and elimination of the drugs. However, most changes occur during the neonatal period and infancy.

Thus, it is necessary that pharmacokinetic parameter sets should be determined at different ages. TCI administration based on adult pharmacokinetics may lead to erroneous predictions. The optimal design of the study should include continuous infusion with

---

[*] [*] Xavier Viviand and Aurélie Bourgoin, Department of Anesthesiology, Hopital Nord, 13915 Marseille-Cedex 20, France

Advances in Modelling and Clinical Application of Intravenous Anaesthesia
Edited by Vuyk and Schraag, Kluwer Academic/Plenum Publishers, 2003

161

early and late arterial samples to obtain an optimal estimation of volumes of distribution and elimination phase. These requirements are compounded by the difficulties and ethical considerations in obtaining sufficient blood samples from children. This explains the reason that the majority of pharmacokinetic models are based on venous samples. Despite these difficulties, several pharmacokinetics are available for propofol and various opioids. One of the criteria for choosing a parameter set for a given I.V. anaesthetic is to take into account the statistical performance of the model as evaluated ideally prospectively or at least through cross-validation. Bias (median prediction error or MDPE) and imprecision (median absolute prediction error or MDAPE) are the most important criteria. [3] The prediction error (PE) is the difference between the measured (C_m) and the target (C_t) concentrations:

$$PE\ (\%) = (C_m - C_t)\ .\ 100\ /\ C_t$$

A bias of 10-20% and an imprecision of 20-30% (but with a maximal value less than 50-60%) are considered acceptable for clinical use.[4]

Table 1. Theoretical and practical constraints associated with TCI in children.

	Theoretical	Practical
• Pharmacokinetics:		
	- dedicated parameter set	• I.V. line management
	- blood-effect transfer parameter ke0	
• Pharmacodynamics:		
	- adequate concentrations	• Lack of marketed device
	- hypnotic-opioid interaction	

2.1 Propofol

Several pharmacokinetics have been determined in children (Table 2).[5-8] The pharmacokinetics of propofol were best described by a three-compartment model. At first glance, volumes of distribution and metabolic clearance are inversely correlated to age. This explains why children require higher infusion rates of propofol than adults to maintain a given blood concentration. [9]

Marsh's and Kataria's pharmacokinetics are weight-proportional. Kataria et al. developed more complex models but without improving the performance of the weight-proportional model. [6] The parameter set proposed by Schüttler and Ihmsen presents several originalities.[10] First, it is based on a mixed population of patients of adults and children. It is mainly composed, for its paediatric part, of the patients studied by Kataria and Marsh.[6, 7] This model is age- and weight-adjusted but with the following difference with the two other models: the relation between pharmacokinetic parameters and weight depends on a power function rather on a proportional function. The use of power function has been found to be useful in normalizing a large number of physiological and pharmacokinetic variables across weight and species.[11]

The performance of the Marsh's and Short's model compares favorably to the performance of the Diprifusor® (Table 2).[12]

Table 2. Comparison of pharmacokinetics of propofol in children and adults. TCI : target-controlled infusion, V1: volume of the central compartment, Vd_{ss}: volume of distribution at steady-state. MDPE : median prediction error, MDAPE : median absolute prediction error.

	Murat[5]	Marsh[7]	Short[8]	Kataria[6]	Schüttler[10]	Diprifusor®
n	12	20	10	53	96	17
Age (yr)	1-3	1-12	4-10	3-11	2-11	> 15 yr
Administration	Bolus	TCI	TCI	bolus (n=20) bolus + infusion otherwise	Bolus bolus + infusion TCI	infusion
Duration of surgery (min)			38			2 hr at least
Sampling site after infusion	venous 12 hr	venous until eye opening	venous 2 hr	venous	venous	arterial 8 hr
V1 (ml.kg^{-1})	1030	343	432	520	380	228
Vd$_{ss}$ (ml.kg^{-1})	8087	3413	446	9720	1470	3594
Metabolic clearance (ml^{-1}.kg^{-1}.min^{-1})	49	34	42	34	28	27
Performance (%): MDPE MDAPE		0.9 20.1	-0.1 21.5			-7.0 18.2
Comments	burned infants (< 12%)				for 5 yr, 20 kg	

2.2. Opioids

Several alfentanil pharmacokinetics are published for children. Two were derived from a single bolus administration.[13,14] The third one was determined by using a TCI administration and took into account the influence of cardiopulmonary bypass.[15] The pharmacokinetics of alfentanil in children were best described by a two-compartment model. Meistelman et al. found that Vd_{ss} and terminal half-life (T ½ β) were lower in children than in adults while metabolic clearance was preserved.[13] In contrast, Goreski et al. reported no major differences between infants and children but a weak negative correlation between age and clearance.[14] However, they both noted a wide inter-individual variation of clearances and Vd_{ss} (2 to 3-fold) as generally encountered in adults. The bias and imprecision of Goreski's model were 24% (<1 yr) or –7% (>1 yr) and 34% (<1 yr) and 32% (>1yr) respectively. For Fiset's model, the bias and the imprecision, evaluated by cross-validation, were 18.4% and –3.0% respectively.[15]

Fentanyl has been administered in children by TCI based on adult pharmacokinetics.[16] Not surprisingly, adult pharmacokinetics resulted in a positive bias. Thus, the authors determined a two-compartment model with age and weight as covariates. The cross-validation resulted in an MDPE of –1.6% and an MDAPE of 21%.

Sufentanil is best dscribed by a two-compartment model in children.[17] Metabolic clearance, terminal half-life and total volume of distribution were greater than in adults.

The pharmacokinetics of remifentanil have been recently studied in children.[18] The volumes of distribution and metabolic clearance were inversely correlated to age but the half-life was similar in all age groups. Remifentanil showed an extremely rapid elimination which was similar to that in adults. At the present time, no generally agreed compartmental model is available for this agent in children and thus remifentanil can not benefit from a TCI administration in this population.

In summary, except for remifentanil, suitable pharmacokinetics with good performance are available in children. Thus, pharmacokinetics are not a bottleneck to the use of TCI in paediatric patients.

3.   PHARMACODYNAMICS

Pharmacodynamic data relevant to TCI administration in children are scarce. This can be explained by the fact that the goal of the few existing studies on TCI in children was to establish and validate pharmacokinetic models. Actually, pharmacological effect is related to the concentration prevailing in a virtual compartment called the effect site or biophase. An equilibrium can be obtained between a given constant blood concentration and the effect site concentration after a certain period. This period depends on the pharmacokinetic parameter k_{e0}.[19] It is generally considered that the equilibrium time requires four to five times the $t_{1/2} k_{e0}$. For propofol, the equilibrium is achieved between approximately 10 and 15 minutes. Unfortunately, appropriate values of the k_{e0} have not been established in children yet. In contrast, some data on plasma concentrations required for adequate anaesthesia have been published.

It was first reported that children require a higher propofol target concentration than adults for induction of anaesthesia (Table 3). For induction, a target concentration between 8 and 14 μg ml^{-1} has been suggested. In unpremedicated adults < 60 years, a target concentration of 6 μg ml^{-1} is adequate. This increase in the target concentrations for induction of anaesthesia can better be explained with pharmacokinetic rather than pharmacodynamic reasons. Indeed, cardiac output is one of the main factors governing the time course of plasma concentrations during the first minutes of administration and consequently the time to loss of consciousness.[20] Unpremedicated paediatric patients may demonstrate increased anxiety and thus a higher cardiac output before induction and target concentrations during the first minutes of administration are probably overestimated. We have found that the target concentrations required for LMA insertion in 50% and 90% unpremedicated children were 7.86 μg ml^{-1} and 10.86 μg ml^{-1} respectively.[21]

TCI administration was based on the pharmacokinetics proposed by Kataria et al. and LMA was inserted after 2 min. These figures are higher than those reported in adults.[22]

In another study the LMA was inserted after 12 minutes of constant target concentration.[†] Propofol venous blood concentrations were measured. EC50 and EC90 were 4.31 μg ml[-1] and 7.17 μg ml[-1] respectively. These concentrations are very similar to the theoretical effect site concentration reported in adults for insertion of LMA.[23]

Table 3. Adequate propofol concentrations for induction and maintenance in children.

	Marsh[7]	Doyle[27]	Short[8]	Aun[29]	Browne[24]
n	10	20	20	38	59
Mean age (yr)	4.8	3	5	6.7	3-12 yr
Procedure	minor RA, N2O	minor RA, N2O	minor RA, N2O	minor RA, N2O, paracetamol	minor Alfentanil, temazepam
Duration (min)		33.3	30.0	31.3	
PK data set	TCI - Marsh	TCI - Marsh	TCI-Short	TCI – Short	Manual infusion
Induction (μg.ml[-1])	14	8-14	8-14	8	
Maintenance (μg.ml[-1])			6.6 (measured)		Alf.: 279 ng ml[-1]: EC50: 1.71 -EC95: 1.95 Alf.:135 ng ml[-1]: EC50: 3.87-EC95: 4.26
End of surgery (μg ml[-1])		5.8 (cited in Aun)			
Recovery Time (min) Conc.(μg ml[-1])		13.5 1.4	40 0.86	40 0.90-0.97	Alf.: 279 ng ml[-1]: 16.8 min Alf.: 135 ng ml[-1]: 13.2 min
Comments			Chinese children	Chinese children	

Adequate propofol target concentrations required for maintenance of anaesthesia also appear to be higher than in adults. Several authors have reported mean target concentrations comprised between 6 and 8 μg ml[-1] (Table 3), greater than the 3-5 μg ml[-1] recommended in adults. However, it should be noted that these concentrations were determined in patients undergoing minor surgery and breathing spontaneously through an LMA. They received nitrous oxide and a regional block for analgesia. Propofol was used for its hypnotic properties (i.e. loss of consciousness and amnesia) but also to allow the child to

---

[†] Viviand X, Bellefleur JP, Lando A, Aubry de la Noé C, Martin C. Venous blood concentration of propofol required for insertion of the laryngeal mask airway in children (abstract). ASA Annual Meeting, New-Orleans, 2001

tolerate the LMA and to correct a potential lack of analgesia. A balanced anaesthesia technique with an opioid decreases the adequate concentrations of propofol. Browne et al. measured the blood concentrations of propofol and alfentanil allowing an adequate level of anaesthesia for body surface surgery.[24] EC_{50} and EC_{95} were 1.92 µg ml^{-1} and 4.26 µg ml^{-1} respectively when alfentanil was maintained at 135 ng ml^{-1}. These values are very similar to those reported in adults.

Yet, pharmacodynamic specificities could play a role in children. As a matter of fact, the MAC of halogenated agents is inversely correlated with age, even in children although preterm neonates and newborns may demonstrate lower MAC.[25] The bispectral index (BIS®) has been used in children as a surrogate endpoint of the pharmacodynamic effect of sevoflurane.[26] Infants (0-2 yr) demonstrated higher BIS® than children (2-10 yr) for a given end-tidal concentration of sevoflurane. Using the same methodology, we found that BIS® were inversely correlated to age (between 2 and 10 yr) for a given measured venous concentration of propofol.[‡] From these data, it can be hypothesized that the higher target concentrations of propofol required in children could also have a pharmacodynamic basis. In a preliminary report, pediatric patients were found to be less sensitive to fentanyl than adults and required higher concentrations for adequate anesthesia.[§] Further studies are mandatory to confirm theses points.

4. RECOVERY

Ideally, at the end of surgery, one should obtain concentrations that are compatible with awakening and spontaneous ventilation while still providing good residual analgesia. Actually, return to consciousness depends on the effect site concentration and not on the blood concentration. However, as discussed above, the estimation of effect site concentration over time during TCI administration is not available in children and we are left with target blood concentrations.

The mean target concentration on eye opening varies between 0.86 µg ml^{-1} and 1.4 µg ml^{-1}.[8,27] These concentrations are near adult values (< 60 yr) (between 1 and 1.5 µg ml^{-1} on average). In our study, the target concentrations of propofol on eye opening were 1.03 µg.ml^{-1} and 0.76 µg.ml^{-1} in unpremedicated and premedicated children respectively.[21] The measured venous concentrations of propofol were 0.86 µg ml^{-1} and 0.60 µg ml^{-1} respectively. The performance (MDPE and MDAPE) of pharmacokinetics was lower during the recovery phase. This finding has also been reported in adults.

Target concentrations at the end of surgery and decrement times are the major factors governing the recovery time.[28] Children demonstrate longer decrement times for propofol, either for 50% decrement (i.e. context sensitive half-time or CHST) or for 80% decrement time (Figure 1). These greater decrement times can explain the delayed recovery reported in some studies. For a propofol target concentration at the end of anaesthesia of 4.9 µg ml^{-1}, the time to eye opening was approximately 40 minutes.[29] Their paediatric patients therefore required a 80% decrement time to obtain a target concentration com-

---

[‡] Viviand X, Bourgoin A, Lacarelle B, Aubry de la Noé C, Martin C. Correlation of BIS with venous blood propofol concentration (abstract). ASA Annual Meeting, Orlando, 2002
[§] Ginsberg B, Margolis J, Pressley AB, Ross AK, Dear G, Glass PSA. Plasma levels of fentanyl in non-cardiac pediatric surgical patients (abstract). *Anesthesiology* **81**:3A (1994).

patible with awakening (0.97 µg ml⁻¹ in this study). This period was very close to what
the theory predicts (Figure 1).

Conversely, children demonstrated a faster CSHT for fentanyl compared with adults
after a TCI administration lasting more than 20 to 55 min.[16] Fiset and colleagues also
found a faster CHST for alfentanil in children.[15]

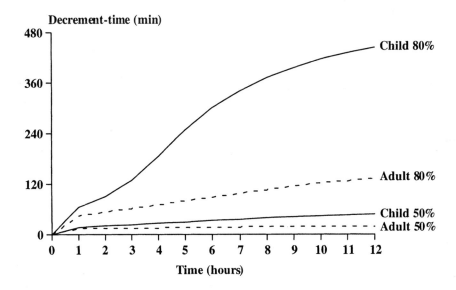

Figure 1. Decrement times of propofol in children and in adults. Calculations were based on the pharmacokinetic parameter set proposed by Kataria et al. for children and on the pharmacokinetics incorporated into the Diprifusor® for adults. [6, 7]

One of the interests of TCI systems is to calculate on line the time required to obtain a
theoretical blood concentration and thus give the anaesthetist an idea of awakening time.
If one desires a rapid awakening in children, the target concentration at the end of surgery
should not be higher than 2 times the theoretical concentration of awakening.

The effect of premedication and the level of residual analgesia on recovery times
should not be neglected. Vuyk et al. have demonstrated that certain hypnotic-opioid combinations are optimal for recovery in adults.[30] The optimal target concentration of propofol varies according to the type of opioid. The data reported by Browne et al. in children
are in favour of such a phenomenon in children.[24] In the high alfentanil concentration
group (279 versus 135 ng ml⁻¹ in the low group), although the propofol concentration
required for maintenance was reduced (EC₉₅: 3.87 µg ml⁻¹ vs. 4.26µg ml⁻¹), the recovery
time was longer (13.2 min vs. 16.8 min).[24] Moreover, the sparing effect of opioid was not
linear (when the alfentanil concentration was double, the propofol concentration decreased by only 9%) which demonstrates that the propofol-alfentanil combination is also
synergistic in children. More studies are necessary to determine the optimal hypnotic-opioid combination, as has been done in adults.

5.   PRACTICAL PROBLEMS

Some practical problems may limit the use of TCI administration in a clinical setting. The placement of I.V. line in conscious children < 2-3 yr may be a challenge even with the use of EMLA cream. The TCI line should be connected close to the I.V. cannula so that administration of anaesthetics does not depend on the infusion rate of the main line.[31] Short connectors designed for TIVA are commercially available and improve administration. In the same sense, the use of a diluted solution for opioids and the insertion of a one-way valve improve the safety of TCI administration in children.

The placement of small catheters (22 G) and high infusion rates ('flash' induction mode) increase the risk of triggering an untimely occlusion alarm, particularly during induction of anaesthesia. Thus, it is recommended that the occlusion threshold alarm be adjusted at its highest value (for example 1000 mmHg) when infusion rates are greater than 300-500 ml/h. Conversely, the alarm should be lower than 500 mmHg during maintenance in order to rapidly detect any cessation in the infusion. Another possibility to minimize this problem is to increase the period of induction ('gradual' induction mode) and consequently the required infusion rate but at the price of a prolonged induction time.

Some Diprifusor® models automatically adjust the occlusion alarm to the infusion rate. These technical constraints explain that propofol TCI induction takes more time than manual bolus. However, in our experience, loss of consciousness can be obtained in less than 1 minute and LMA can be inserted at 2 minutes without triggering an occlusion alarm.[21] This period compares favourably with inhalational induction. Thus, full stomach and crash-induction remain contraindications to TCI induction in small children

At present, the lack of a marketed device limits the use of TCI in children. The Diprifusor® can not be used in children < 16 yr and < 30 kg. Its use in children leads to gross overprediction.[7, 9] Several groups worldwide have developed custom made software allowing TCI administration of several drugs. Some of these systems incorporate paediatric pharmacokinetics for propofol and opioids. These systems are not approved for clinical use and are only dedicated to research.

6.   CONCLUSION

In conclusion, TCI administration of I.V. anaesthetic drugs can be used in children. TIVA-TCI is mainly reserved for children > 2 years. Opioid TCI combined with halogenated agents could be an interesting technique in infants. More clinical studies are mandatory in children.[32] We can also express the wish that specific TCI systems should be marketed in the near future. Finally, TCI administration should be considered as a great opportunity to extend our knowledge of the pharmacokinetics and the pharmacodynamics of intravenous anaesthetics in children.

7.   REFERENCES

1. X. Viviand and M. Leone, Induction and maintenance of intravenous anaesthesia using target-controlled infusion systems, *Best Practice & Research Clinical Anaesthesiology* **15**(1):19-33 (2001).
2. M. van den Niewenhuyzen, F. Engbers, J. Vuyk and A. Burm, Target-controlled infusion systems: role in anaesthesia and analgesia, *Clin. Pharmacokinet.* **38**:181-190 (2000).

3. J. R. Varvel, D. L. Donoho and S. L. Shafer, Measuring the predictive performance of computer-controlled infusion pumps, *J. Pharmacokinet. Biopharm.* **20**:63-94 (1992).
4. J. Schüttler, S. Kloos, H. Schwilden and H. Stoeckel, Total intravenous anaesthesia with propofol and alfentanil by computer-assisted infusion, *Anaesthesia* **43**(suppl):2-7 (1988).
5. I. Murat, V. Billard, J. Vernois, M. Zaouter, P. Marsol, R. Souron and R. Farinotti, Pharmacokinetics of propofol after a single dose in children aged 1-3 years with minor burns. Comparison of three data analysis approaches, *Anesthesiology* **84**:526-532 (1996).
6. B. Kataria, S. Ved, H. Nicodemus, G. Hoy, D. Lea, M. Dubois, J. Mandema and S. Shafer, The pharmacokinetics of propofol in children using three different data analysis approaches, *Anesthesiology* **80**:104-122 (1994).
7. B. Marsh, M. White, N. Morton and G. Kenny, Pharmacokinetic model driven infusion of propofol in children, *Br. J. Anaesth.* **67**:41-48 (1991).
8. T. G. Short, C. S. Aun, P. Tan, J. Wong, Y. H. Tam and T. E. Oh, A prospective evaluation of pharmacokinetic model controlled infusion of propofol in paediatric patients, *Br. J. Anaesth.* **72**:302-306 (1994).
9. C. S. McFarlan, B. J. Anderson and T. G. Short, The use of propofol infusions in paediatric anaesthesia: a practical guide, *Paediatric Anaesthesia* **9**:209-216 (1999).
10. J. Schüttler and H. Ihmsen, Population pharmacokinetics of propofol, *Anesthesiology* **92**:727-738 (2000).
11. B. Anderson and G. Meakin, Scaling for size: some implications for paediatric anaesthesia dosing, *Paediatric Anaesthesia* **12**:205-219 (2002).
12. J. Coetzee, J. Glen, C. Wium and L. Boshoff, Pharmacokinetic model selection for target controlled infusions of propofol. Assessment of three parameter sets, *Anesthesiology* **82**:1328-1345 (1995).
13. C. Meistelman, C. Saint-Maurice, M. Lepaul, J. Levron, J. Loose and K. Mac Gee, A comparison of alfentanil pharmacokinetics in children and adults, *Anesthesiology* **66**:13-16 (1987).
14. G. Goresky, G. Koren, M. Sabourin, J. Sale and L. Strunin, The pharmacokinetics of alfentanil in children, *Anesthesiology* **67**:654-659 (1987).
15. P. Fiset, L. Mathers, R. Engstrom, D. Fitzgerald, S. C. Brand, F. Hsu and S. L. Shafer, Pharmacokinetics of computer-controlled alfentanil administration in children undergoing cardiac surgery, *Anesthesiology* **83**:944-55 (1995).
16. B. Ginsberg, S. Howell, P. S. Glass, J. O. Margolis, A. K. Ross, G. L. Dear and S. L. Shafer, Pharmacokinetic model-driven infusion of fentanyl in children, *Anesthesiology* **85**:1268-75 (1996).
17. J. Guay, P. Gaudreault, T. Alexander, B. Goulet and F. Varin, Pharmacokinetics of sufentanil in normal children, *Can. J. Anaesth.* **39**:14-20 (1992).
18. K. Ross, P. Davis, G. L. Dear, B. Ginsberg, F. McGowan, R. Stiller, L. Henson, C. Huffman and K. Muir, Pharmacokinetics of remifentanil in anesthetized pediatric patients undergoing elective surgery or diagnostic procedures, *Anesth. Analg.* **93**:1393-1401 (2001).
19. L. Sheiner, D. Stanski, S. Vozeh, R. Miller and J. Ham, Simultaneous modeling of pharmacokinetics and pharmacodynamics: application to d-tubocurarine, *Clin. Pharmcol. Ther.* **25**:358-371 (1979).
20. T. Krejcie and M. Avram, What determines anesthetic induction dose? It's the front-end kinetics, Doctor ! *Anesth. Analg.* **89**:541-544 (1999).
21. X. Viviand, L. Berdugo, C. Aubry de la Noé, A. Lando and C. Martin, Target concentration of propofol required to insert the laryngeal mask airway in children, *Paediatric Anaesthesia* (accepted for publication)
22. I. Taylor and G. Kenny, Requirements for target-controlled infusion of propofol to insert the laryngeal mask airway, *Anaesthesia* **53**:222-226 (1998).
23. A. Casati, G. Fanelli, E. Casaletti, V. Cedrati, F. Veglia and G. Torri, The target plasma concentration of propofol required to place the laryngeal mask versus cuffed oropharyngeal airway, *Anesth. Analg.* **88**:917-920 (1999).
24. B. L. Browne, C. Prys_Roberts and A. R. Wolf, Propofol and alfentanil in children: infusion technique and dose requirement for total i.v. anaesthesia, *Br. J. Anaesth.* **69**:570-576 (1992).
25. W. Mapleson, Effect of age on MAC in humans : a meta-analysis, *Br. J. Anaesth.* **76**:179-185 (1996).
26. W. Denman, E. Swanson, D. Rosow, K. Ezbicki, P. Connors and C. Rosow, Pediatric evaluation of the bispectral index (BIS) monitor and correlation of BIS with end-tidal sevoflurane concentration in infants and children, *Anesth. Analg.* **90**:872-877 (2000).
27. E. Doyle, W. McFadzean and N. S. Morton, IV anaesthesia with propofol using a target-controlled infusion system: comparison with inhalation anaesthesia for general surgical procedures in children, *Br. J. Anaesth.* **70**:542-545 (1993).
28. M. Hugues, P. Glass and J. Jacobs, Context-sensitive half-time in multicompartment pharmacokinetic models for intravenous anesthetic drugs, *Anesthesiology* **76**:334-341 (1992).

29. C. S. Aun, T. G. Short, M. O'Meara, D. Leung, Y. Rowbottom and T. E. Oh, Recovery after propofol infusion anaesthesia in children: comparison with propofol, thiopentone or halothane induction followed by halothane maintenance, *Br. J. Anaesth.* **72**:554-558 (1994).

30. J. Vuyk, M. Mertens, E. Olofsen, A. Burm and J. Bovill, Propofol anesthesia and rational opioid selection: determination of optimal EC50-EC95 propofol-opioid concentrations that assure adequate anesthesia and a rapid return of consciousness, *Anesthesiology* **87**:1547-1569 (1997).

31. F. Engbers, Practical use of 'Diprifusor' systems, *Anaesthesia* **53** (Suppl. 1):28-34 (1998).

32. M. Schreiner and W. Greeley: Pediatric clinical trials: shall we take a lead? *Anesth. Analg.* **94**:1-3 (2001).

REMIFENTANIL FOR CARDIAC ANAESTHESIA

Luc Barvais and Nicholas Sutcliffe[*]

1. INTRODUCTION

Total intravenous anaesthesia (TIVA) incorporating high dose opioid is the mainstay of modern anaesthesia for cardiac surgery. High dose opioids attenuate the sympathetic and somatic responses to noxious stimulation. They have minimal negative effects on the contractility, the coronary circulation and the myocardial metabolism and can be given even in patients with impaired cardiac function.

Remifentanil has a rapid onset of action with a $T\frac{1}{2}k_{e0}$ of 1 to 3 minutes and a very short duration of action with a context-sensitive half-ime of 3-7 minutes whatever the duration of infusion. It is rapidly inactivated by esterases in both blood and tissues, resulting in this unique pharmacokinetic profile. These characteristics facilitate the titration of dose to effect and also allow the use of very high doses without prolonging recovery. The duration of action of remifentanil has been found to be short, even in patients with renal or hepatic failure, although only low doses have been used in the studies published to date. The hydrolysis of remifentanil produces a metabolite with very weak opioid receptor activity that does not contribute significantly to the effects of remifentanil. All these characteristics make remifentanil an easy opioid drug to titrate with a good predictability of awakening and early extubation. The potential problems of such a technique are the risks of bradycardia, thoracic rigidity and the need to mix the lyophilized drug with a diluent. Other possible disadvantages of remifentanil include; the need for administration as a continuous infusion, risk of rapid loss of analgesic and anaesthetic effects if the infusion is interrupted accidentally and also the difficulty in judging the dose of a longer lasting opioid that will be required to control postoperative pain without producing excessive ventilatory depression. Remifentanil is likely to be more expensive than other opioids, but its use may reduce overall costs if prompt

[*] Luc Barvais; Erasmus hospital, 808 Lennikstreet, Brussels, Belgium. Nicholas Sutcliffe; HCI Hospital, Clydebank Glasgow, UK

Advances in Modelling and Clinical Application of Intravenous Anaesthesia
Edited by Vuyk and Schraag, Kluwer Academic/Plenum Publishers, 2003

171

recovery from its effects results in shorter stays and a more rapid turn-over in the operating room, recovery and intensive care unit (ICU). There will also be a cost saving effect from a reduced dose of hypnotic agent used with this technique.

This chapter will focus on remifentanil and cardiac anaesthesia with a particular emphasis on:

- fast track cardiac anaesthesia
- patients with poor cardiac function
- its use during cardiopulmonary bypass
- the administration technique
- the transition period for the optimal management of postoperative analgesia
- the combination with regional techniques.

2. REMIFENTANIL AND FAST TRACK CARDIAC ANAESTHESIA

In a prospective, randomised, controlled clinical trial, Cheng et al have evaluated the morbidity outcomes and safety of a modified anaesthetic technique (15 μg/kg fentanyl + propofol) to provide shorter sedation and early extubation (1 to 6 hours) than those of the conventional anaesthetic protocol (50 μg/kg fentanyl + midazolam) in 120 patients after coronary artery bypass grafting.[1] Postoperative time before extubation, ICU time and hospital length of stay were shorter in the early extubation group. Between both groups, there was no difference with respect to myocardial ischaemia, CPK-Mb and atelectasis at 48 hours after operation. The authors concluded that early extubation after CABG surgery was safe and did not increase perioperative morbidity.[1] Moreover, there was an improvement in post-extubation intrapulmonary shunt fraction and a reduction in ICU and hospital lengths of stay.

Since this study, fast-track programs have become popular when postoperative haemodynamic and pulmonary conditions are acceptable in an attempt to decrease the costs of cardiac surgery and several studies have been performed to evaluate the place of remifentanil in fast track cardiac anaesthesia technique.

Howie et al.[2] have compared 304 ASA III or IV patients with an ejection fraction greater than 30 % and a BMI within 50%. Patients were anaesthetised using either, a fentanyl/isoflurane/propofol or, a remifentanil/isoflurane/propofol regimen for fast-track cardiac anaesthesia in a prospective, randomised, double-blinded study on patients undergoing elective coronary artery bypass graft surgery. There were no differences between the groups in extubation time, time to discharge from the surgical intensive care unit, ST segment and other ECG changes, catecholamine levels, or cardiac enzymes. The remifentanil-based anaesthetic (consisting of a bolus followed by a continuous infusion) resulted in significantly less responses to surgical stimulation and less need for anaesthetic interventions compared with the fentanyl regimen (consisting of an initial bolus, and followed by subsequent boluses only to treat haemodynamic responses). Both drug regimens allowed early extubation. More patients in the fentanyl group experienced hypertension during skin incision and maximal sternal spread compared to the remifentanil group.

In a multi-centre, parallel group, randomised, double-blind study, Molhoff et al.[3] have compared the efficacy and safety of high-dose remifentanil administered by continuous infusion with an intermittent bolus low dose of fentanyl regimen, when given in combination with propofol for general anaesthesia in 321 patients undergoing elective coronary artery bypass graft surgery. A significantly lower proportion of the patients who received remifentanil had responses to maximal sternal spread (the primary efficacy endpoint) compared with those who received fentanyl (11% vs. 52%; $P < 0.001$).[3] However, the median time to extubation was longer in the subjects who received remifentanil than for those who received fentanyl (5.1 vs. 4.2 h; $P = 0.006$). Overall, the incidence of adverse events was similar but greater in the remifentanil group with respect to shivering and hypertension. There were no drug-related adverse cardiac outcomes and no deaths from cardiac causes before hospital discharge in either treatment group.

Fifty patients scheduled for elective cardiac surgery were anaesthetized by combining TCI of propofol (1.5-2 µg/ml) and remifentanil (1 µg/kg followed by 0.25 to 1 µg/kg/min) with a morphine transition of 0.1 mg/kg, 30 min before end of surgery. This technique resulted in haemodynamic stability, good postoperative analgesia and allows physicians to schedule the time of extubation in patients undergoing cardiac anaesthesia.[4]

Engoren et al.[5] have compared the effects of fentanyl-based, sufentanil-based, or remifentanil-based anaesthetic techniques. Ninety adult patients undergoing cardiac surgery were randomised. Pain scores at 30 min after extubation and at 6:30 am were similar in all three groups ($P > 0.05$). Median ventilator times, intensive care unit stays and hospital stays did not differ among the three groups. Two patients in the sufentanil group and one in the fentanyl group needed endotracheal re-intubation. Median anaesthetic costs were largest in the remifentanil group and smallest in the fentanyl group but hospital costs were similar. The authors concluded that any of these opioid drugs can be recommended for fast-track cardiac surgery.

Remifentanil, when used in off-pump bypass surgery, was associated with an increased likelihood of extubation in the operating room but length of stay and total hospital costs remained unchanged.[6]

In summary, the results of the fast track techniques vary according to the different studies, the protocol used and the experience of the anaesthesiologist involved. The classical cardiac anaesthesia techniques of high opioid doses of fentanyl, sufentanil and alfentanil delayed the extubation time compared to a high dose remifentanil. Anaesthetic techniques using lower dose opioid regimens of fentanyl, sufentanil or alfentanil used for fast tracking did not delay the extubation time compared to a high dose remifentanil technique. Using remifentanil, a high dose opioid technique can still be used with a rapid recovery. Anaesthesia with this technique is no longer a limiting factor for fast track cardiac surgery. Haemodynamic stability, hypoxemia, haemorrhage and hypothermia are now the more important factors prolonging the recovery period after cardiac surgery.

3. REMIFENTANIL AND PATIENTS WITH POOR CARDIAC FUNCTION

The direct myocardial effects of cumulative concentrations of remifentanil on inotropic and lusitropic variables of isolated human myocardium were compared in vitro with a control group. Remifentanil did not modify active isometric force, peak of the positive force derivative and did not alter lusitropic variables.[7]

In vivo, the effects of remifentanil on myocardial blood flow, metabolism and systemic haemodynamic variables were investigated in patients with coronary artery disease scheduled for elective coronary artery bypass grafting.[8] Systemic haemodynamic variables, myocardial blood flow and metabolism were measured when patients were awake and when they were anaesthetized with high-dose remifentanil (2.0 μg.kg^{-1}.min^{-1}), or with remifentanil 0.5 μg.kg^{-1}.min^{-1} combined with propofol (target-controlled infusion aiming at a plasma concentration of 2.0 μg.ml^{-1}). In this study of Kazmaier et al, heart rate, mean arterial pressure, myocardial blood flow and myocardial oxygen uptake were significantly reduced using either very high dose of remifentanil or using the remifentanil/propofol anaesthesia technique.

In the clinical practice of anaesthesia for patients with severely reduced left ventricular function, TIVA using remifentanil and propofol was performed in 20 patients undergoing first-time implantation of an implantable cardioverter-defibrillator.[9] Remifentanil/propofol anaesthesia was safe, well-controllable, and allowed early extubation after implantation of an ICD in patients with severely reduced left ventricular function. Because patients without complications did not need postoperative intensive care, costs may be considerably reduced with this regimen.[9] In summary, remifentanil appears to be a suitable choice for perioperative analgesia in patients with poor cardiac function.

4. REMIFENTANIL AND ITS USE DURING CARDIOPULMONARY BYPASS

The cardiopulmonary bypass (CPB) may influence the pharmacokinetics of remifentanil and alter drug requirements because of its high clearance and rapid tissue distribution. Michelsen et al. have administered remifentanil by continuous infusion to 68 patients having coronary artery bypass graft surgery with CPB and hypothermia to describe the effects of these interventions on its pharmacokinetics.[10] Remifentanil concentrations were measured before, during, and after CPB. Disposition was best described by a two-compartment model. The volume of distribution increased by 86% with institution of CPB and remained increased after CPB. Elimination clearance decreased by 6.4% for each degree Celsius decrease below 37 degrees Celsius. In the clinical practice, remifentanil concentrations decrease with the institution of CPB because of an increase in the volume of distribution. The decrease in elimination clearance with hypothermia results in increased total remifentanil concentrations during CPB if the infusion rate is not altered. More constant blood remifentanil levels may be obtained by reducing the remifentanil infusion rate by 30% for each 5 degrees Celsius decrease in temperature.

Duthie et al. have measured the apparent blood clearance and pulmonary extraction ratio of remifentanil in 10 adult patients undergoing elective myocardial revascularization with hypothermic CPB.[11] Patients received continuous infusions of remifentanil 1.0, 1.5 or 2.0 μg.kg^{-1}.min^{-1}. After surgery, remifentanil was infused at 1.0 μg.kg^{-1}.min^{-1} in all patients. Remifentanil concentrations were measured in pulmonary and radial artery blood by gas chromatography with high resolution mass spectrometry before and after CPB. Remifentanil concentrations in pulmonary and radial artery blood were related directly to infusion rate, but not to duration of infusion. There was no evidence of accumulation or sequestration. Mean apparent blood remifentanil clearance was 2 L/min. Increased tissue perfusion increased blood remifentanil clearance. Duthie et al found predictable blood remifentanil levels with no evidence of accumulation or pulmonary extraction.[11]

In the study of Russell et al.,[12] 16 patients undergoing coronary revascularization requiring CPB, received remifentanil 2 µg.kg^{-1} or 5 µg.kg^{-1} by infusion over 1 min after sternotomy but before commencing CPB, during hypothermic CPB and during CPB after re-warming. Hypothermic CPB reduced the clearance of remifentanil by an average of 20%, and this was attributed to the effect of temperature on blood and tissue esterase activity. Reductions in arterial pressure occurred with administration of both doses during normothermia only. In summary, the metabolism of remifentanil decreases when the body temperature drops but there is no remifentanil accumulation or extraction in the lungs during CPB.

Table 1. Comparison of the pharmacokinetics of the phenylpiperidines derivatives.

	Fentanyl	Alfentanil	Sufentanil	Remifentanil
Potency	+++	+	+++++	++
PKa	8,4	6,5	8,0	7,1
% non ionised at pH 7,4	<10	90	20	67
Vdss (L/kg)	3-5	0,4-1	2,5-3	0,3-0,4
Clearance (mL/min/kg)	10-20	10-15	4-9	40-60
T½ k$_{e0}$ (min)	5	1,5	5-6	1-3 (20-80 yr)
T½β (hours)	2-4	1-2	2-3	0,1

5. REMIFENTANIL AND ITS ADMINISTRATION TECHNIQUE

The phenylpiperidines derivatives have the same pharmacodynamic profile as morphine but differ essentially in their potency and pharmacokinetic properties (Table 1). The elimination half lives of alfentanil, sufentanil and fentanyl are much longer than that of remifentanil. Shafer et al. have demonstrated that sufentanil and alfentanil have intermediate context-sensitive half-times but the time required to get a 50% or 80% decrease of fentanyl concentration increases rapidly if it is administered by continuous infusion.[13] Beside the duration of infusion, the level of the opioid concentration at the end of infusion is also of prime importance because opioid concentrations associated with spontaneous ventilation are often 80 to 90 % less than those obtained during high opioid anaesthesia techniques.

The haemodynamic stability of fentanyl, sufentanil and alfentanil administration for cardiac anaesthesia has been compared in three separate studies.[14-16] No one drug proved to be superior in this respect. A variable continuous infusion is associated with good haemodynamic stability in patients undergoing coronary revascularization.[17] Computer assisted continuous infusion decreases the requirements of vasoactive agents and the number of episodes of hypo- or hypertension compared to a repeated opioid bolus technique.[18]

   The fast onset and short duration of action of remifentanil are the main reasons that remifentanil is the easiest opioid drug to titrate to effect. However, Minto et al have identified an effect of age on the pharmacokinetics and pharmacodynamics of remifentanil (Table 2), an effect of lean body mass on the pharmacokinetic parameters and no influence of gender on any pharmacokinetic or pharmacodynamic parameter.[19] As a result, elderly patients may occasionally have a slower emergence from anaesthesia than expected but the decrease of the effect site and plasma concentrations of remifentanil remains always faster than the decrease of fentanyl, alfentanil and sufentanil concentrations. For the daily clinical practice of cardiac anaesthesia using remifentanil, infusion rates between 0.05 and 0.5 µg/kg/min are generally prescribed. Infusion rates of remifentanil greater than 1 µg/kg/min do not improve peroperative haemodynamic stability and are not recommended.[20] To avoid accumulation of large doses of remifentanil in the dead space of the infusion line, the authors recommend a remifentanil solution of 20 µg/ml. At this dilution, 0.5 µg/kg/min corresponds to the weight of the patient multiplied by 1.5. That means that for a patient weighing 70 kg, 0.5 µg/kg/min is equal to 105 ml/h and 0.1 µg/kg/min to 21 ml/h.

Table 2. Clearance and T½ Keo of remifentanil according to age.

	20 year	50 year	80 year
Clearance (L/min)	2.9	2.4	2.0
T½ k_{e0} (min)	0.94	1.32	2.2

   Figure 1 compares the plasma and effect site concentrations of remifentanil generated by the same infusion scheme of 0.5 µg/kg/min during 5 minutes followed by 0.25 µg/kg/min either in a young patient (age 24 year, weight 65 kg, height 180 cm) or in an elderly obese patient (age 76 year, weight 110 kg, height 160 cm). The pharmacokinetic simulation of this infusion scheme yields a peak plasma concentration of 7.5 ng/ml and a plateau concentration of 6 ng/ml in the young patient. In the elderly obese patient, this same infusion regimen is associated with a peak plasma concentration of 20 ng/ml and a plateau level of 14 ng/ml. Consequently, in the daily clinical practice, a manual infusion regimen of remifentanil must be adjusted to the age and habitus of the patient as well as to be titrated to the intensity of the surgical stimulus.

   Remifentanil in common with other opioid drugs reduces the hypnotic requirements for loss of consciousness[21] but remifentanil cannot be used as the sole anaesthetic agent to induce cardiac anaesthesia.[20] For this reason, the analgesic and hypnotic titration must be progressive and independent.

   Figure 2 suggests different remifentanil infusion regimens according to age and ASA status. In a young healthy patient, a loading bolus of 1 µg/kg followed by 0.25 µg/kg/min rapidly generates a concentration of 5 ng/ml in the effect site. In a 50 year old patient a loading infusion rate of 0.5 µg/kg/min administered over a period of 2 minutes followed by 0.2 µg/kg/min generates and maintains the same level of 5 ng/ml of remifentanil effect site concentration. In an 80-year-old patient, an infusion rate of 0.25 µg/kg/min during 2 minutes followed by 0.1 µg/kg/min achieves a progressively increasing remifentanil effect site concentration up to 4 ng/ml. These proposed remifentanil administration schemes must always be combined with an appropriate dose of the hypnotic component. If remifentanil and propofol are administered by target controlled infusion, 1.5-2.5 µg/ml propofol and 6-12 ng/ml remifentanil without epidural anaesthesia and about 4-6 ng/ml remifentanil with epidural anaesthesia are recommended.

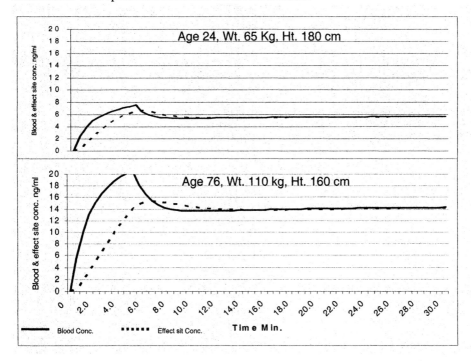

Figure 1. Comparison of the blood and effect site concentrations of remifentanil generated by the same infusion scheme of 0.5 µg/kg/min for 5 minutes followed by 0.25 µg/kg/min in a young patient (age 24 years, weight 65 kg, height 180 cm) or in an elderly (age 76 years, weight 110 kg, height 160 cm).

Figure 3 shows an example of a variable profile of remifentanil target concentrations during the successive steps of routine cardiac surgery. A stable propofol target concentration will help to prevent any episode of implicit or explicit memories. The analgesic and hypnotic regimens must also be adapted to the premedication, the measurement of EEG parameters such as the BIS, movements and the autonomic signs. In contrast, haemodynamics do not reliably reflect depth of anaesthesia in cardiac patients because the adjuvant drugs such as the β-blockers can attenuate the haemodynamic responses and they can be unreliable when myocardial function is poor.

In summary, 0.05 to 0.5 µg/kg/min is the most common range of remifentanil infusion used during cardiac anaesthesia. The remifentanil infusion regimen must be adapted to the age and the cardiac function of the patient and titrated to the intensity of the surgical stimulation with appropriate adjustments for concomitant techniques such as locoregional analgesia.

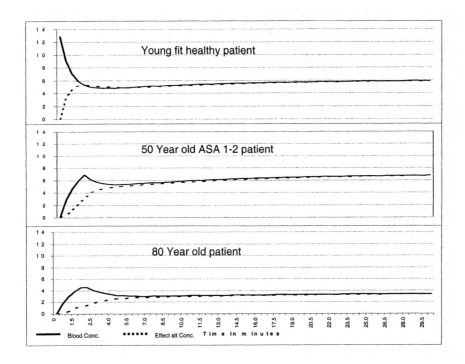

Figure 2. Suggested remifentanil infusion regimens tailored to the age of the patient. Top graph a young healthy patient, a loading bolus of 1 µg/kg followed by 0.25 µg/kg/min rapidly generates a concentration of 5 ng/ml in the effect site. In a 50 year old patient a loading infusion rate of 0.5 µg/kg/min administered over a period of 2 minutes followed by 0.2 µg/kg/min generates and maintains the same level of 5 ng/ml of remifentanil effect site concentration (middle graph). In a 80 year old patient, an infusion rate of 0.25 µg/kg/min for 2 minutes followed by 0.1 µg/kg/min results in a progressively increasing remifentanil effect site concentration rising to around 4 ng/ml (bottom graph).

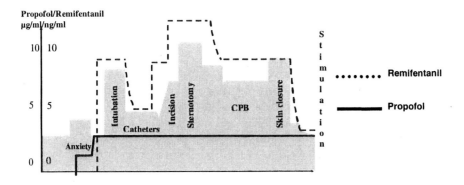

Figure 3. Variable profile of remifentanil target concentrations during the successive steps of routine cardiac surgery associated with a stable propofol target concentration.

6. THE TRANSITION TO POSTOPERATIVE ANALGESIA

Apitzsch et al. studied 52 patients with coronary artery disease or with risk factors for coronary heart disease scheduled for elective extraperitoneal and extrathoracic operation. A balanced anaesthetic technique with high dose remifentanil was associated with a more pronounced sympatho-adrenergic stimulation in the recovery period compared to alfentanil.[22] The incidence of shivering and requirements for analgesics and cardiac medications were higher in the remifentanil group because of the more rapid clearance of the analgesic effect requiring more analgesics and medications for the control of the haemodynamic parameters. Because of these specific pharmacological effects, the abrupt cessation of remifentanil without an alternative analgesic regimen in place will be associated with marked postoperative pain. This may be particularly critical for cardiac patients (Figure 4).

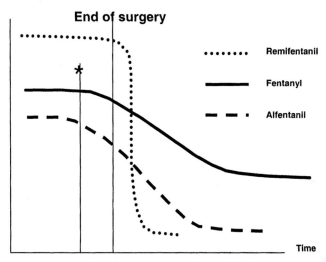

Figure 4. Comparison of the decrease of plasma concentrations of remifentanil, alfentanil and fentanyl at the end of surgery. The abrupt decline of remifentanil requires an anticipated loading dose of a long acting analgesic drug before the end of surgery or a locoregional analgesic technique.

Studies in experimental animals have demonstrated a rapidly developing acute tolerance to the analgesic effect of opioids administered by continuous infusion. In adult volunteers, tolerance to analgesia during remifentanil infusion exists and develops rapidly.[23] Relatively large-dose intraoperative remifentanil has been associated with increased postoperative pain and morphine consumption which has been attributed to acute opioid tolerance.[24]

The transition from remifentanil intraoperative anaesthesia to postoperative analgesia must be planned carefully due to the short duration of action of remifentanil. Continuous remifentanil infusion at a low infusion rate started at 0.05 μg.kg^{-1}.min^{-1} in the immediate postextubation period has been demonstrated to provide safe and effective postoperative analgesia.[25] In this multicenter, double-blind, double-dummy study including 150 patients who had received open-label remifentanil and propofol for intraoperative anaesthesia, postoperative remifentanil infusion provided more effective postoperative analgesia than did intraoperative treatment with morphine (0.15 mg/kg) followed by morphine boluses of 2 mg. However, the effects of remifentanil dissipated rapidly after ending the infusion, and alternate analgesia was required. Median recovery times from the end of surgery were similar in the groups receiving either a remifentanil infusion or morphine boluses. Transient respiratory depression, apnoea, or both were the most frequent adverse events (14% for the remifentanil group vs. 6% for the morphine group).

The use of an infusion of remifentanil to provide postoperative analgesia during recovery from total intravenous anaesthesia with remifentanil and propofol after major surgery was also evaluated in 157 patients from seven medical centers.[26] Remifentanil was titrated in an attempt to limit pain scores to 0 or 1 on a 0-3 scale. At the end of the 30-min titration period, 78% of infusion rates were in the range of 0.05 to 0.15 μg.kg^{-1}.min^{-1}. Respiratory adverse events (oxygen saturation by pulse oximetry [Spo2] < 90% or respiratory rate < 12) affected 29% of patients. Apnoea occurred in 11 patients (7 %). There was a large variation in the incidence of respiratory depression between the centres, ranging from 0 to 75%. The explanation for the large variability in respiratory outcome was not evident.[26]

In summary, at the end of surgery, remifentanil could be continued but only under constant supervision in a recovery or ICU unit. An abrupt cessation of remifentanil infusion is often associated with pain and sympathetic responses. The recommended infusion rate to treat postoperative pain is around 0.05 μg.kg^{-1}.min^{-1}. This infusion rate must be adapted according to the age of the patient, the type of surgery and the peroperative opioid requirements. A one-way valve with a small dead space is mandatory. The co-administration of minor analgesics such as paracetamol, and none steroidal anti-inflammatory drugs can be helpful. The infusion rate of remifentanil has to be progressively decreased and boluses of morphine titrated according to the patient's demand. A loading dose of a long acting opioid is generally given at the end of surgery. If a rapid recovery or fast track extubation is programmed, the morphine loading dose has to be low and analgesia can be titrated by using a low rate remifentanil infusion. In contrast, if fast track is not scheduled a larger loading dose can be given to provide profound analgesia but this may result in prolonged extubation times.

7. REMIFENTANIL AND LOCOREGIONAL TECHNIQUES

The use of central regional anaesthesia alone or in combination with general anaesthesia has much to recommend it. Not only do patients benefit from a superior quality of analgesia, there is also a proven reduction in thromboembolic events in certain types of surgery. There is also the suggestion that blocking sympathetic reflexes to intense surgical stimulus may be beneficial. The later may be particularly appropriate for patients undergoing cardiac surgery. Unfortunately these potential benefits have largely been denied to this surgical population due to the fear of epidural haematoma in patients undergoing full heparinisation. This is particularly problematic if the patient is kept intubated and ventilated for a prolonged period postoperatively, making neurological assessment difficult. However, recently this debate has been re-opened by the publication of a number of randomised controlled trials suggesting that the advantages of thoracic epidural anaesthesia may outweigh these theoretical objections.

7.1 Benefits of Regional Anaesthesia

Post operative myocardial ischaemia as diagnosed by electrocardiography and or transoesophageal echocardiography occurs in 25-38% of cardiac surgical cases, and is related to outcome.[27,28] Such ischaemia is most commonly observed in the immediate postoperative period, thus any treatment designed to reduce its incidence must be continued postoperatively. Regional anaesthetic techniques may serve to reduce myocardial ischaemia by a number of mechanisms. Firstly, aggressive control of postoperative analgesia may beneficially affect outcome, this can be achieved with high dose long acting intravenous opioids.[29] However, such regimens necessarily increase extubation times and are not compatible with fast tracking techniques. Regional anaesthesia can be helpful in this respect. The use of remifentanil combined with intrathecal (IT) morphine as an alternative to sufentanil during desflurane anaesthesia with respect to postoperative pain control was evaluated in another cardiac fast-track study.[30] Prior to entering the operating room, patients in the remifentanil group (n = 20) received morphine, 8 μg/kg IT. Anaesthesia was induced using a standardized anaesthetic technique in all patients. In the remifentanil group, anaesthesia was maintained with 0.1 μg.kg^{-1}.min^{-1} remifentanil in combination with desflurane 3-10%. In the sufentanil group (n = 20), patients received 0.3 μg.kg^{-1}.h^{-1} sufentanil and desflurane 3-10%. There were no differences between the two groups with respect to time from arrival in the intensive care unit to tracheal extubation. After extubation, patients in the remifentanil group had significantly lower visual analogue pain scores, reduced patient-controlled analgesic requirements, and greater satisfaction with their perioperative pain management, compared with patients in the sufentanil group. The authors concluded that as part of a cardiac fast-tracking program involving desflurane anaesthesia, the use of intrathecal morphine in combination with a remifentanil infusion provided improved postoperative pain control, compared with IV sufentanil alone. On the contrary, in a comparable prospective, randomised, non blinded study design, the use of remifentanil in combination with intrathecal morphine did not facilitate earlier tracheal extubation or improve intraoperative haemodynamic stability compared with sufentanil alone for fast-track cardiac anaesthesia.[31]

A number of authors have shown improved postoperative analgesia and early extubation times with both intrathecal[30] and thoracic epidural anaesthesia (TEA).[32,33] The implementation of an ultra-fast-track anaesthetic technique conducted with propofol, remifentanil, vecuronium, and thoracic epidural analgesia compared to thiopental, fentanyl, pancuronium, and isoflurane in the control group and using an active temperature control, provided adequate haemodynamic control and facilitated operating room extubation in all patients. No difference was found in ICU and hospital length of stay.[34]

An uninhibited stress response perioperatively in cardiac surgery patients may be detrimental; adverse haemodynamic changes like tachycardia, hypertension and vasoconstriction will further increase myocardial ischaemia. Whilst metabolic, immunologic and haemostatic consequences of the stress response may further compromise the situation. Again, regional anaesthesia has the potential to attenuate such responses. TEA using local anaesthetics has been shown to significantly attenuate the stress response in cardiac surgery patients.[35-37]

A third benefit from regional anaesthesia is an effective cardiac sympathectomy. The myocardium is supplied by sympathetic nerves from T1-T5, activity in these nerves results in coronary artery vasoconstriction.[38] Blocking this nerve supply has the potential to increase coronary blood flow. TEA with local anaesthetics can effectively block the cardiac sympathetic nerve supply.[39] TEA has also been shown to be effective in the management of angina,[40] improves left ventricular function[41] and improves collateral blood flow during myocardial ischaemia.[42]

7.2 Problems associated with regional anaesthesia

Many of the above potential benefits can be achieved with both intrathecal (IT) or epidural anaesthesia. However, whilst IT opioid can be effective in achieving dense postoperative analgesia such techniques can be associated with over-sedation and respiratory depression.[43] Furthermore, to produce effective stress response attenuation and cardiac sympathectomy, requires the use of local anaesthetic drugs. To produce these effects via the intrathecal route may produce profound hypotension which is unacceptable in cardiac surgery patients.[44,45,36] The use of opioids in both the intrathecal and epidural route can be associated with pruritus, nausea, urinary retention and respiratory depression. The risk appears higher with the intrathecal route. Further, other supplements to TEA with local anaesthetics may be employed without the risk of sedation or respiratory depression. Scott et al have described the use of low dose clonidine supplementation to good effect in cardiac surgery patients.[46]

The biggest barrier to the use of regional techniques in cardiac anaesthesia is the potential risk of thoracic epidural haematoma (THE) formation. The risk of this life threatening complication is difficult to assess. The estimated incidence after epidural anaesthesia is around 1:150,000.[47] THE can occur spontaneously without epidural instrumentation but most occur either during epidural catheter placement or removal in anti-coagulated patients.[47,48] The risk is increased with traumatic placement therefore experience of the clinician may be of major importance. Many strategies are described to reduce the incidence of this complication; certainly normal coagulation status should be confirmed preoperatively. Many authors insert catheters well in advance of proposed surgery and full heparinisation is usually delayed for at least 1 hour post-insertion. It seems prudent to delay surgery for at least several hours and perhaps as much as 24 hrs following a "bloody tap". The true risk of THE is difficult to assess but every centre using this technique must have an appropriate method in place for detecting and treating THE. First, all patients must be assessed neurologically within the first few hours post-operatively, thus a suitable general anaesthetic technique must be used to allow such assessment. Even in patients unsuitable for extubation, because of pulmonary problems or bleeding, this regimen facilitates rapid titration of sedation, to allow gross neurological assessment of limb movement at regular intervals and thus exclude significant THE. If there is any doubt about the neurological status of these patients urgent MRI of the thoracic spine is required, and ultimately availability of a neurosurgical team to perform spinal decompression within 12 hrs, should this be required.

Currently there is insufficient data to make clear the clinical benefits of TEA. Many studies are poorly controlled or have insufficient numbers to show a benefit in clinical outcome. Scott et al. have reported a randomised prospective study of 420 patients having coronary artery bypass surgery.[46] There were significantly fewer episodes of supraventricular arrhythmias, respiratory tract infections, confusion, and renal failure in the TEA group compared to controls. In this study there was no significant difference in mortality, however, it may be that the observed reduced complication rates may translate into a reduced mortality if larger numbers had been studied. Also extubation times were shorter in the TEA group a finding confirmed by many authors this field.

In summary, it appears clear that regional anaesthesia in cardiac patients has many attractions such as better analgesia and faster extubation times. Evidence is starting to build suggesting that these advantages may also lead to improved outcome. However, more data from larger studies are required to demonstrate that these advantages outweigh the potential complications associated with the technique.

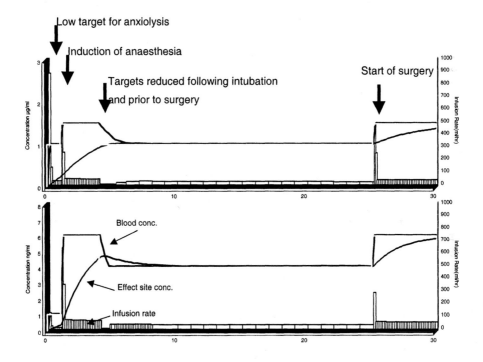

Figure 5. Calculated blood and effect site concentrations of propofol (upper panel in μg/ml) and remifentanil (lower panel in ng/ml) for induction of anaesthesia and initial titration up to start of surgery in a patient with thoracic epidural blockade with 10 ml 0.5% levobupivacaine.

8. CONCLUSIONS

Remifentanil with its fast onset and short duration of action is now the most titrable opioid drug. It's use by a variable rate of infusion is a modern and controllable way to rapidly adapt the analgesia level to the events of cardiac surgery. Compared to the classical phenylpiperidine derivatives, its risk of prolonged respiratory depression is reduced. The recommended infusion rates are below 0.5 μg/kg/min with a reduction for the elderly patient.

Theoretically, the ideal cardiac anaesthetic would combine deep anaesthesia and analgesia during surgery with rapid recovery and profound analgesia in the postoperative period. This ideal can now be achieved with the combination of TIVA using rapidly metabolised drugs such as propofol and remifentanil in combination with TEA. At the end of the remifentanil infusion, the remifentanil transition must be smooth and progressive. Postoperative pain therapy must be anticipated either by a long acting morphine derivative or a loco-regional block. Paracetamol, NSAIDs or the new generation of anticox 2 agents can be added to the analgesic protocol. The transition technique after remifentanil analgesia is a major determinant of the rapidity and quality of the recovery and of the postoperative comfort. The use of a one-way valve or a dedicated line is recommended for iv infusion of remifentanil.

In the future, titration of cardiac anaesthesia and sedation can be facilitated by the use of Target Controlled Infusion (TCI). Delayed extubation should only occur as required for surgical bleeding or concurrent disease and complications. Figures 5 and 6 show a typical example from the practice of propofol and remifentanil TCI combined with thoracic epidural blockade for anaesthesia induction (Figure 5) or for the period of transfer to ICU and sedation in the early postoperative phase (Figure 6). When the patient's temperature and other conditions are suitable, sedation can be titrated down to allow extubation in a controlled fashion.

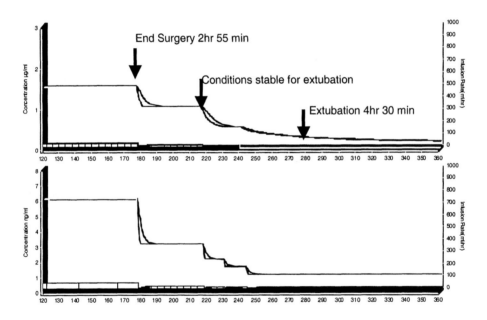

Figure 6. Calculated blood and effect site concentrations of propofol (upper panel in μg/ml) and remifentanil (lower panel in ng/ml) during the transition from end of surgery to postoperative sedation in a patient with thoracic epidural blockade with 10 ml 0.5% levobupivacaine.

9. REFERENCES

1. D.C. Cheng, Karski J, Peniston C, Asokumar B, Raveendran G, Carroll J, Nierenberg H, Roger S, Mickle D, Tong J, Zelovitsky J, David T, Sandler A., Morbidity outcome in early versus conventional tracheal extubation after coronary artery bypass grafting: a prospective randomized controlled trial, *J Thorac Cardiovasc Surg* **112** (3):755-64 (1996).
2. M.B. Howie, Cheng D, Newman MF, Pierce ET, Hogue C, Hillel Z, Bowdle TA, Bukenya D., A randomized double-blinded multicenter comparison of remifentanil versus fentanyl when combined with isoflurane/propofol for early extubation in coronary artery bypass graft surgery, *Anesth Analg* May **92** (5): 1084-93 (2001).
3. T. Mollhoff, Herregods L, Moerman A, Blake D, MacAdams C, Demeyere R, Kirno K, Dybvik T, Shaikh S, Remifentanil Study Group. Comparative efficacy and safety of remifentanil and fentanyl in 'fast track' coronary artery bypass graft surgery: a randomized, double-blind study. *Br J Anaesth* **87** (5): 718-26 (2001).
4. P. Olivier, Sirieix D, Dassier P, D'Attellis N, Baron JF, Continuous infusion of remifentanil and target-controlled infusion of propofol for patients undergoing cardiac surgery: a new approach for scheduled early extubation, *J Cardiothorac Vasc Anesth* **14**: 29-35 (2000).
5. M. Engoren, Luther G, Fenn-Buderer N, A comparison of fentanyl, sufentanil, and remifentanil for fast-track cardiac anesthesia. *Anesth Analg* **93**: 859-64 (2001).
6. P. Reddy, Feret BM, Kulicki L, Donahue S, Quercia RA, Cost analysis of fentanyl and remifentanil in coronary artery bypass graft surgery without cardiopulmonary bypass. *J Clin Pharm Ther* **27**: 127-132 (2002).
7. J.L. Hanouz, Yvon A, Guesne G, Eustratiades C, Babatasi G, Rouet R, Ducouret P, Khayat A, Bricard H, Gerard JL., The in vitro effects of remifentanil, sufentanil, fentanyl, and alfentanil on isolated human right atria. *Anesth Analg* **93**: 543-9 (2001).
8. S. Kazmaier, Hanekop GG, Buhre W, Weyland A, Busch T, Radke OC, Zoelffel R, Sonntag H., Myocardial consequences of remifentanil in patients with coronary artery disease, *Br J Anaesth* **84**: 578-83 (2000).
9. A. Lehmann, Boldt J, Zeitler C, Thaler E, Werling C., Total intravenous anesthesia with remifentanil and propofol for implantation of cardioverter-defibrillators in patients with severely reduced left ventricular function. *J Cardiothorac Vasc Anesth* **13** (1):15-9 (1999).
10. L.G. Michelsen, Holford NH, Lu W, Hoke JF, Hug CC, Bailey JM, The pharmacokinetics of remifentanil in patients undergoing coronary artery bypass grafting with cardiopulmonary bypass, *Anesth Analg* **93**: 1100-5 (2001).
11. D.J. Duthie, Stevens JJ, Doyle AR, Baddoo HH, Gupta SK, Muir KT, Kirkham AJ., Remifentanil and pulmonary extraction during and after cardiac anesthesia, *Anesth Analg* **84**: 740-4 (1997).
12. D. Russell, Royston D, Rees PH, Gupta SK, Kenny GN, Effect of temperature and cardiopulmonary bypass on the pharmacokinetics of remifentanil, *Br J Anaesth* **79**: 456-9 (1997).
13. S.L. Shafer, Varvel JR., Pharmacokinetics, pharmacodynamics and rationale opioid selection. *Anesthesiology* **74**: 53-62 (1991).
14. J.G. Bovill, Warren PJ, Schuller J et al., Comparison of fentanyl, sufentanil and alfentanil anesthesia in patients undergoing valvular heart surgery. *Anesth Analg* **63**: 1081-85 (1984).
15. Th. Stanley, de Lange S, Comparison of sufentanil-O2 and fentanyl-O2 anesthesia for mitral and aortic valvular surgery, *J. Cardiothorac Anesth* **2**: 6-12 (1988).
16. H.M. Mathews, Furness G, Carsonn IW et al., Comparison of sufentanil-O2 and fentanyl-O2 anesthesia for CABG, *Br J Anaesth* **60**: 530-536 (1988).
17. C.C. Hug, Hall RI, Angert KC, Reeder DA, Moldenhauer CC, Alfentanil plasma concentration v. effect relationships in cardiac surgical patients, *Br. J. Anaesth* **61**: 435-440, (1988).
18. M. Alvis, Reves JG, Govier AV, Menkhaus PG, Henling CE, Spain JA, Bradley E., Computer-assisted continuous infusions of fentanyl during cardiac anesthesia: comparison with a manual method. *Anesthesiology* **63**: 41-49, (1985).
19. C.F. Minto, Schnider TW, Egan TD, Youngs E, Lemmens HJ, Gambus PL, Billard V, Hoke JF, Moore KH, Hermann DJ, Muir KT, Mandema JW, Shafer SL., Influence of age and gender on the pharmacokinetics and pharmacodynamics of remifentanil. I. Model development, *Anesthesiology* **86**: 10-23 (1997).
20. D. Royston, Kirkham A, Van Aken H, et al, Remifentanil based total intravenous anesthesia in primary CABG patients : use as a sole induction agent and hemodynamic responses throughout surgery. *Anesthesiology* **85**, 3A, A83 (1996).

21. J. Vuyk, Engbers FH, Burm AGL, Vletter AA, Griever GER, Olofsen E, Bovill JG, Pharmacodynamic interaction between propofol and alfentanil when given for induction of anesthesia. *Anesthesiology* **84**: 288-299 (1996).
22. H. Apitzsch, Olthoff D, Thieme V, Wiegel M, Bohne V, Vetter B., Remifentanil and alfentanil: Sympathetic-adrenergic effect in the first postoperative phase in patients at cardiovascular risk, *Anaesthesist* **48**: 301-9 (1999).
23. H.R. Vinik, Kissin I., Rapid development of tolerance to analgesia during remifentanil infusion in humans, *Anesth Analg* **86**: 1307-11 (1998).
24. B. Guignard, Bossard AE, Coste C, Sessler DI, Lebrault C, Alfonsi P, Fletcher D, Chauvin M, Acute opioid tolerance: intraoperative remifentanil increases postoperative pain and morphine requirement, *Anesthesiology* **93**: 409-17 (2000).
25. J. Yarmush, D'Angelo R, Kirkhart B, O'Leary C, Pitts MC 2nd, Graf G, Sebel P, Watkins WD, Miguel R, Streisand J, Maysick LK, Vujic D.. A comparison of remifentanil and morphine sulfate for acute postoperative analgesia after total intravenous anesthesia with remifentanil and propofol, *Anesthesiology* **87**: 235-43 (1997).
26. T.A. Bowdle, Camporesi EM, Maysick L, Hogue CW Jr, Miguel RV, Pitts M, Streisand JB., A multicenter evaluation of remifentanil for early postoperative analgesia, *Anesth Analg* **83**: 1292-7 (1996).
27. R.C. Smith, Leung JM, Mangano DT. Postoperative myocardial ischemia in patients undergoing coronary artery bypass graft surgery. S.P.I. *Anesthesiology* **74**:464-73 (1991).
28. J.M. Leung, O'Kelly B, Browner WS, et al., Prognostic importance of postbypass regional wall-motion abnormalities in patients undergoing coronary artery bypass graft surgery. *Anesthesiology* **93**: 409-17 (2000).
29. D.T. Mangano, Siliciano D, Hollenberg M, et al., Postoperative myocardial ischemia. Therapeutic trials using intensive analgesia following surgery. *Anesthesiology* **76**:342-53 (1992).
30. E. Zarate, Latham P, White PF, Bossard R, Morse L, Douning LK, Shi C, Chi L., Fast-track cardiac anesthesia: use of remifentanil combined with intrathecal morphine as an alternative to sufentanil during desflurane anesthesia, *Anesth Analg* **91**: 283-7 (2000).
31. P. Latham, Zarate E, White PF, Bossard R, Shi C, Morse LS, Douning LK, Chi L., Fast-track cardiac anesthesia: a comparison of remifentanil plus intrathecal morphine with sufentanil in a desflurane-based anesthetic, *J Cardiothorac Vasc Anesth* **14** : 645-51 (2000).
32. H.M. Loick, Mollhoff T, Erren M et al. Thoracic epidural anesthesia lowers catecholamine and TNFa release after CABG in humans, *Anesth Analg* **86**: S81 (1998).
33. J.R. Shayevitz, Merkel S, O'Kelly SW, Reynolds PI, Gutstein HB, Lumbar epidural morphine infusions for children undergoing cardiac surgery. *J Cardiothorac Vasc Anesth* **10**:217-24 (1996).
34. G.N. Djaiani, Ali M, Heinrich L, Bruce J, Carroll J, Karski J, Cusimano RJ, Cheng DC., Ultra-fast-track anesthetic technique facilitates operating room extubation in patients undergoing off-pump coronary revascularization surgery. *J Cardiothorac Vasc Anesth* **15**: 152-7 (2001).
35. C.M. Moore, Cross MH, Desborough JP, Burrin JM, Macdonald IA, Hall GM, Hormonal effects of thoracic extradural analgesia for cardiac surgery. *Br J Anaest* **75**:387-93 (1995).
36. R. Stenseth, Bjella L, Berg EM, et al, Thoracic epidural analgesia in aortocoronary bypass surgery. II: Effects on the endocrine metabolic response, *Acta Anaesthesiol Scand.* **38**:834-9 (1994).
37. T.H. Liem, Booij LH, Gielen MJ, Hasenbos MA, van Egmond J, Coronary artery bypass grafting using two different anesthetic techniques: Part 3: Adrenergic responses. *J Cardiothorac Vasc Anesth* **6**:162-7 (1992).
38. D.D. Lee, Kimura S, DeQuattro V., Noradrenergic activity and silent ischaemia in hypertensive patients with stable angina: effect of metoprolol. *Lancet* **1**: 403-6 (1989).
39. S. Liu, Carpenter RL, Neal JM, Epidural anesthesia and analgesia. Their role in postoperative outcome. *Anesthesiolog* **82**:1474-506 (1995).
40. D.A. Birkett, Althoep GH, Chamberlain DA, et al, Bilateral upper thoracic sympathectomy in angina pectoris:results in 52 cases. *Br Med J* **2**: 187-90 (1965).
41. M. Kock, Blomberg S, Emanuelsson H, Lomsky M, Stromblad SO, Ricksten SE., Thoracic epidural anesthesia improves global and regional left ventricular function during stress-induced myocardial ischemia in patients with coronary artery disease. *Anesth Analg* **71**: 625-30 (1990).
42. G.A. Klassen, Bramwell RS, Bromage PR, Zborowska-Sluis DT, Effect of acute sympathectomy by epidural anesthesia on the canine coronary circulation. *Anesthesiology* **52**:8-15 (1980).
43. M. Behar, Magora F, Olshwang D, Davidson JT. Epidural morphine in treatment of pain. *Lancet* **1**: (8115): 527-9 (1979).
44. A. Tenling, Joachimsson PO, Tyden H, Wegenius G, Hedenstierna G, Thoracic epidural anesthesia as an adjunct to general anesthesia for cardiac surgery: effects on ventilation-perfusion relationships, *J Cardiothorac Vasc Anesth* **13**: 258-64 (1999).

45. K. Kirno, Friberg P, Grzegorczyk A, Milocco I, Ricksten SE, Lundin S., Thoracic epidural anesthesia during coronary artery bypass surgery: effects on cardiac sympathetic activity, myocardial blood flow and metabolism, and central hemodynamics. *Anesth Analg* **79**: 1075-81 (1994).

46. N.B. Scott, Turfrey DJ, Ray DA, Nzewi O, Sutcliffe NP, Lal AB, Norrie J, Nagels WJ, Ramayya GP. A prospective randomized study of the potential benefits of thoracic epidural anesthesia and analgesia in patients undergoing coronary artery bypass grafting. *Anesth Analg* **93**:528-35 (2001).

47. E.P. Vandermeulen, Van Aken H, Vermylen J. Anticoagulants and spinal-epidural anesthesia. *Anesth Analg* **79**:1165-77 (1994).

48. J.W. Markham, Lynge HN, Stahlman GE. The syndrome on spontaneous spinal epidural hematoma. Report of three cases. *J Neurosurg* **26**: 334-42 (1967).

SECTION 3

EFFECT SITES OF ANALGESIC AND ANAESTHETIC ACTION

THE NMDA RECEPTOR: BEYOND ANAESTHETIC ACTION

Francesc X. Sureda and Jordi Mallol[*]

1. INTRODUCTION

Since 1970, ketamine has been used as an intravenous anaesthetic agent and has found a niche in several anaesthesia and emergency medicine procedures. Although it has been shown to interact with several neurotransmitter receptors, it is well established that its anaesthetic and psychotomimetic effects are related to its ability to block NMDA receptors,[1, 2, 3] a particular type of the family of glutamate-activated receptors. In this review, we shall not only summarize the pharmacological basis of the activation of NMDA receptors, but also explore the role of NMDA receptors in anaesthesia and analgesia, as well as in the excitotoxic process, one of the underlying causes of several neurodegenerative disorders.

2. THE NMDA RECEPTOR

Acting through different types of receptors, glutamate, and possibly aspartate, function as excitatory neurotransmitters in the central nervous system. After a presynaptic stimulus, glutamate is released in high concentrations to the synaptic cleft, binds to its receptors and is then cleared out by very effective selective carriers. In this way, glutamate mediates sensory, noxious and motoneuron stimuli, and has an important role in learning and memory.[4, 5] Four different types of receptors mediate the actions of glutamate: three ionotropic receptors and one family of G-protein coupled receptors, the so-called metabotropic receptors (Figure 1). The ionotropic receptors (channel-forming receptors) are subdivided into three receptor classes that receive their name from their

[*] Unitat de Farmacologia. Departament de Ciències Mèdiques Bàsiques. Facultat de Medicina i Ciències de la Salut. Universitat Rovira i Virgili. c./St. Llorenç 21 43201 Reus (Tarragona) Spain.

Advances in Modelling and Clinical Application of Intravenous Anaesthesia
Edited by Vuyk and Schraag, Kluwer Academic/Plenum Publishers, 2003

selective agonists: AMPA (α-amino-3-hydroxy-5-methyl-4-isoxazolepropionic acid) receptors, kainate receptors and NMDA (N-methyl-D-aspartate) receptors.

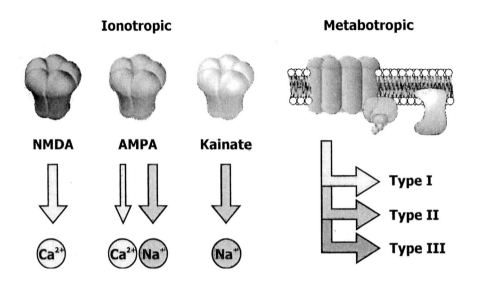

Figure 1. The family of glutamate receptors.

AMPA and kainate receptors trigger rapid excitatory neurotransmission in the CNS by promoting entry of Na^+ (and Ca^{2+} in several areas of the brain). NMDA receptors are associated with a high-conductance Ca^{2+} channel that in resting, non-depolarising conditions is blocked by Mg^{2+} in a voltage-dependent manner. Their activation is secondary to AMPA- or kainate-receptor activation, which depolarises the neuron, and releases the Mg^{2+} blockade. Calcium entry through the NMDA receptor activates a number of Ca^{2+}-dependent enzymes that influence a wide variety of cellular components, such as cytoskeletal proteins or second-messenger synthases. For example, cytoskeletal proteins must be activated if new synapses are to be formed. Moreover, long-term potentiation, a process believed to be responsible for the acquisition of information, is highly dependent on calcium entry, since several calcium-activated enzymes are required if this phenomenon is to occur. In fact, the physiological role of the NMDA receptor is related to synaptic plasticity, including pro-nociceptive sensitization.[6]

However, apart from their physiological action, NMDA receptors play a critical role in the excitotoxic process. Continuous release of glutamate, which leads to excessive activation of glutamatergic receptors, causes neuronal cell death, and it is well known that enhanced activation of glutamate receptors is involved in many neurodegenerative disorders. The toxic effects of glutamate have been known since 1957, when degenerative changes were found in the retina of mice which had been administered monosodium glutamate subcutaneously.[7] However, at that time the role of glutamic acid as an excitatory neurotransmitter was still not clear. It was several years later that John W. Olney described the neurotoxic effects of monosodium glutamate on infant mice.[8] Today, we use the term excitotoxicity to describe the phenomenon that causes neuronal death due to excessive release of glutamate, and which has necrotic or apoptotic features depending of the intensity and duration of the stimulus.

3. THE NMDA RECEPTOR AND ANAESTHETIC ACTION

As stated above, ketamine has been used for more than three decades as an intravenous anaesthetic drug. Although it can bind to several types of receptors, it is now clear that its anaesthetic action is due to its interaction with the calcium-channel associated with the NMDA receptor. As a matter of fact, more specific antagonists at the NMDA receptor share not only the anaesthetic action but also the psychotomimetic effects.[9, 10] Blockers at the NMDA receptor have a dissociative anaesthetic effect that has been described as a functional and electrophysiological dissociation between the limbic system and the thalamus-neocortex. Ketamine acts as a non-competitive blocker, since its binding pocket at the NMDA receptor is in the associated calcium channel, not in the glutamate binding site. In this manner, ketamine only enters the channel while it is in an open state (use-dependent blockade). Other antagonists at the NMDA receptor might show some anaesthetic effect. For instance, the competitive antagonist CPP reduces in a dose-dependent manner the halothane minimum alveolar concentration (MAC) in rats.[11]

4. ANALGESIC EFFECTS THROUGH NMDA RECEPTOR BLOCKADE

After noxious stimulation, glutamate is the major excitatory neurotransmitter released at central terminals of primary afferent nociceptive neurons. In fact, glutamate concentration increases in the ipsilateral spinal dorsal horn after chronic constriction injury of the sciatic nerve, an experimental model of neuropathic pain.[12] Several reports suggest that the NMDA receptor is crucial in nerve injury-induced central sensitisation (for detailed review, see Fisher et al.[13] and Sang [14]), and NMDA antagonists, administered before or after the noxious stimuli, have been shown to have analgesic properties.[15, 16, 17] Ketamine also has analgesic effects at low doses, and some studies claim that it is useful in pre-emptive analgesia[18] and in postoperative pain.[19, 20]

However, the use of ketamine or other NMDA receptor antagonists is restricted because of their psychotomimetic side-effects. In fact, ketamine is used as a substance of abuse. Considerable effort is being made to dissociate the hallucinatory and sedative effects from the analgesic in newly designed drugs. In particular, the antagonists that are selective for the NR2B-containing NMDA receptors (a particular type of NMDA receptor mainly located in pain-related structures) seem to be the most promising (see section 6).[6]

5. THE NMDA RECEPTOR AND EXCITOTOXICITY

As mentioned above, the excessive release of glutamate, or the reduced capacity of glutamate removal, causes a process of neuronal death known as excitotoxicity. In physiological conditions, the presence of the excitatory amino acid in the synapse is regulated by very active ATP-dependent transporters in neurons and glia.[21] Although glutamate can diffuse passively to other areas, there are no other mechanisms (for instance, catabolic enzymes) designed for removing glutamate from the synaptic cleft, so removal is highly dependent on intracellular ATP levels. If ATP levels decrease due to impaired synthesis in the neuron, NMDA or other glutamate receptors may be overactivated. This can happen in two main ways. Firstly, the increased production of free radicals interferes with enzymes in the mitochondrial respiratory chain, which impairs the capacity of the neuron to produce ATP. Secondly, neurons are highly dependent on glucose for ATP production, and when glucose levels decrease due to a reduced blood flow, as occurs during cardiac arrest or stroke, the production of ATP is also hampered.

5.1. Intracellular Events After Excessive NMDA Activation

When NMDA receptors are overactivated, there is an excessive entry of Ca^{2+} that initiates a series of cytoplasmic and nuclear processes that promote neuronal cell death. For instance, Ca^{2+}-activated proteolytic enzymes, such as calpains, can degrade essential proteins. Moreover, Ca^{2+}/calmodulin kinase II (CaM-KII) is activated, and a number of enzymes are phosphorylated, which increases their activity. Transcription factors such as c-fos, c-jun or c-myc are also expressed. Furthermore, Ca^{2+}-dependent endonucleases can degrade DNA. All these mechanisms, together with enhanced oxidative stress, can induce cell death through necrosis as well as apoptosis, a type of programmed cell death. This is what has been called "strong excitotoxicity", a relatively rapid phenomenon evoked by a massive and continuous release of glutamate.

One of the most important consequences of NMDA receptor overactivation is oxidative stress.[22] It is well known that reactive oxygen species (ROS) and "free radicals", are harmful to cells. These highly reactive compounds are able to oxidize a number of essential constituents of cells, such as proteins or membrane phospholipids. In fact, free radicals are the basis of several neurodegenerative diseases. After NMDA receptors have been overactivated, with the resulting increase in intracellular calcium, calcium is stored in the endoplasmic reticulum and mitochondria. Mitochondria have a very important role in regulating the intracellular calcium concentration. An increased entry of Ca^{2+} into the mitochondria is believed to enhance the mitochondrial electron transport, increasing the production of reactive oxygen species such as superoxide anion. Although mitochondria are the main source of free radicals in the excitotoxic process, there are many enzymatic systems that primarily or secondarily increase the presence of these compounds in the CNS after calcium overload. Calcium-dependent enzymes convert xanthine dehydrogenase to xanthine oxidase, leading to the production of superoxide anions and hydrogen peroxide. Moreover, Ca^{2+} activates the enzyme phospholipase A_2. This produces arachidonic acid, which in turn is transformed by cyclooxygenases to increase the formation of superoxide anions. Calcium also activates nitric oxide(NO)-synthase, increasing the amount of NO in the neuron and also in surrounding areas. Nitric oxide has a role as a second messenger, activating guanylylcyclases, but also reacts with superoxide to form the highly toxic compound peroxynitrite. This is a strong oxidizing agent that causes nitration of proteins and oxidation of lipids, proteins and DNA, leading to a form of cell death that has the characteristics of apoptosis. Lipid peroxidation alters the structure of lipidic membranes, and leakage occurs in the cytoplasmic membrane. As well as the loss of ionic gradients, the release of glutamate from presynaptic terminals is enhanced, which exacerbates all these effects, and worsens the situation.

We have already mentioned the role of mitochondria in regulating the intracellular calcium concentration, and their importance in controlling the excessive calcium influx after NMDA receptor overactivation in "strong excitotoxicity". In fact, this increased calcium accumulation is believed to be the cause of greater free radical production. This, of course, can lead to oxidative stress and lead to neuronal death. However, several years ago, it was postulated that mitochondria have an important role in glutamate-mediated apoptosis. Complexes I, III and IV of the mitochondrial respiratory chain pump protons from the mitochondria to the cytoplasm, allowing for a mitochondrial membrane potential. Uptake of increasing amounts of calcium can impair this membrane potential and this opens up a megapore known as the *permeability transition pore* and releases small mitochondrial proteins called Apoptotic Inducing Factors. These proteins, as their name indicates, signal the initiation of apoptosis. This makes it possible to hypothesize that normal activation of glutamate receptors could be lethal in a population of neurons with a bioenergetic defect due to mitochondrial dysfunction. This process has been termed "weak excitotoxicity", and would explain the selective loss of neurons found in some neurodegenerative diseases.

5.2. Glutamate Receptors and Epilepsy

Since 1952 it has been known that applying glutamate to the cortex of animals causes convulsions. The hypothesis that glutamate is involved in the aetiology of epilepsy was strengthened by the fact that in experimental epileptic seizures, there is an enhanced release of glutamate (see Chapman[23] for review). Moreover, histological findings after prolonged *status epilepticus* in humans are very similar to what is observed in experimental models of enhanced glutamate release. Most remarkably, antagonists at the NMDA or other glutamate receptors protect rodents from convulsions. In fact, there are two antiepileptic drugs on the market (felbamate and topiramate) that are claimed to act by inhibiting glutamate receptors and this may be the reason, at least in part, for their anticonvulsant effects.

5.3. Glutamate Receptors and Stroke

In ischaemic stroke and in post-traumatic lesions, the involvement of excitotoxicity is well established.[24] In these particular pathological situations a reduction in the levels of glucose causes a decrease in ATP production and impairs glutamate uptake. Moreover, the membrane potential of presynaptic neurons is lost and efflux of excitatory amino acids occurs, contributing to the excessive activation of post-synaptic glutamate receptors. Again, cerebral lesions after ischaemia are similar to the lesions caused by increased glutamate release and glutamate receptor antagonists are protective in experimental models of ischaemia. In this case, it is believed that there is a process of fast or strong excitotoxicity. Here, both NMDA and AMPA/kainate antagonists could be useful for treating this highly incapacitating disorder.

5.4. Excitotoxicity In Chronic Neurodegenerative Disorders

In pathologies like Parkinson's or Alzheimer's disease, Huntington's chorea or amyotrophic lateral sclerosis (ALS), it has been postulated that weak excitotoxicity plays a role. Although the aetiology of these diseases is not fully understood, glutamate synapses seem to be involved.[25] In Parkinson's disease, dopamine deficiency causes overactivity of the subthalamic nucleus. Neurons that project from the subthalamic nucleus to the globus pallidum and the substantia nigra are glutamatergic, so overactivation of these projections results in enhanced release of glutamate in the target structures. In this case, excitotoxicity may contribute to the progression of the disease. Several findings have confirmed that excitotoxicity has a role in Parkinson's disease.[26] Firstly, NMDA antagonists or glutamate-release inhibitors are protective in animal models of Parkinsonism. Secondly, ablation of the subthalamic nucleus (and decrease of glutamatergic output) is beneficial in these models. And finally, in Parkinson's disease there is a selective defect in complex I of the mitochondrial respiratory chain. This could provide a basis for particular susceptibility to glutamate toxicity, as the weak excitotoxicity hypothesis predicts.

In Alzheimer's disease, the situation may be quite different. It is interesting to note that with advancing age the NMDA receptor system becomes hypoactive, and that chronic administration of NMDA antagonists causes a neurodegeneration in cerebrocortical areas that is similar to histological findings in Alzheimer's disease. Olney and co-workers have hypothesized that hypofunction of NMDA receptors decreases inhibitory systems, in such a way that other excitatory neurotransmitters (acetylcholine or glutamate itself) would be released excessively.[27]

Other neurodegenerative diseases affecting motoneurons have been related to excessive activation of glutamatergic receptors. Lathyrism and Guam disease are caused by oral intake of excitotoxins. They resemble the neurodegenerative disease known as amyotrophic lateral sclerosis, in which several findings indicate that there is a dysfunction in glutamate neurotransmission.[28] On this basis, clinical studies were initiated with the glutamate release inhibitor, riluzole. Nowadays, riluzole is used to treat this severe disease, although its protective effect is quite modest.

Administration of nitropropionic acid in animals is a well-established experimental model of Huntington's disease. It is interesting to note that nitropropionic acid is a mitochondrial excitotoxin, and that the lesions it produces are compatible with a process of weak excitotoxicity, which as mentioned earlier, impairs mitochondrial respiration. Moreover, there is a selective loss of NMDA receptors in the putamen area of patients. Although the relation between the gene of Huntington's disease and excitotoxicity is still being studied, various experimental models indicate that NMDA antagonists may act as neuroprotective drugs. Finally, in HIV-induced neuronal injury, there is also a process of weak excitotoxicity. Chronic inflammation of microglia results in continued release of platelet-activating factor and Tumor Necrosis Factor-α (TNF-α). The platelet-activating factor enhances excitatory neurotransmission because it acts as an NMDA agonist, and TNF-α and arachidonic acid inhibit glutamate uptake by astrocytes. It should be pointed out that NMDA antagonists have been shown to reduce this toxic process. However, due to the chronic nature of the infection, the best therapeutic approach would be to combine NMDA antagonists with chemotherapy, antioxidant therapy and antagonists of inflammatory mediators.[29]

6. THE NMDA RECEPTOR AS A PHARMACOLOGICAL TARGET

Due to the importance of the processes mediated through glutamate receptors, the diseases mentioned and the lack of effective treatment, research in the field of glutamate receptor ligands in recent decades has been extremely active. The NMDA receptor has attracted most of the attention because it is highly permeable to calcium and the possibility to act at different sites of the receptor. In fact, several reports show that ketamine and other NMDA antagonists have neuroprotective effects in different experimental models.[30, 31]

The NMDA receptor brings exceptional opportunities to modulate its activity through the interaction at different binding sites (Figure 2). Some drugs are competitive antagonists, some block the associated channel, and others interact with modulatory sites such as the glycine site or the polyamine site. At high glutamate concentrations, when the channel is more likely to be open, drugs that block the passage of calcium at this level have a theoretical advantage over drugs that compete with glutamate. The channel blocker dizocilpine is able to block glutamate-induced death in neuronal cultures. The effect is robust and is also evident *in vivo*. However, dizocilpine was withdrawn from clinical trials due to vacuolization in neurons and psychotomimetic side effects. This is a common feature of other NMDA antagonists, so tolerability has proved to be the cornerstone in the development of drugs acting at the NMDA receptor. Fortunately, other channel-blocking drugs seem to be better tolerated than dizocilpine. Memantine has been applied clinically for over 15 years to treat dementia and has shown few side effects. For several years its mechanism of action was unknown, but Riederer and colleagues have demonstrated that memantine and other analogues act at the same site as dizocilpine and Mg^{2+}.[32] However, no psychotomimetic effects have been reported. It is accepted that a good NMDA antagonist should block the pathological actions of glutamate through the NMDA receptor but not disturb its physiological function. Although memantine binds to the same site as dizocilpine, its fast offset kinetics mean that the receptor is still permeable to calcium when glutamate is released in high concentrations but transiently.

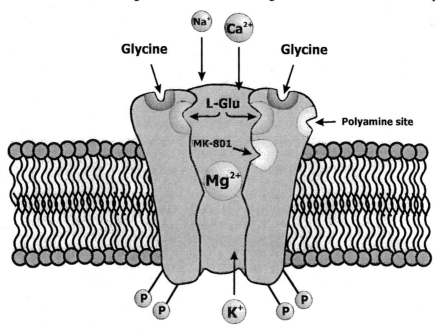

Figure 2. Modulatory sites at the NMDA receptor

However, when glutamate is released at lower concentrations but stays in the synapse for a longer time, memantine is able to act as a blocker at the receptor-associated calcium channel.

Glycine-site or polyamine-site ligands are also claimed to have fewer side effects. This may be partly due to partial agonist capabilities. The ligand for the glycine receptor ACPC (1-amino-cyclopropane carboxilic acid) proved to act as a functional antagonist at the NMDA receptor.[33] In the presence of ACPC, the increase in intracellular calcium is approximately 30% lower. This compound and other glycine-site ligands have proved to be neuroprotective in animal models of ischaemia, and better tolerated than other NMDA antagonists.[34] Although the search for compounds that can act at NMDA receptors continues, other drugs like glutamate-release inhibitors or non-NMDA receptor antagonists are being developed. Probably the best therapeutic approach in ischaemia or other neurodegenerative diseases would be to combine drugs that act at different levels.

Another important issue is the development of new drugs that can act on a particular subtype of NMDA receptor. There are regional differences in the composition of the receptor throughout the central nervous system and the periphery. The NMDA receptor consists of five different subunits that combine to form the channel-forming receptor. Eliprodil and ifenprodil show relative selectivity for NMDA receptors that contain the NR2B subunit. In fact, these ligands have properties that are different from those of non-selective subtype NMDA receptor antagonists.[6] Hopefully, in the coming years we shall see the development of new NMDA receptor ligands which will have different pharmacological profiles, showing a clear separation between analgesic, anaesthetic or neuroprotective actions.

7. CONCLUSIONS

The NMDA receptor brings new therapeutic opportunities other than the anaesthetic and analgesic actions that have been discovered as a result of ketamine development and clinical use. Moreover, antagonists acting at the NMDA receptor may be useful as neuroprotective drugs in disorders where an excitotoxic process exists. Excitotoxicity is a phenomenon that is involved in various acute and chronic neurodegenerative diseases. It may be the cause, as has been shown in ischaemia, or an important contributing factor, as in Parkinson's or Huntington's diseases. New antagonists with better tolerability are still being developed and some promising compounds have been produced. The medical community, however, is still expecting potent, safe neuroprotective drugs to treat diseases that have so far been untreatable.

8. REFERENCES

1. J. G. Bovill, Mechanism of action of anaesthetic drugs. *Minerva Anestesiol.* **65**, 210-214 (1999).
2. L. C. Daniell, The noncompetitive N-methyl-D-aspartate antagonists, MK-801, phencyclidine and ketamine, increase the potency of general anesthetics. *Pharmacol. Biochem. Behav.* **36**, 111-115 (1990).
3. A. C. Lahti, B. Koffel, D. LaPorte and C. A. Tamminga, Subanesthetic doses of ketamine stimulate psychosis in schizophrenia. *Neuropsychopharmacology.* **13**, 9-19 (1995).
4. P. M. Headley and S. Grillner, Excitatory amino acids and sinaptic transmission – the evidence for a physiological function. *Trends Pharmacol. Sci.* **11**, 205-211 (1990).

5. B. S. Meldrum, Glutamate as a neurotransmitter in the brain: review of physiology and pathology. *J. Nutr.* **130**(4S Suppl), 1007S-15S (2000).

6. B. A. Chizh, P. M. Headley and T. M. Tzschentke, NMDA receptor antagonists as analgesics: focus on the NR2B subtype. *Trends Pharmacol. Sci.* **22**(12), 646-642 (2001).

7. D. R. Lucas and J. P. Newhouse. *Amer. Med. Assoc. Arch. Ophtal.*, **58**,193 (1957).

8. J. W. Olney and O. L. Ho, Brain damage in infant mice following oral intake of glutamate, aspartate or cysteine. *Nature.* **227**, 609-611 (1970).

9. W. J. Perkins and D. R. Morrow, Correlation between anesthetic potency and receptor binding constant for noncompetitive N-methyl-D-aspartate receptor antagonists. Anesthesiology **77**(3A), A742 (1992).

10. T. H. Svensson, Dysfunctional brain dopamine systems induced by psychotomimetic NMDA-receptor antagonists and the effects of antipsychotic drugs. *Brain Res. Brain Res. Rev.* **31**(2-3), 320-329 (2000).

11. W. J. Perkins and D. R. Morrow, A dose dependent reduction in halothane M.A.C. in rats with a competitive N-methyl-D-aspartate (NMDA) receptor antagonist. *Anesth. Analg.* **74**, S234 (1992).

12. M. Kawamata and K. Omote, Involvement of increased excitatory amino acids and intracellular Ca^{2+} concentration in the spinal dorsal horn in an animal model of neuropathic pain. *Pain.* **68**, 85-96 (1996).

13. K. Fisher, T. J. Coderre and N. A. Hagen, Targeting the N-methyl-D-aspartate receptor for chronic pain management. Preclinical animal studies, recent clinical experience and future research directions. *J. Pain Symptom Manage.* **20**, 358-373 (2000).

14. C. N. Sang, NMDA-receptor antagonists in neuropathic pain: experimental methods to clinical trials. *J. Pain Symptom Manage.* **19**(1 Suppl), S21-25 (2000).

15. G. Davar, A. Hama, A. Deykin, B. Vos and R. Maciewicz, MK-801 blocks the development of thermal hyperalgesia in a rat model of experimental painful neuropathy. *Brain Res.* **553**, 327-330 (1991).

16. J. Mao, D. D. Price, D. J. Mayer, J. Lu and R. L. Hayes, Intrathecal MK-801 and local nerve anesthesia synergistically reduce nociceptive behaviors in rats with experimental peripheral mononeuropathy. *Brain Res.* **576**, 254-262 (1992).

17. R. Suzuki, E. A. Matthews and A. H. Dickenson, Comparison of the effects of MK-801, ketamine and memantine on responses of spinal dorsal horn neurones in a rat model of mononeuropathy. *Pain.* **91**(1-2):101-109 (2001).

18. M. Tverskoy, Y. Oz, A. Isakson, J. Finger, E. L. Bradley Jr. and I. Kissin, Preemptive effect of fentanyl and ketamine on postoperative pain and wound hyperalgesia. *Anesth. Analg.* **78**, 205-209 (1994).

19. J. O. Dich-Nielsen, L. B. Svendsen and P. Berthelsen, Intramuscular low-dose ketamine versus pethidine for postoperative pain treatment after thoracic surgery. *Acta Anaesthesiol. Scand.* **36**, 583-587 (1992).

20. R. L. Schmid, A. N. Sandler and J. Katz, Use and efficacy of low-dose ketamine in the management of acute postoperative pain: a review of current techniques and outcomes. *Pain.* **82**:111-125 (1999).

21. R. P. Seal and S.G. Amara, Excitatory amino acid transporters: a family in flux. *Annu. Rev. Pharmacol. Toxicol.* **39**, 431-456 (1999).

22. M. Gerlach, H. Desser, M. B. H. Youdim and P. Riederer, New horizons in molecular mechanisms underlying Parkinson's disease and in our understanding of the neuroprotective effects of selegiline. *J. Neural Transm.* **48**(Suppl), 7-21 (1996).

23. A. G. Chapman, Glutamate and epilepsy. *J. Nutr.* **130**(4S Suppl), 1043S-1045S (2000).

24. J. M. Lee, G. J. Zipfel and D. W. Choi, The changing landscape of ischaemic brain injury mechanisms. Nature. **399**(Suppl), A7-A14 (1999)

25. J. Hugon, J. M. Vallat, and M. Dumas, Rôle du glutamate et de l'excitotoxicité dans les maladies neurologiques. *Rev. Neurol. (Paris).* **152**(4), 239-248 (1996).

26. M. C. Rodriguez, J. A. Obeso and C. W. Olanow, Subthalamic nucleus-mediated excitotoxicity in Parkinson's disease: A target for neuroprotection. *Ann. Neurol.* **44**(suppl 1), S175-S188 (1998).

27. J. W. Olney, D.F. Wozniak and N. B. Farber, Excitotoxic neurodegeneration in Alzheimer disease. New hypothesis and new therapeutic strategies. *Arch. Neurol.* **54**, 1234-1240 (1997).

28. P. J. Shaw, Glutamate, excitotoxicity and amyotrophic lateral sclerosis. *J. Neurol.* **244**(Suppl 2), 3-14 (1977).

29. L. G. Epstein and H. A. Gelbard, HIV-1-induced neuronal injury in the developing brain. *J. Leukoc. Biol.* **65**, 453-457 (1999).

30. P. Hans and V. Bonhomme, The cerebral protective effect of anaesthetics. *Curr. Anaesth. Crit. Care.* **11**, 326-330 (2000).

31. M. Proescholdt, A. Heimann and O. Kempski, Neuroprotection of S(+) ketamine isomer in global forebrain ischemia. *Brain Res.* **904**, 245-251 (2001).

32. W. Berger, J. Deckert, J. Hartmann, C. Krotzer, J. Kornhuber, R. Ransmayr, H. Heinsen, H. Beckmann and P. Riederer, Memantine inhibits [^{3}H]MK-801 binding to human hippocampal NMDA receptors. *Neuroreport.* **5**, 1237-1240 (1994).

33. F. X. Sureda, E. Viu, A. Zapata, J. L. Capdevila, A. Camins, E. Escubedo, J. Camarasa, and R. Trullas, Modulation of NMDA-induced cytosolic calcium levels by ACPC in cultured cerebellar granule cells. *Neuroreport.* **7**, 1824-1828 (1996).
34. M. F. Stromberg, J. R. Volpicelli, C. P. O'Brien and S. A. Mackler, The NMDA receptor partial agonist, 1-aminocyclopropanecarboxylic acid (ACPC), reduces ethanol consumption in the rat. *Pharmacol. Biochem. Behav.* **64**, 585-590 (1999).

PHARMACOLOGY AND CLINICAL ACTION OF COX-2 SELECTIVE NSAIDS

James G. Bovill[*]

1. INTRODUCTION

The non-steroidal anti-inflammatory analgesics (NSAIDs) are a heterogeneous group of compounds with analgesic, anti-inflammatory and antipyretic properties. Since the experimental observations of Horton in 1963[1] and the subsequent work of Vane[2], Smith and Willis[3] and Ferreira[4] it has been recognised that the principle mechanism by which the NSAIDs produce their pharmacological effects is inhibition of the enzyme cyclooxygenase. Cyclooxygenase (COX), also known as prostaglandin H2 synthase, catalyses the first two steps in the synthesis of prostaglandins, thromboxane and prostacyclin (collectively known as prostanoids), from arachidonic acid (Figure 1). Prostaglandins are involved in many homeostatic processes and are important mediators of inflammation. COX is a bifunctional enzyme which catalyses both the oxidation of arachidonic acid to the cyclic endoperoxide PGG2 and the peroxidative reduction of PGG2 to PGH2. PGH2 is then converted to a variety of prostaglandins and other compounds by cellular synthetases. Inhibition of cyclooxygenase can explain all of the pharmacological and most of the adverse effects of NSAIDs.

The variability in the inhibitory properties of NSAIDs in different tissues of the body and the apparent discrepancy between the clinical efficacy of some NSAIDs and their inhibitory potency on COX suggested that there might be different forms of the enzyme. For example, changes in prostaglandin production were not always associated with similar changes in prostaglandin synthase mRNA. The issue was resolved in 1991 when two distinct COX enzymes were described, COX-1 and COX-2.[5-7] COX-1 is the constitutive form responsible for the production of prostaglandins involved in cell-cell

[*] Department of Anaesthesiology, Leiden University Medical Centre, P.O. Box 9600, 2300 RC Leiden, The Netherlands.

Advances in Modelling and Clinical Application of Intravenous Anaesthesia
Edited by Vuyk and Schraag, Kluwer Academic/Plenum Publishers, 2003

signalling and cellular "house-keeping" functions such as the regulation of vascular homeostasis and co-ordinating the actions of circulating hormones. COX-2 is induced in cells activated by exposure to mediators of inflammation such as cytokines and endotoxin, and is responsible for the production of prostanoids that mediate inflammation, pain and fever. COX-2 is also constitutively expressed in the kidneys and in parts of the central nervous system (CNS).

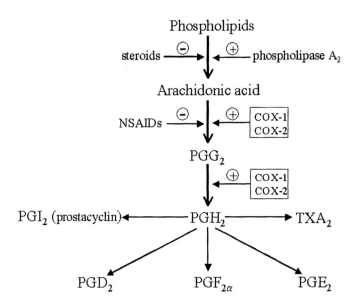

Figure 1. The arachidonic cascade. The sites where NSAIDs inhibit COX-1 and COX-2 are shown.

After peripheral tissue injury or inflammation, the prostaglandins synthesised by COX-2 sensitise peripheral receptors through activation of nociceptors on peripheral nerve terminals. This results in exaggerated pain behaviour, including hyperalgesia (an increased responsiveness to noxious stimuli) and allodynia (pain elicited in response to normally innocuous stimuli). This contributes to heightened sensitivity at the site of tissue damage (primary hyperalgesia) through protein kinase A-mediated phosphorylation of sodium channels in nociceptive terminals.[8] The analgesic effects of NSAIDs have long been thought to be mediated primarily through inhibition of prostaglandins in the periphery, recent evidence suggests that actions in the CNS may also contribute to their analgesic activity.[9] Although CNS levels of COX-2 are normally low, the enzyme is upregulated in the spinal cord by peripheral inflammation, leading to the production of prostaglandin E2 (PGE2). PGE2 may facilitate nociceptive transmission through alteration of dorsal horn neuronal excitability.[10-12] The increase in spinal PGE2 and the hyperalgesia induced by peripheral inflammation are attenuated in animals by intrathecally administered NSAIDs.[13-15]

2. MOLECULAR PHARMACOLOGY OF COX

The COX-1 and COX-2 isoforms are derived from different genes, which in humans are located on chromosomes 9 and 1 respectively. The intron/exon arrangements are identical, except that exons 1 and 2 of COX-1 are condensed into a single exon in COX-2. Both enzymes have about 60-80% of their amino acid sequence in common, depending on the species, but the active site residues are highly conserved and differ only at two locations. The active arachidonic acid binding site for COX is located in the upper half of a long, narrow, hydrophobic channel extending from the outer surface of the membrane, which allows arachidonic acid to gain access to the catalytic sites directly from the membrane (Figure 2).

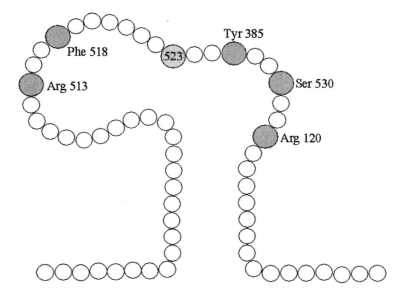

Figure 2. Diagram representing the apex of the COX channel showing the location of the amino acids involved in binding arachidonic acid and in the catalytic process, as well as the side channel involved in COX-2 activity. The amino acid at position 523 is isoleucine in COX-1 and valine in COX-2.

Arachidonic acid, released from damaged membranes, is sucked into the channel, two oxygen atoms are inserted and a free radical extracted, resulting in the five-carbon ring that characterises prostaglandins.[16] In COX-1 NSAIDs block this channel about halfway along. This blocking occurs by hydrogen bonding to the polar arginine at position 120 (Figure 2). It is the nearby amino acid at position 523, however, that is critical for selectivity. In COX-1 the amino acid at position 523 isoleucine while in COX-2 the isoleucine is replaced by valine (smaller by a single methyl group) at this position. The smaller valine molecule in COX-2 leaves a gap in the wall of the channel, giving access to a side-pocket, which is thought to be the binding site for COX-2 selective drugs. The bulkier isoleucine at position 523 in COX-1 is large enough to block access to this side-pocket. The single amino acid substitution of isoleucine for valine allows the COX-1 enzyme to be inhibited by COX-2 selective agents.[17] The apex of the channel contains a tyrosine at position 385, which is thought to be actively involved in oxygenase activity of COX (Figure 2). Serine at position 530 and arginine at position 120 are sites where arachidonic acid binds to the enzyme. Aspirin irreversibly inhibits cyclooxygenase by acetylating Ser 530, which lies just below Tyr 385, preventing arachidonic acid from contacting Tyr 385.[18]

All current selective COX-2 inhibitors lack the carboxylic acid group present in COX-1 inhibitors, but have a specific branched sulphur-containing side chain, either a sulphonamide, sulphonyl or a sulphone group. These rigid side-extensions can access the COX-2 side channel.[16]

While both COX isoforms use the same substrate, arachidonic acid, and form the same products by the same catalytic reaction, they differ markedly in their pathophysiological functions. While COX-1 activity is restricted to arachidonic acid, COX-2 is able to metabolise a wider range of substrates, including many fatty acids. COX-1 is continuously expressed in almost all tissues whereas COX-2 is an inducible enzyme that is almost undetectable in most tissues under physiological conditions. It is constitutively expressed, however, in small amounts in gastric mucosa, in neurones, and in the kidneys. COX-2 is localised to the renal vasculature, the cortical macula densa and the medullary interstitial cells, and appears to be linked to renin production.[19] By contrast COX-1 is found in the vasculature, the collecting ducts and the thin loop of Henle.[20] In several human tissues both isoforms are expressed to a similar extent.[21]

While COX-1 expression may increase by 2-3 fold above baseline during stimulation, that of COX-2 can increase by 20-80 fold when induced by bacterial products such as endotoxin, cytokines (e.g. IL-1 and TNF-α) and growth factors important for the healing process.[22] The induction of COX-2 is characterised by bursts of large quantities of prostaglandin production for relatively short periods. COX-2 expression starts about 1 hour, peaks at 3 hours and subsides at 6 hours.[23] COX-2 induction is suppressed by anti-inflammatory steroids, and by those cytokines that inhibit inflammation.

3. SELECTIVE COX-2 INHIBITORS

There are wide differences in the selectivity of conventional NSAIDs for the two isoforms (Table 1). Some, such as aspirin, indomethacin and ibuprofen are more potent inhibitors of COX-1 than COX-2. Diclofenac, paracetamol and naproxen are equipotent inhibitors of both types. Nimesulide and meloxicam are relatively selective COX-2 inhibitors.[24, 25] The new generation of COX-2-selective drugs, the coxibs, have little or no activity against COX-1.

Selectivity for COX-2 has been measured using a variety of assays, which often give very different values for COX-2:COX-1 selectivity ratios. Biochemical assays using recombinant enzymes give much higher ratios, but these do not necessarily reflect the complexity of drug-enzyme interactions *in vivo*. Whole blood assays have been developed that probably reflect more accurately the true selectivity in patients. These are based on the production of thromboxane B2 during blood clotting (an index of platelet COX-1 activity) and the production of prostaglandin E2 by bacterial lipopolysaccharide (LPS) in whole blood (an index of monocyte COX-2 activity).[26, 27]

Table 1: Concentrations (μM) of various NSAIDs that produce 50% inhibition (IC_{50}) of COX-1 or COX-2 activity in human whole blood assays.

Drug	IC_{50} COX-1	IC_{50} COX-2	COX-2 selectivity	Reference
Celecoxib	6.3	0.96	6.6	41
Celecoxib	6.7	0.87	7.6	57
Celecoxib	1.2	0.83	1.5	88
Rofecoxib	18.8	0.53	35.5	53
Valdecoxib	25.4	0.89	28.5	53
Etoricoxib	116	1.1	105	57
Meloxicam	1.4	0.7	2.0	41
Nimesulide	4.1	0.56	7.3	57
Nimesulide	10	7.9	5.26	88
Diclofenac	0.15	0.05	3.0	41
Ibubrofen	4.8	24.3	0.2	57
Pirocoxam	0.76	9.0	0.08	57

These procedures have shown that rofecoxib and celecoxib have no significant effects on COX-1 activity at recommended therapeutic doses. Celecoxib, however, may inhibit COX-1-mediated TXB2 production when administered in excess of the therapeutic doses.[28]

The first selective COX-2 inhibitors, the coxibs celecoxib, rofecoxib and parecoxib (Figure 3), are available for clinical use. Valdecoxib[29] and etoricoxib[30] are currently undergoing clinical trials. The extremely short time span (about a decade) between the identification of the COX-2 isoform and the development of these drugs is a remarkable achievement.

3.1. Celecoxib

Celecoxib, the first specific COX-2 inhibitor to be approved for clinical use, is about 7-fold more specific for COX-2 than COX-1. It is only available for oral administration. Celecoxib is highly lipophilic with a large volume of distribution (> 400 L). It is metabolised by hepatic cytochrome CYP 2C9 enzymes to inactive metabolites. The oral bioavailability is 22-40 % and the elimination half-life approximately 11 hours. Protein binding is greater than 97%.[26]

In Europe and the USA celecoxib is approved for the treatment of osteoarthritis and rheumatoid arthritis. In the USA it is also approved for the treatment of patients with familial adenomatous polyposis in an attempt to minimise the risk that they will develop colorectal cancer.[31] The results of one study showed a significant reduction in adenoma burden in familial adenomatous polyposis patients who received celecoxib.[32] Although celecoxib has not been associated with upper gastrointestinal symptoms when given in the recommended doses, it has been associated with gastrointestinal bleeding.[33] Although several studies suggest that the coxibs may be well tolerated in patients with aspirin-induced asthma[34-36], allergic reactions to the sulphomamide group in celecoxib have been reported.[36, 37] In a large clinical trial to investigate the gastrointestinal safety of celecoxib (CLASS study), the incidence of skin rash was more than double that of comparable NSAIDs.[38] Thus on the present evidence celecoxib should be considered as contraindicated in patients with a known sulphonamide allergy.

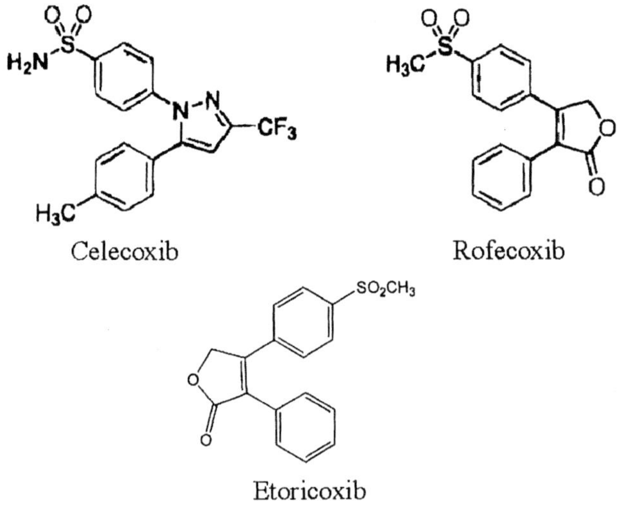

Figure 3. Chemical structures of celecoxib, rofecoxib and etoricoxib

There is limited experience with celecoxib for the treatment of postoperative pain. In patients with moderate to severe pain acute pain after ambulatory orthopaedic surgery single doses of celecoxib 200 mg produced comparable analgesia to hydrocodone 10 mg/paracetamol 1000 mg over 8 hours.[39] Over a 5-day period, oral doses of celecoxib 200 mg taken 3 times a day demonstrated superior analgesia and tolerability compared with hydrocodone 10 mg/paracetamol 1000 mg taken 3 times a day. Most patients required no more than 2 daily doses of celecoxib 200 mg for the control of pain after orthopaedic surgery.[39] Celecoxib 200 mg and rofecoxib 50 mg both decreased patient-controlled analgesia (PCA) morphine use in patients after spinal fusion surgery. Celecoxib resulted in decreased morphine use for the first 8 h after surgery, whereas rofecoxib demonstrated less morphine use throughout the 24-h study period.[40]

3.2. Rofecoxib

Rofecoxib, the second coxib to be approved for clinical use, is a selective COX-2 inhibitor which *in vivo* studies have shown to have no appreciable effect on COX-1 in doses up to 1000 mg per day. In both *in vitro* and *in vivo* studies it has a higher COX-2 selectivity than celecoxib and meloxicam.[41] Like celecoxib, it is only available for oral administration. The oral bioavailability is about 90%, and maximum plasma concentrations are reached within 2-3 hours. Rofecoxib is metabolised in the liver by cytosolic reduction, by flavoprotein reductase, a pathway independent of cytochrome

P450. The elimination half-life is 10-17 hours. Rofecoxib can result in an 8-10% increase in the INR in patients taking warfarin. This may reflect increased plasma concentrations of the biologically less active R(+) warfarin.[42] The small increase in INR at steady state with warfarin co-administered with rofecoxib is not likely to be clinically important in most patients taking warfarin. However, for patients receiving warfarin, standard monitoring of INR values should be conducted when therapy with rofecoxib is initiated or changed, particularly in the first few days. Like other NSAIDs it can reduce the effectiveness of hypertensive therapy.[43] Coadministration of rofecoxib with the cytochrome P-450 enzyme inducer rifampicin has resulted in a 50% decrease in the plasma concentration of rofecoxib, and an increase in the initial dose should be considered in patients taking enzyme inducers.[44]

In controlled clinical trials rofecoxib was more effective than celecoxib, and similar to conventional NSAIDs, in the treatment of osteoarthritis and rheumatoid arthritis. It was also associated with significantly lower incidences of endoscopically confirmed gastroduodenal ulceration and gastrointestinal adverse events than conventional NSAIDs.[44, 45] Rofecoxib has been evaluated for the treatment of pain after orthopaedic surgery[46, 47], spinal fusion surgery[48] and radical prostatectomy.[49] Rofecoxib was more efficacious than celecoxib in patients with pain after spinal fusion surgery, although the dose of celecoxib in this study may have been subtherapeutic. Ehrich et al.[50] compared the analgesic efficacy of rofecoxib to placebo and ibuprofen in 102 patients with dental pain. In the dental pain study, pain relief over the 6 hours after dosing was similar between 50 mg and 500 mg rofecoxib and 400 mg ibuprofen.

3.3. Parecoxib

Parecoxib sodium is a water-soluble pro-drug of valdecoxib (Figure 4), a potent and selective inhibitor of COX-2.[51] It has recently been approved for clinical use in Europe. Parecoxib is the only COX-2 inhibitor available for intravenous or intramuscular administration. In humans and rats parecoxib undergoes rapid and complete amide hydrolysis to valdecoxib.[52] The time to maximum plasma concentrations of valdecoxib are about 0.5 hours after intravenous administration of parecoxib, and about 1.5 hours after intramuscular administration.[51] Valdecoxib, the active metabolite of parecoxib, is 28 000 times more selective for COX-2 than COX-1 in assays using human recombinant COX enzymes.[53] In human ex vivo whole blood assay, the IC_{50} values for LPS-induced PGE_2 production (a function of COX-2 activity) and TBX_2 production (a function of COX-1 activity) were 0.89 ± 0.033 μM and 25.4 ± 1.2 μM, a COX-2 selectivity of 28.5. Valdecoxib is metabolised primarily by hepatic cytochrome P450 enzymes, CYP 2C9 and CYP 3A4.

Both parecoxib and valdecoxib are inhibitors of CYP2C9 [54] and there is therefore a potential for them to interact with other similarly metabolised drugs, such as propofol. Ibrahim et al.[55] demonstrated that parecoxib, in doses to be used perioperatively, does not alter the disposition or the magnitude or time course of clinical effects of propofol. Parecoxib in doses between 20-80 mg intravenously produced effective analgesia when given before oral surgery.[56] There were no significant differences between the 40- and 80-mg doses, suggesting that the analgesic effect of preoperatively administered parecoxib reaches a plateau at 40 mg in this model. Parecoxib, in doses up to 100 mg, has also been evaluated in single-dose and multiple-dose studies for the treatment of acute postoperative pain after a variety of surgical procedures.[51] Parecoxib 40 mg was comparable with keterolac 30 mg in onset, peak effect and duration of analgesia, but with fewer side effects. Parecoxib 40 mg was superior to morphine 4 mg.

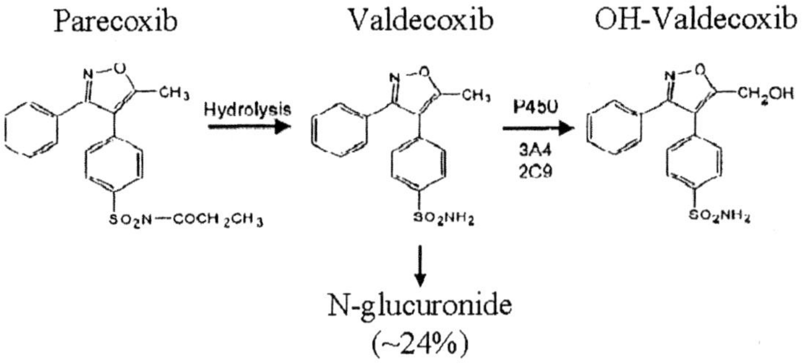

Figure 4. Metabolic pathway for the formation of valdecoxib from the prodrug, parecoxib. Metabolism of valdecoxib occurs via glucuronidation of the sulphonamide group and P 450-mediated hydroxylation of the methyl group to form the minor metabolite (SC-66905), which also has COX-2 inhibitory activity.

3.4. Etoricoxib

Etoricoxib is a potent, rapid-acting second-generation coxib currently undergoing clinical trial. It has the highest COX-2 selectivity of all the coxibs. In the whole blood assay the selectivity ratio for the inhibition of COX-2 was 106, making etoricoxib approximately three times more selective than rofecoxib and valdecoxib, and 15 times more selective than celecoxib.[57]

4. HOW SAFE ARE SELECTIVE COX-2 INHIBITORS?

Selective COX-2 inhibitors have been hailed as "better aspirins" without the side effects associated with conventional NSAIDs.[58] This claim was based on the premise that they do not interfere with COX-1 related physiological functions. Toxicity associated with NSAID therapy is largely due to inhibition of COX-1, whereas therapeutic benefit derives from inhibition of the inducible enzyme, COX-2. Compounds that selectively inhibit COX-2 are analgesic and anti-inflammatory with less of the gastric or renal toxicity normally associated with NSAIDs. There is considerable evidence that selective COX-2 inhibitors cause significantly fewer gastrointestinal complications compared with non-selective NSAIDs.[31] Also, because the only isoform present in platelets is COX-1, selective COX-2 inhibitors should have no effect on haemostasis. However, although the preponderance of evidence suggests that selective inhibition of COX-2 will be largely beneficial, evidence is emerging that inhibiting the physiological functions of prostaglandins may not be as innocuous as previously thought. The idea that here is a clear distinction between the physiological and pathological roles of the two COX isoforms is becoming less tenable and that indeed their activities overlap to a considerable degree.[59] Indeed in some circumstances prostaglandins may be beneficial in the resolution of inflammation and tissue damage.[60-62] Thus, while selective COX-2 inhibitors are efficacious in acute inflammation, they may exacerbate a late phase characterized by the generation of anti-inflammatory prostaglandins by cyclooxygenase.

Recent studies have shown that COX-2 is constitutively expressed in neurones and gastric epithelial cells and may be important in neural transmission and gastric protection. COX-2 in vascular endothelium may also be important in vasoprotection.[63] A recent study suggests that COX-2 may play a crucial role in protecting the gastric mucosa from injury.[64] Prostaglandins play an important role in healing stomach ulcers and COX-2 mRNA is strongly induced in gastric mucosa in the vicinity of an ulcer.[65] In the rat COX-2 inhibition had a negative influence on gastric ulcer healing.[66] Celecoxib and rofecoxib given to rats for 5 days did not produce lesions in healthy gastrointestinal mucosa. In contrast, when administered to rats with damaged gastrointestinal mucosa, they aggravated and complicated gastric ulcers as well as producing necrosis in the small intestine.[67]

It may be that complete inhibition of COX-2 may carry as yet unknown risks in humans. Prostaglandins have an important physiological role in the kidneys, maintaining renal perfusion especially in the face of reduced perfusion pressure or plasma volume. In susceptible patients, NSAIDS can induce disturbances of renal haemodynamics, leading to acute renal failure. Prostaglandins also modulate ADH release and their inhibition can result in salt retention, oedema and a reduction of the antihypertensive effects of diuretics. While the adverse renal effects have largely been attributed to inhibition of COX-1, it is now recognised that COX-2 has a physiological role in renal homeostasis. COX-2 is the only COX isoform that has been detected in the macula densa and its expression is triggered by salt restriction.[68] It may also have a developmental role since COX-2 'knock-out' mice develop a progressive nephropathy as they age.[69, 70] To date there is no firm evidence for adverse renal effects in humans with the presently available COX-2 selective NSAIDs. However, there is as yet only limited experience with these drugs and caution is advised with their use in susceptible patients.[71] NSAIDs, in part due to their actions on renal function, can destabilize blood pressure control in patients treated for hypertension. Patients taking antihypertensive therapy, especially ACE-inhibitors, and receiving cyclooxygenase-2-specific inhibitors should be monitored for the development of cardiorenal events. Patients receiving celecoxib experienced less oedema and less destabilization of blood pressure control compared with those receiving rofecoxib.[72]

COX-2 'knock-out' mice also develop cardiac fibrosis and die early. Females are infertile. Prostaglandins are involved in several stages of pregnancy. Both COX-1 and COX-2 are thought to be important for implantation of the ovum and for the angiogenesis needed for the establishment of the placenta.[73] COX-2 expression increases significantly in the amnion and placenta immediately before the start of labour.[74] and COX-2 derived prostaglandins are thought to be necessary for the initiation of labour.[75]

5. ALTERNATIVE THERAPEUTIC APPLICATIONS

5.1. Cancer

There is overwhelming evidence that COX-2 is involved in the pathogenesis of cancer, particularly colon cancer. Major epidemiological studies have found a negative correlation between chronic use of NSAIDs and the incidence of colorectal cancer, with a 40-50% decrease in the relative risk of cancer in individuals taking chronic NSAIDs.[76-78] The mechanisms responsible for these effects are not completely understood, but it is likely that NSAIDs target several steps in the carcinogenesis pathway. Cox-2, but not

COX-1 expression is upregulated by up to 50% in many human cancers, including colon, breast, prostate and skin.[79] COX-2 selective drugs are thus likely to be more effective in cancer prevention.[80] This may be associated with an increased resistance of the cancer cells to apoptosis, and with the generation of prostaglandins and related compounds that support carcinogenesis. Blocking this overexpression by COX-2 selective NSAIDs might induce apoptosis and tumour regression. NSAIDs also inhibit angiogenesis, which is important for tumour growth and metastasis.[81]

5.2. Alzheimer's disease

This disease is characterised by inflammatory cascades involving local production of pro-inflammatory cytokines, which are potent inducers of COX-2. As with colon cancer, epidemiological studies have shown a reduced prevalence of Alzheimer's disease in patients on long-term NSAID therapy.[82-84] NSAIDs may influence this inflammatory response by inhibiting COX-1 and COX-2 and by activation of the perioxisome proliferator γ (PPARγ) nuclear transcription factor.[85] NSAIDs may also directly affect amyloid pathology in the brain by reducing the levels of the highly amyloidogenic Aβ42 peptide by a mechanism independent of COX activity.[86] Non-selective COX inhibitors, with their risk of gastrointestinal damage and platelet dysfunction, are unlikely to find a role in the preventive therapy of asymptomatic subjects genetically at risk for this disease. Selective COX-2 inhibitors could have a prophylactic role.[87]

6. REFERENCES

1. E.W. Horton, Action of PGE1 on tissues which respond to bradykinin, *Nature* **200**, 982-987 (1963).
2. J.R. Vane, Inhibition of prostaglandin synthesis as a mechanism of action for aspirin-like drug,. *Nat. New Biol.* **231**, 232-235 (1971).
3. Smith J.B, and A.L Willis, Aspirin selectively inhibits prostaglandin production in human platelets, *Nat. New Biol.* **231,** 235-237 (1971).
4. S.H. Ferriera, Prostaglandins, aspirin-like drugs and analgesia, *Nature* **240**,1139-1142 (1972).
5. W.Y.L. Wong, and J.C. Richards, Evidence for two antigenically distinct molecular weight variants of prostaglandin H synthase in the rat ovary, *Mol. Endocrino.l* **5**,1269-1279 (1991).
6. J.Y. Fu, J.L.Masferrer, K. Seibert, A. Raz, and P. Needleman, The induction and suppression of prostaglandin H2 synthase (cyclooxygenase) in human monocytes, *J. Biol. Chem.* **265**, 16737-16740 (1990).
7. J.L. Masferrer, B.S. Zweifel, K. Seibert, and P. Needleman, Selective regulation of cellular cyclooxygenase by dexamethasone and endotoxin in mice, *J. Clin. Inves.t.* **86**, 1375-1379 (1990).
8. E.W. McCleskey, and M.S. Gold, Ion channels of nociception, *Annu. Rev. Physiology* **61**,833-56 (1999).
9. U.S. Muth-Selbach, I. Tegeder, K. Brune, and G.Geisslinger, Acetaminophen inhibits spinal prostaglandin E2 release after peripheral noxious stimulation, *Anesthesiology* **91**, 231-9 (1999).
10. D.M. Dirig, and T.L.Yaksh, In vitro prostanoid release from spinal cord following peripheral inflammation: effects of substance P, NMDA and capsaicin, *Br. J. Pharmacol.* **126**,1333-40 (1999).
11. H. Baba, T. Kohno, K.A. Moore, and C.J.Woolf, Direct activation of rat spinal dorsal horn neurons by prostaglandin E2, *J. Neurosci.* **21**,1750-6 (2001).
12. T.A. Samad, K.A. Moore, Sapirstein A, S. Billet, A. Allchome, S. Poole, J. V.Bonventre, and C. J. Woolf, Interleukin 1β-mediated induction of Cox 2 in the central nervous system contributes to inflammatory pain hypersensitivity, *Nature* **410**, 471-475 (2001).
13. A.B. Malmberg, and T.L. Yaksh, Antinociceptive actions of spinal nonsteroidal anti-inflammatory agents on the formalin test in the rat, *J. Pharmaco.l Exp. Ther.* **263**,136-146 (1992).
14. A.B. Malmberg, and T.L. Yaksh, Cyclooxygenase inhibition and the spinal release of prostaglandin E2 and amino acids evoked by paw formalin injection: a microdialysis study in unanesthetized rats, *J. Neurosci.* **15**,2768-2776 (1995).

15. T. Yamamoto, and N. Nozaki-Taguchi, Role of spinal cyclooxygenase (COX)-2 on thermal hyperalgesia evoked by carageenan injection in the rat, *Neuro. Report* **8**,2179-2182 (1997).
16. C.J. Hawkey, COX-2 inhibitors. *Lancet* **353**, 307-314 (1999).
17. J.K. Gierse, J.J. McDonald, S.D. Hauser, S. H. Rangwala, P. C. Isakson, and K. Seibert, A single amino acid difference between cyclooxygenase-1 (COX-1) and -2 (COX-2) reverses the selectivity of COX-2 specific inhibitors, *J. Biol. Chem.* **271**, 15810-15814 (1996).
18. D. Picot, P.J. Loll, and R.M.Garavito, The X-ray crystal structure of the membrane protein prostaglandin H2 synthase-1, *Nature* **367**, 243-249 (1994).
19. M.C. Kammerl, R.M. Nusing, F. Schweda, D. Endemann, M. Stubanus, F. Kees, K. J. Lackner, M. Fischereder, and B. K. Kramer, Low sodium and furosemide-induced stimulation of the renin system in man is mediated by cyclooxygenase 2, *Clin. Pharmacol. Ther.* **70**, 468-474 (2001).
20. F. Nantel, E. Meadows, D. Denis, B. Conolly, K. M. Metters, and A. Giaid, Immunolocalization of cyclooxygenase-2 in the macula densa of human elderly, *F.E.B.S. Lett.* **457**, 475-477 (1999).
21. G.P. O'Neill, and A.W. Ford-Hutchinson, Expression of mRNA for cyclooxygenase-1 and cyclooxygenase-2 in human tissues, *F.E.B.S. Lett.* **330**,156-160 (1993).
22. J-Y. Jouzeau, B. Terlain, A. Abid, E. Nedelec, and P. Netter, Cyclo-oxygenase isoenzymes. How recent findings affect thinking about nonsteroidal anti-inflammatory drugs, *Drugs* **53**,563-582 (1997).
23. K. K-Y.Wu, Biochemical pharmacology of nonsteroidal anti-inflammatory drugs, *Biochem. Pharmacol.* **55**,543-547 (1998).
24. J.P. Famaey, In vitro and in vivo pharmacological evidence of selective cyclooxygenase-2 inhibition by nimesulide: an overview, *Inflamm. Res.* **46**,437-446 (1997).
25. S. Noble, and J.A. Balfour, Meloxicam. *Drugs* **51**,424-430 (1996).
26. G.A. FitzGerald, and C. Patrono, The coxibs, selective inhibitors of cyclooxygenase-2, *N. Engl. J. Med.* **345**,433-442 (2001).
27. P. Brooks, P. Emery, J.F. Evans, H. Fenner, C. J. Hawkey, C. Patrono, J. Smolen, F. Breedveld, R. Day, M. Dougados, E. W. Ehrich, J. Gijon-Banos, T. K. Kvien, M. H. Van Rijswijk, T. Warner, and H. Zeidler, Interpreting the clinical significance of the differential inhibition of cyclooxygenase-1 and cyclooxygenase-2, *Rheumatology* **38**,779-788 (1999).
28. B.F. McAdam, F. Catella-Lawson, I.A. Mardini, S. Kapoor, J. A. Lawson, and G. A. Fitzgerald, Systemic biosynthesis of prostacyclin by cyclooxygenase (COX)-2: The human pharmacology of a selective inhibitor of COX-2, *Proc. Natl. Acad. Sci. USA.* **96**,272-277 (1999).
29. J.J. Talley, D.L. Brown, J.S. Carter, M. J. Graneto, C. M. Koboldt, J. L. Masferrer, W. E. Perkins, R. S. Rogers A. F. Shaffer, Y.Y. Zhang, B. S. Zweifel, and K. Seibert, 4-[5-Methyl-3-phenylisoxazol-4-yl]-benzenesulfonamide, valdecoxib: a potent and selective inhibitor of COX-2, *J. Med. Chem.* **43**,775-777 (2000).
30. D. Riendeau, M.D. Percival, C. Brideau, S. Charleson, D. Dube, D. Ethier, J. P. Falgueyret, R. W. Friesen, R. Gordon, G. Greig, J. Guay, J. Mancini, M. Ouellet, E. Wong, L. Xu, S. Boyce, D. Visco, Y. Girard, P. Prasit, R. Zamboni, I. W. Rodger, M. Gresser, A. W. Ford-Hutchinson, R. N. Young, and C-C. Chan, Etoricoxib (MK-0663): preclinical profile and comparison with other agents that selectively inhibit cyclooxygenase-2, *J. Pharmacol. Exp. The.r* **296**,558-566 (2001).
31. R.W. McMurray, and K.J. Hardy, COX-2 inhibitors: Today and tomorrow, *Am. J. Med. Sc.i* **323**,181-189 (2002).
32. P.M. Lynch, COX-2 inhibition in clinical cancer prevention, *Oncology (Huntingt)* **15(Suppl 5)**, 21-26 (2001).
33. S. Mohammed, and D.W. Croom, Gastropathy due to celecoxib, a Cox-2 inhibitor, *N. Engl. J. Med.* **340**,2005-2006 (1999).
34. P.V. Dicpinigaitis, Effect of the cyclooxygenase-2 inhibitor celecoxib on bronchial responsiveness and cough reflex sensitivity in asthmatics, *Pulm. Pharmacol. Ther.* **14**, 93-97 (2001).
35. D.D. Stevenson, and R.A. Simon, Lack of cross-reactivity between rofecoxib and aspirin in aspirin-sensitive patients with asthma, *J. Allergy Clin. Immuno.l* **108**,47-51 (2001).
36. R. Patterson, A.E. Bello, and J. Lefkowith, Immunologic tolerability profile of celecoxib, *Clin. Ther.* **21**,2065-2079 (1999).
37. M.V. Galan, S.C. Gordon, and A.L. Silverman, Celecoxib-induced cholestatic hepatitis, *Ann. Intern. Med.* **134**, 254 (2001).
38. F.E. Silverstein, G. Faich, J.L. Goldstein, L. S. Simon, T. Pincus, A. Whelton, R. Makuch, G. Eisen, N. M. Agarwal, W. F. Stenson, A. M. Burr, W. W. Zhao, J. D. Kent, J. B. Lefkowith, K. M. Verburg, and G. S. Geis, Gastrointestinal toxicity with celecoxib vs nonsteroidal anti-inflammatory drugs for osteoarthritis and rheumatoid arthritis: the CLASS study: A randomized controlled trial. Celecoxib Long-term Arthritis Safety Study, *J.A.M.A.* **284**,1247-1255 (2000).

39. J.S. Gimbel, A. Brugger, W. Zhao, K.M. Verburg, and G.S. Geis, Efficacy and tolerability of celecoxib versus hydrocodone/acetaminophen in the treatment of pain after ambulatory orthopedic surgery in adults, *Clin. Ther.* **23**,228-241 (2001).
40. S.S. Reuben, and N.R. Connelly, Postoperative analgesic effects of celecoxib or rofecoxib after spinal fusion surgery, *Anesth. Analg.* **91**,1221-1225 (2000).
41. C.C. Chan, S. Boyce, C. Brideau, S. Charlson, W. Cromlish, D. Ethier, J. Evans, A. W. Ford-Hutchinson, J. Y. Gauthier, R, Gordon, J. Guay, M. Gresser, S. Kargman, B. Kennedy, Y. Leblanc, S. Leger, J. Mancini, G. P. O'Neill, M. Ouillet, M. D. Percival, H. Perrier, D. Riendeau, I. Rodger, R. Zamboni, et al., Rofecoxib [Vioxx, MK-0966 4-(4'-methylsulfonylphenyl)-3-phenyl-2-(5H)-furanone]: a potent and orally active cyclooxygenase-2 inhibitor. Pharmacological and biochemical profiles, *J. Pharmacol. Exp. Ther.* **290**,551-560 (1999).
42. J.I. Schwartz, K.J. Bugianesi, D.L. Ebel, M. De Smet, R. Haesen, P. J. Larson, A. Ko, R. Verbesselt, T. L. Hunt, R. Lins, S. Lens, A. G. Porras, J. Diek, B. Keymeulen, and B. J. Gertz, The effect of rofecoxib on the pharmacodynamics and pharmcokinetics of warfarin, *Clin. Pharmacol. Ther.* **68**,626-636 (2000).
43. A. Whelton, J.G. Fort, J.A. Puma, D. Normandin, A. E. Bello, and K. M. Verburg, Cyclooxygenase-2-specific inhibitors and cardiorenal function: a randomized, controlled trial of celecoxib and rofecoxib in older hypertensive osteoarthritis patients, *Am. J. Ther.* **8**, 85-95 (2001).
44. A.J. Matheson, and D.P.Figgitt, Rofecoxib - A review of its use in the management of osteoarthritis, acute pain and rheumatoid arthritis, *Drugs* 2001 61 , 833-65.
45. L.J. Scott, and H.M. Lamb, Rofecoxib, *Drugs* **58**, 499-505 (1999).
46. A. Reicin, J. Brown, M. Jove, J. R. deAndrade, M. Bourne, D. Krupa, D. Walters, and B. Seidenberg, Efficacy of single-dose and multidose rofecoxib in the treatment of post-orthopedic surgery pain, *Am. J. Orthop.* **30**, 40-8 (2001).
47. S.S. Reuben, H. Maciolek, R.K. Parker, et al., Evaluation of the safety and efficacy of the preoperative administration of rocecoxib for total knee arthroplasty, *Reg. Anesth. Pain Med.* **26 (Suppl)**, 48 (2001).
48. S.S. Reuben, and N.R.Connelly, Postoperative analgesic effects of celecoxib or rofecoxib after spinal fusion surgery, *Anesth. Analg.* **91**,1221-1225 (2000).
49. J.J. Huang, A.Taguchi, H. Hsu, G.L. Andriole Jr, and A. Kurz, Preoperative oral rofecoxib does not decrease postoperative pain or morphine consumption in patients after radical prostatectomy: a prospective, randomized, double-blinded, placebo-controlled trial, *J. Clin. Anesth.* **13**, 94-97 (2001).
50. E.W. Ehrich, A. Dallob, I. De Lepeleire, A. Van Hecken, D. Riendeau, W. Yuan, A. Porras, J. Wittreich, J. R. Seibold, P. De Schepper, D. R. Mehlisch, and B. J. Gertz, Characterization of rofecoxib as a cyclooxygenase-2 isoform inhibitor and demonstration of analgesia in the dental pain model, *Clin. Pharmacol. Ther.* **65**, 336-347 (1999).
51. S.M. Cheer, and K.L. Goa, Parecoxib (parecoxib sodium). *Drugs* **61**,1133-1141 (2001).
52. J.J. Talley, S.R. Bertenshaw, D.L. Brown, J. S. Carter, M. J. Graneto, M. S. Kellogg, C. M. Koboldt, J. Yuan, Y.Y. Zhang, and K. Seibert, N-[[(5-methyl-3-phenylisoxazol-4-yl)-phenyl]sulfonyl]propanamide, sodium salt, parecoxib sodium: A potent and selective inhibitor of COX-2 for parenteral administration, *J. Med. Chem.* **43**, 1661-1663 (2000).
53. J.J. Talley, D.L. Brown, J.S. Carter, M. J. Graneto, C. M. Koboldt, J. L. Masferrer, W. E. Perkins, R. S. Rogers, A. F. Shaffer, Y.Y. Zhang, B. S. Zweifel, and K. Seibert, 4-[5-Methyl-3-phenylisoxazol-4-yl]-benzenesulfonamide, valdecoxib: A Potent and Selective Inhibitor of COX-2, *J. Med. Chem.* **43**, 775-777 (2000).
54. A. Karim, A. Laurent, M.E. Slater, M. E. Kuss, J. Quian, S. L. Crosby-Sessoms, and R. C. Hubbard, A pharmacokinetic study of intramuscular (IM) parecoxib sodium in normal subjects, *J. Clin. Pharmacol.* **41**, 1–9 (2001).
55. A. Ibrahim, S. Park, F. Feldman, A. Karim, and E.D. Kharasch, Effects of parecoxib, a parenteral COX-2–specific inhibitor, on the pharmacokinetics and pharmacodynamics of propofol, *Anesthesiology* **96**,88-95 (2002).
56. P.J. Desjardins, E.H. Grossman, M.E. Kuss, S. Talwalker, S. Dhadda, D. Baum, and R. C. Hubbard, The injectable cyclooxygenase-2-specific inhibitor parecoxib sodium has analgesic efficacy when administered preoperatively, *Anesth. Analg.* **93**, 721-727 (2001).
57. D. Riendeau, M. D. Percival, P.C. Brideau, S. Charleson, D. Dube, D. Ehtier, J. P. Falgueyret, R. W. Friesen, R. Gordon, G. Greig, J. Guay, J. Mancini, M. Ouellet, E. Wong, L. Xu, S. Boyce, D. Visco, Y. Girard, P. Prasit, R. Zamboni, I. W. Rodger, M. Gresser, A. W. Ford-Hutchinson, R. N. Young, and C. C. Chan, Etoricoxib (MK-0663): Preclinical profile and comparison with other agents that selectively inhibit cyclooxygenase-2, *J. Pharmacol. Exp. Ther.* **296**,558-566 (2001).
58. J.Vane, Towards a better aspirin, *Nature* **367**,215-216 (1994).
59. J.L. Wallace, Selective COX-2 inhibitors: is the water becoming muddy? *Trends Pharmacol. Sci.* **20**,4-6 (1999).

60. D.W. Gilroy, P.R. Colville-Nash, D. Willis, J. Chivers, M. J. Paul-Clark, and D. A. Willoghby, Inducible cyclooxygenase may have anti-inflammatory properties, *Nature Med.* **5**,698-701 (1999).

61. H. Mizuno, C. Sakamoto, K. Matsuda, K. Wada, T. Uchida, H. Noguchi, T. Akamatsu, and M. Kasuga, Induction of cyclooxygenase 2 in gastric mucosal lesions and its inhibition by the specific antagonist delays healing in mice, *Gastroenterology* **112**,387-397 (1997).

62. K. Seibert, J. Lefkowith, C. Tripp, P. Iskson, and P. Needleman, COX-2 inhibitors – Is there cause for concern? *Nature Med.* **5**,621-622 (1999).

63. K. K.-Y. Wu, Biochemical pharmacology of nonsteroidal anti-inflammatory drugs, *Biochem. Pharmacol.* **55**,543-547 (1998).

64. B. Gretzer, K. Ehrlich, N. Maricic, N. Lambrecht, M. Respondek, and B. M. Peskar, Selective cyclooxygenase-2 inhibitors and their influence on the protective effect of a mild irritant in the rat stomach, *Br. J. Pharmacol.* **123**,927-935 (1998).

65. H. Mizuno, C. Sakamoto, K. Matsuda, K. Wada, T. Uchida, H. Noguchi, T. Akamatsu, and M. Kasuga, Induction of cyclooxygenase 2 in gastric mucosal lesions and its inhibition by the specific antagonist delays healing in mice, *Gastroenterology* **112**,387-397 (1997).

66. A. Schmassmann, B.M. Peskar, C. Stettler, P. Netzer, T. Stroff, B. Flogerzi, and F. Halter, Effects of inhibition of prostaglandin endoperoxide synthase-2 in chronic gastro-intestinal ulcer models in rats, *Br. J. Pharmacol.* **123**,795-804 (1998).

67. O.M. Laudanno, J.A. Cesolari, J. Esnarriaga, L. Rista, G. Piombo, C. Maglione, L. Aramberry, J. Sambrano, A. Godoy, and A. Rocaspana, Gastrointestinal damage induced by celecoxib and rofecoxib in rats, *Dig. Dis. Sci.* **46**,779-84 (2001)

68. R.C. Harris, J.A. McKanna, Y. Akai, H. R. Jacobson, R. N. Dubois, and M. D. Breyer, Cyclooxygenase-2 is associated with the macula densa of rat kidney and increases with salt restriction, *J. Clin. Invest.* **94**,2504-2510 (1994)

69. S.G. Morham, R. Langenbach, C.D. Loftin, H. F. Tiano, N. Vouloumanos, J. C. Jenette, J. F. Mahler, K. D. Kluckman, A. Ledford, C. A. Lee, et al., Prostaglandin synthase-2 gene disruption causes severe renal pathology in the mouse, *Cell* **83**,473-482 (1995).

70. J.E. Dinchuk, B.D. Car, R.J. Focht, J. J. Johnston, B. D. Jaffee, M. B. Covington, N. R. Contel, V. M. Eng, R. J. Collins, P. M. Czerniak, et al., Renal abnormalities and an altered inflammatory response in mice lacking cyclooxygenase II, *Nature* **378**, 406-409 (1995).

71. D.C. Brater, C. Harris, J.S. Redfern, and B.J. Gertz, Renal effects of COX-2-selective inhibitors, *Am. J. Nephrol.* **21**,1-15 (2001).

72. A. Whelton, J.G. Fort, J.A. Puma, D. Normandin, A.E. Bello, and K.M..Verburg, Cyclooxygenase-2-specific inhibitors and cardiorenal function: a randomized, controlled trial of celecoxib and rofecoxib in older hypertensive osteoarthritis patients, *Am. J. Ther.* **8**,85-95 (2001).

73. I. Chakraborty, S.K. Das, J. Wang, and S.K. Dey, Developmental expression of the cyclo-oxygenase-1 and cyclo-oxygenase-2 genes in the peri-implantation mouse uterus and their differential regulation by the blastocyst and ovarian steroids, *J. Mol. Endocrinol.* **16**,107-122 (1996).

74. A. Fuentes, E.P. Spaziani, and W.F. O'Brien, The expression of cyclooxygenase-2 (COX-2) in amnion and decidua following spontaneous labor, *Prostaglandins* **52**,261-267 (1996).

75. W. Gibb, and M. Sun, Localization of prostaglandin H synthase type 2 protein and mRNA in term human fetal membranes and deciduas, *J. Endocrinol.* **150**,497-503 (1996)

76. E. Giovannucci, K.M. Egan, D.J. Hunter, M. J. Stampfer, G. A. Colditz, W. C. Willett, and F. E. Speizer, Aspirin and the risk of colorectal cancer in women, *N. Engl. J. Med.* **333**, 609-614 (1995).

77. M,J, Thun, NSAID use and decreased risk of gastrointestinal cancers, *Gastroenterol. Clin. North Am.* **25**,333-348 (1996)

78. E. Giovannucci, E.B. Rimm, M.J. Stampfer, G. A. Colditz, A. Ascheiro, and W. C. Willett, Aspirin use and the risk for colorectal cancer and adenoma in male health professionals, *Ann. Intern. Med.* **121**,241-246 (1994).

79. Eberhart CE, Coffey RJ, Radhika A, F. M. Giardiello, S. Ferrenbach, and R. N. DuBois, Up-regulation of cyclooxygenase 2 gene expression in human colorectal adenomas and adenocarcinomas, *Gastroenterology* **107**,1183-1188 (1994).

80. T. Kawamori, and C.V. Rao, Chemopreventive activity of celecoxib, a specific cyclooxygenase-2 inhibitor, against colon carcinogenesis, *Cancer Res.* **58**,409-412 (1998).

81. M.K. Jones, H. Wang, B.M. Peskar, et al., Inhibition of angiogenesis by NSAIDs: Insight into the mechanisms and implications for cancer growth and ulcer healing. *Nature Med.* **5**,1418-1423 (1999).

82. J.C. Breitner. The role of anti-inflammatory drugs in the prevention and treatment of Alzheimer's disease, *Annu. Rev. Med.* **47**,401-411 (1996).

83. W.F. Stewart, C. Kawas, M. Corrada, and E.J. Metter, Risk of Alzheimer's disease and duration of NSAID use, *Neurology* **48**,626-632 (1997).

84. B.A. in't Veld, A. Ruitenberg, A. Hofman, L. J. Launer, C. M. van Duijn, T. Stijnen, M. M. Breteler, and B. H. Stricker, Nonsteroidal antiinflammatory drugs and the risk of Alzheimer's disease, *N. Engl. J. Med.* **345**,1515-1521 (2001).

85. J.M. Lehmann, J.M. Lenhard, B.B. Oliver, G.M. Ringold, and S.A. Kliewer, Perioxisome proliferator-activated receptors alpha and gamma are activated by indomethacin and other non-steroidal anti-inflammatory drugs, *J. Biol. Chem.* **272**,3406-3410 (1997).

86. S. Weggan, J.L. Eriksen, P. Das, S. A. Sagi, R. Wang, C. U. Pietrzik, K. A. Findlay, T. E. Smith, M. P. Murphy, T. Bulter, D. E. Kang, N. Marquez-Sterling, T. E. Golde, and E. H. Koo, A subset of NSAIDs lower amyloidogenic Aβ42 independently of cyclooxygenase activity, *Nature* **414**,212-216 (2001).

87. J. Fricker. NSAIDs may reduce the risk of Alzheimer's disease. *Lancet* **347**,958 (1996).

88. T.D. Warner, F. Giuliano, I. Vojnovic, A. Bukasa, J.A. Mitchell, and J.R. Vane, Nonsteroid drug selectivities for cyclo-oxygenase-1 rather than cyclo-oxygenase-2 are associated with human gastrointestinal toxicity: A full in vitro analysis, *Proc. Natl. Acad. Sci USA* **96,** 7563-7568 (1999).

NEUROMODULATORY ACTIONS OF ENDOCANNABINOIDS IN PAIN AND SEDATION

Luciano De Petrocellis, Tiziana Bisogno, and Vincenzo Di Marzo[*]

1. INTRODUCTION

Endocannabinoids[1] are endogenous substances that bind to and activate at least one of the two high affinity membrane receptors discovered for marijuana's psychoactive principle, (-)-$\square^9$-tetrahydrocannabinol (THC). Three types of endocannabinoids have been described so far in both nervous and non-nervous tissues: 1) the anandamides,[1] i.e. amides of ethanolamine with polyunsaturated fatty acids with at least twenty carbon atoms and three 1,4-diene double bonds, of which the C20: 4 homologue, arachidonoylethanolamide (AEA)[2, 3] has been most thoroughly studied; 2) 2-arachidonoyl glycerol (2-AG)[4,5]; and 3) the recently described 2-arachidonyl glyceryl ether, or noladin ether,[6] whose pharmacological activity as an endocannabinoid has not yet been thoroughly assessed. An entirely saturated AEA congener, palmitoylethanolamide (PEA), was proposed to act as an endocannabinoid at yet-to-be-characterized receptors, but the precise mechanism(s) underlying the THC-like anti-inflammatory and analgesic activity of this compound is(are) still a matter for speculation.[7]

2. METABOLIC PATHWAYS AND MOLECULAR TARGETS

Biochemical mechanisms for the synthesis and inactivation have been described so far for AEA, PEA and 2-AG.[8] Endocannabinoids are not stored in vescicles like other mediators but are produced "on demand". This peculiarity is the result of a biosynthetic mechanism relying on the existence of phospholipid precursors for these compounds, and

[*] *Endocannabinoid Research Group*, Institutes di Biomolecular Chemistry and Cybernetics, Consiglio Nazionale delle Ricerche – Via Campi Flegrei 34, Comprensorio Olivetti, Fabbr. 70, 80078 Pozzuoli (Napoli), Italy

of Ca^{2+}-sensitive phosphodiesterases for the conversion of these precursors into endocannabinoids. The biosynthesis of endocannabinoids is immediately followed by their release, which occurs through the cell membrane according to the gradient of concentration across the membrane, and in a way probably facilitated by a selective membrane transporter (see below). Most importantly, the cell (or mitochondrial) membrane-dependent biosynthetic mechanism of AEA and 2-AG allows them to be produced from both axons and somas in neurons, and hence to activate receptors located either pre- or post-synaptically. In particular, AEA is produced from the hydrolysis of *N*-arachidonoyl-phosphatidylethanolamine (NarPE)[9] catalyzed by a specific phospholipase D-like enzyme, which has been recently partially purified and characterized.[10, 11] The same enzyme also catalyzes the formation of other acylethanolamides, including PEA, from the corresponding *N*-acyl-phosphatidyl-ethanolamines (NAPEs).[12] NarPE and other NAPEs are produced in turn from the *N*-acylation of phosphatidylethanolamine using as acyl donors the fatty acids coming from the *sn*-1 position of most phospholipids. This reaction is catalyzed by a *trans*-acylase, or *N*-acyl-transferase. Both the phospholipase D and, particularly, the *N*-acyl-transferase are Ca^{2+}-sensitive enzymes, which explains why AEA biosynthesis is triggered by Ca^{2+}-ionophores and neuronal membrane depolarization.

The biosynthesis of 2-AG occurs from the hydrolysis of *sn*-2-arachidonate-containing diacylglycerols, catalyzed by a *sn*-1-selective diacylglycerol lipase. The formation of these diacylglycerols relies on different types of phospholipid precursors and occurs via Ca^{2+}-sensitive phospholipases C or $Ca^{2+}(Mg^{2+})$-sensitive phosphatidic acid hydrolase.[13-15]

Once released by stimulated cells, endocannabinoids act primarily at cannabinoid receptors for THC. Although evidence is accumulating for the existence of more than two subtypes of such receptors, the only G-protein-coupled membrane proteins characterized so far that are capable of being activated by AEA and, particularly, 2-AG are the CB_1 and CB_2 cannabinoid receptors.[16] AEA is almost functionally inactive at CB_2 receptors, whereas 2-AG is equi-efficacious at both receptor subtypes. While CB_2 receptors seem to be expressed almost uniquely in immune cells, detectable levels of CB_1 receptors are found not only in central and peripheral (both sensory and autonomic) neuronal cells, but also in a number of other cell types occurring in several organs.[16]

In the brain, CB_1 is densest in areas controlling motor, cognitive, emotional and sensory functions, i.e. the hippocampus, basal ganglia, cerebellum, cortex, thalamus, amygdala and olfactory bulb. However, CB_1 receptors are also found in areas controlling pain, body temperature, sleep-wake cycles and hormone function, such as small nuclei in the brainstem, medulla, and hypothalamus, as well as in the pituitary gland.[17]

Apart from cannabinoid receptors, some membrane cation channels seem to be directly modulated specifically by AEA at sub-micromolar concentrations. In particular, TASK-1 K^+ channels [18] and T-type Ca^{2+} channels [19] are blocked by AEA, whereas vanilloid type 1 receptors (VR1), the sites of action of the pungent component of 'hot' red peppers, capsaicin, are activated by this endocannabinoid.[20,21] In heterologous expression systems the potency of AEA to induce typical VR_1-mediated effects (*e.g.* cation currents, Ca^{2+}-influx and cell depolarization) is 5-20 fold lower than its average potency at CB_1 receptors. However, recent data, reviewed in, [22, 23] indicate that several *in vitro* and *ex vivo* pharmacological actions of AEA are due to activation of native vanilloid receptors, possibly under conditions of inflammation. Interestingly, the effects of AEA on both VR1 receptors and T-type Ca^{2+} channels seem to be exerted by binding to sites on the cytosolic side of these membrane proteins.[19, 24]

Mechanisms for the inactivation of endocannabinoids have been identified.[9,25] When AEA and 2-AG act by binding to sites on the extracellular side, one simple way of inactivating them is by means of their cellular uptake. This is achieved by means of a transporter named "anandamide membrane transporter" (AMT). The AMT has been only partially characterized from many neuronal and non-neuronal cells as a temperature-sensitive, saturable and Na^+-insensitive selective carrier protein for the facilitated transport across the membrane (see [26] for a comprehensive review). Recently it has been shown that the AMT also mediates the cellular uptake of noladin ether in both glioma C6 and basophilic RBL-2H3 cells.[27]

Since this(ese) protein(s) transport(s) endocannabinoids according to the gradient of concentrations across the membrane, the AMT has been suggested to: (i) facilitate also AEA *release* from neurons immediately after AEA biosynthesis, by working in the opposite direction to cellular uptake (28), and (ii) require intracellular metabolism to carry on clearing AEA (and possibly 2-AG) from the extracellular milieu. Indeed, both AEA and 2-AG are subject to intracellular metabolism, mostly through hydrolysis of their amide or ester bond, respectively, which can be catalyzed by the enzyme "fatty acid amide hydrolase" (FAAH).[29, 30] This enzyme is distributed in CNS neurons post-synaptically to CB_1 receptors, in support of its role as an endocannabinoid inactivating enzyme, a role further confirmed by recent studies carried out in FAAH "knockout" mice.[31]

As the biochemical pathways underlying endocannabinoid formation, action and inactivation are being revealed, synthetic tools for the manipulation of endocannabinoid levels and activity, through selective inhibition of either the metabolic enzymes or the molecular targets of AEA and 2-AG, are needed. Selective inhibitors of endocannabinoid, particularly AEA, inactivation, e.g. AMT competitive inhibitors and FAAH reversible and irreversible inhibitors, as well as selective agonists and antagonists for CB_1 and CB_2 receptors are now available.[32] On the other hand, the development of specific inhibitors of endocannabinoid biosynthesis still awaits a serious investment of energies and resources. Of these compounds, those that mimic or strengthen a putative tonic beneficial action on pain and sleep by endocannabinoids, could provide valid therapeutic avenues for novel efficacious analgesic or anesthetic drugs.

3.   NEUROMODULATORY EFFECTS OF ENDOCANNABINOIDS

By being coupled to $G_{i/o}$ proteins, the cannabinoid receptors trigger several intracellular signals in both excitable and non-excitable cells (see [33] for a recent review). Common to both CB_1 and CB_2 receptors is the inhibition of adenylate cyclase and the stimulation of both p38 and ERK1/ERK2 mitogen activated protein kinases. Possibly by acting at phospholipase C or A_2 enzymes, it has also been suggested that CB_1 receptors induce intracellular Ca^{2+} mobilization and eicosanoid formation, respectively. In the CNS, these effects lead to the postsynaptic interference by endocannabinoids on the activity of other neuromodulators as well as to the modulation of neuronal plasticity. But probably more relevant to the proposed role of endocannabinoids as neuromodulators[34, 35] are their effects on K^+ and voltage-dependent Ca^{2+} channels.[33] In fact, since CB_1 receptors appear to be mostly located on presynaptic neurons, their activation with subsequent Gi-mediated inhibition of N-, P- and Q-type channels and/or stimulation of inwardly rectifying K^+

channels would result in neuronal hyperpolarization and, hence, in a reduced probability of neurotransmitter release into the synapse.

The intracellular effects induced by presynaptic CB_1 receptor stimulation underlie in most cases the inhibitory effect on either glutamate or GABA release observed in either CNS or peripheral neurons, or in nervous tissue slices, after treatment with CB_1 agonists, including in many instances, AEA and 2-AG.[34,35] CB_1-mediated inhibition of glutamatergic transmission has been found in rat cerebellar slices,[36] substantia nigra pars reticulata,[37] and substantia gelatinosa neurons of the spinal cord,[38] in mouse nucleus accumbens[39] in slices of the rat periaqueductal gray[40] and in rat prefrontal cortex pyramidal neurons.[41]

By contrast, *in vivo* microdialysis in rat prefrontal cortex revealed that *i.p.* injection of WIN55.212-2 led to a release of glutamate, which was counteracted by SR141716A.[42] On the other hand, the inhibition of glutamate, but not GABA, release from mouse hippocampal neurons was recently suggested to be due to a non-CB_1 receptor.[43] Inhibition of GABA release has been observed in rat substantia nigra pars reticulata neurons (44), hippocampal inter-neurons,[45,46] rostral ventromedial medulla neurons (47), and superficial medullary dorsal horn neurons.[48] Interestingly, however, CB_1 receptor agonists have also been shown to enhance GABAergic signalling by inhibiting GABA reuptake in the globus pallidus.[49,50] Finally, both synthetic cannabinoids and endocannabinoids have been shown to inhibit the release of other neurotransmitters, namely acetylcholine and noradrenaline, in CNS and peripheral neurons (see [34, 35] for reviews).

The CB_1-mediated inhibition of glutamate and GABA release has been recently correlated with the capability of endocannabinoids to act as fundamental retrograde mediators of depolarization-induced inhibition of excitatory (DSE) or inhibitory (DSI) postsynaptic currents, respectively, in cerebellar Purkinje cells and/or hippocampal CA1 pyramidal neurons.[51-56] It was shown that blockade[51-54] or genetic deletion[55,56] of CB_1 receptors prevent the observation of DSE and DSI, whereas treatment with CB_1 agonists occludes these two phenomena.

Furthermore, in one case[51] it was found that inhibition of endocannabinoid cellular uptake leads to an enhancement of DSE. These findings prompted that the endocannabinoids are synthesized by the soma of the post-synaptic neuron following depolarization and Ca^{2+} influx, and act backwards on the pre-synaptic neuron to inhibit the release of either glutamate or GABA, thus leading to DSE or DSI, respectively.

In a more recent article it was also suggested that endocannabinoids acting as retrograde effectors of DSE are produced independently from Ca^{2+} influx and following metabotropic glutamate receptor stimulation.[56] However, no direct data exist as yet on the production of endocannabinoids during DSE or DSI, and on the nature of endocannabinoid involved in this phenomenon.

4. ENDOCANNABINOIDS AND PAIN

Extensive studies[57,58] have been carried out suggesting the involvement of endocannabinoids and CB_1 receptors in the control of nociception and, in particular, chronic and inflammatory pain. CB_1 receptor knockout mice do not seem to show consistently altered nociception, thus arguing against a possible tonic action of the endocannabinoid system in the control of pain perception.[59, 60] On the other hand, FAAH knockout mice do exhibit lower sensitivity to nociception as compared to wild type mice, thus indicating that enhanced endocannabinoid levels in those nervous areas involved in the control of pain can lead to analgesia.[31] Electrical stimulation of the periaqueductal grey (PAG) induces CB_1-mediated analgesia concomitantly to the release of AEA in microdialysates from this region of the brainstem.[61] Also the injection of formalin into the paw induced a nociceptive response concomitantly to the release of AEA from the PAG, thus establishing a correlation between nociception and supra-spinal endocannabinoid release.[61] Furthermore, an earlier investigation had suggested that an endocannabinoid tone may down-modulate pain perception via CB_1 receptors in another nucleus of the medulla/brainstem, the rostral ventromedial medulla, through the same neural circuit known to participate in the pain-suppressing effects of morphine.[62]

The existence of an endocannabinoid tone down-modulating the nociceptive response also at the spinal level was proposed on the basis of the observation that blockade of the action or expression of spinal CB_1 receptors by the selective antagonist, SR141716A, or a CB_1 receptor anti-sense oligonucleotide, respectively, leads to glutamate-mediated hyperalgesia.[63] The neurochemical substrate for the analgesic effects of endocannabinoids at the spinal and supra-spinal level is provided by the recent findings that CB_1 receptor stimulation inhibits glutamate release from both the substantia gelatinosa neurons of the spinal cord [38] and slices of the periaqueductal gray.[40] Finally, indirect evidence for the presence of CB_1 receptors in peripheral sensory afferents in the skin, and for their involvement in the control of inflammatory pain, was also gained.[64] It was proposed[65] that tonic activation of these as well as CB_2 receptors[2,3] by endocannabinoids control pain at the peripheral level based on the observation that, in the formalin test carried out in mice, local administration of either CB_1 or CB_2 receptor antagonists leads to hyperalgesia,[65] whereas exogenous AEA and PEA [65] or a selective CB_2 receptor agonist [66] block the painful response. However, no difference in the amounts of AEA, PEA and 2-AG in the hind paw of rats can be found between vehicle- and formalin-treated rat paws during the maximal nociceptive response.[67]   Furthermore, no hyperalgesic effect of CB_1/CB_2-receptor antagonists was found when the formalin test carried out in rats[67] More recently, PEA was shown to exert analgesic effects in several rodent models of inflammatory peripheral pain.[68, 69] Despite the fact that PEA does not bind to or activate appreciably either CB_1 or CB_2 receptors, these effects were attenuated by the CB_2 antagonist, SR144528. This led the authors to propose the existence of CB_2-like receptors for this mediator. However, no pharmacological or molecular characterization of the putative CB_2-like receptors for PEA has been reported to date.

There is considerable interest in determining the role, if any, that opioids play in cannabinoid-induced antinociception. THC stimulates the release of endogenous opioids, which thus contribute to the analgesia caused by this compound.[70] More recently, it was shown that cannabinoids and opioids act in a synergistic way to control pain perception, a finding that may result in attractive novel therapeutic strategies for the control of pain.[71] However, AEA does not elicit antinociception through the same mechanism as THC, which appears to trigger the release of dynorphin A or other □- opioid receptor agonists.[72] Furthermore, the analgesic effect of intrathecal AEA, unlike that of THC, is not totally blocked by SR141716A,[72, 73] thus pointing to the existence of non-CB_1 receptors for AEA in the spinal cord.

Further evidence for the role of non-CB_1 receptors in AEA-induced antinociception came from studies on some analogues of capsaicin. By acting at a recently identified type of nociceptor, the vanilloid VR1 receptor, these synthetic substances induce hyperalgesic responses, followed by rapid tachyphylaxis and insensitivity to painful stimuli. It was originally reasoned that substances that could activate VR1 and CB_1 receptors simultaneously would exert ultra-potent analgesic effects. Thus the AEA/capsaicin 'hybrid', *N*-vanillyl-arachidamide (arvanil),[73] was synthesized and shown to be an extremely potent analgesic in mice when using the hot-plate test and intrathecal or intra-cerebroventricular administration (EC_{50}=30-40 ng/mouse).[73] However, the analgesic effect of arvanil was not blocked by either SR141716A or the vanilloid receptor antagonist capsazepine, which instead reversed the analogous effects of THC or capsaicin, respectively.[73] This finding, together with the observation that capsaicin was more potent in the hot-plate test when latency was measured 24 hours after administration, while arvanil and AEA analgesic effects were maximal 3 min after injection, led to suggest that non-CB_1, non-vanilloid receptors underlie the analgesic effect induced in mice by AEA and, more efficaciously, arvanil. This hypothesis was confirmed by the finding that the very potent effect exhibited by arvanil in the formalin test carried out in rats (EC_{50} ~0.1 mg/kg) was not attenuated by either capsazepine or SR141716A (74). Whatever their mechanism of action, "hybrid" VR1/CB_1 agonists are likely to represent a useful template for the development of novel potent analgesic drugs.

Finally, the recent discovery that AEA, but not 2-AG, acts as a full agonist at VR1 receptors [20, 21] deserves special consideration. Although the potency of this endocannabinoid at vanilloid receptors is lower than its potency at CB_1 receptors, its efficacy is comparable to that of capsaicin. Furthermore, several regulatory factors can enhance AEA potency at VR1.[22] Via VR1, AEA can induce the release of nociceptive/inflammatory neuropeptides from sensory neurons, including dorsal root ganglia (DRG) neurons. In order to observe this effect, however, high concentrations of AEA are normally required, whereas lower doses exert an *inhibitory* action on neuropeptide release that is mediated by CB_1 receptors.[63, 75] These findings correlate with electrophysiological and/or in vivo studies showing that AEA, at high doses (up to 800 nmol), activates, via VR1, nociceptive afferents innervating rat knee joints in both normal and arthritic animal,[76] whereas at lower doses (up to 144 nmol) inhibits, via CB_1, spinal neuronal responses in non-inflamed and carrageenan-inflamed rats.[77] Additionally, low concentrations of AEA reduce, and high concentrations increase, the frequency of glutamatergic miniature excitatory postsynaptic currents recorded from the neurons of substantia gelatinosa in the spinal cord.[78] Thus, exogenous AEA can induce either pro- or anti-nociceptive effects depending on its concentration and, possibly, the presence or absence of cannabinoid CB_1 receptors on sensory fibers. Indeed, CB_1 and VR1 receptors are co-localized to a great extent in DRG neurons in culture and in the spinal cord, but only in a minority of peripheral (e.g. skin) sensory afferents.[78, 79] However, there is still no evidence supporting the possibility that endogenous AEA exerts tonic VR1-mediated nociceptive (or, after VR1 desensitization, anti-nociceptive) actions under pathological conditions, in addition to it CB_1-mediated anti-nociceptive effects.

5. ENDOCANNABINOIDS AND SEDATION

Apart from the sedative effects of marijuana, little is known on the possible role of the endocannabinoid system in the control of the sleep-wake cycle, or in its pathological aspects. However, another fatty acid amide, oleamide,[7, 80] was shown to be produced in the cerebrospinal fluid of sleep-deprived mammals and to induce sleep in rats. Although several non-CB_1, non-CB_2 sites of action ([81], and [82] for review), and a pattern of sleep induction different from that of AEA, have been demonstrated for oleamide,[83] there is evidence that at least part of oleamide hypnotic effects are due to the intermediacy of endocannabinoids. [84, 85] In fact, oleamide is a substrate for FAAH and can efficiently inhibit AEA hydrolysis competitively, as well as enhance AEA actions both in vivo and in vitro, possibly by increasing AEA endogenous levels.[7, 86] Accordingly, the CB_1 antagonist, SR141716A, attenuates the sedative effects of oleamide,[84, 85] even though the latter compound does not activate CB_1 or CB_2 receptors. Furthermore, SR141716A administered *per se* increases the time spent awake by rats.[87] These data suggest that endocannabinoids, acting at CB_1 receptors and reinforced by oleamide, might tonically regulate the sleep-wake cycle. This hypothesis is supported by the recent preliminary findings of diurnal variations of AEA levels in rat CSF and brain,[88] and of increases of CB_1 receptor expression with sleep rebound,[89] as well as by the proven capability of both oleamide [82, 90, 91] and AEA (see above) to modulate, via different mechanisms, GABAergic and serotoninergic signaling. However, it remains to be established whether these findings might result in the development of novel sedatives and anesthetics from AEA, 2-AG and oleamide.

6. CONCLUSIONS

As reviewed in this article, it is very likely that the endocannabinoid system, comprising CB_1, CB_2 and yet-to-be discovered cannabinoid receptors, their endogenous ligands, and the enzymes and proteins responsible for endocannabinoid biosynthesis and inactivation, will provide new therapeutic agents useful as anesthetics or for the treatment of pain in general. Agents that activate the cannabinoid receptors, by modulating neurotransmitter and inflammatory mediator release and action, might prove efficacious analgesics. Undesired marijuana-like effects of CB_1 receptor agonists might be prevented by the use of CB_2-selective agents or of yet-to-be-developed analogs that do not cross the blood brain barrier, although both these strategies may also lead to a decreased efficacy of the analgesic effect. If the existence of an endogenous anti-nociceptive tone by endocannabinoids is confirmed by further experiments, then selective inhibitors of endocannabinoid cellular uptake or enzymatic hydrolysis, by enhancing this tone, might provide analgesic drugs devoid of psychotropic effects. Finally, selective endocannabinoid-based CB_1 receptor agonists, such as arachidonoyl-2-chloro-ethylamide, alone or in concert with oleamide analogs, are likely to exert analgesic as well as hypnotic effects with little potential for physical dependence[92] and only few of the immune-suppressive side effects typical of THC.[93] However, the possible cardiovascular actions of these compounds[94] might represent a complicating factor if they are to be used systemically in surgery. At any rate, the great advantage of the possible future use in clinical anaesthesia of endocannabinoid-based drugs over conventional anesthetics might reside in their capability of simultaneously inhibiting pain perception and inducing sedation and hypomotility, with no neurotoxic and hepatotoxic effects.

6. REFERENCES

1. V. Di Marzo, 'Endocannabinoids' and other fatty acid derivatives with cannabimimetic properties: biochemistry and possble physiopathological relevance, *Biochim. Biophys. Acta* **1392**:153 (1998).

2. W. A. Devane, L. Hanus, A. Breuer, R. G. Pertwee, L. A. Stevenson, G. Griffin, D. Gibson, A. Mandelbaum, A. Etinger, and R. Mechoulam, Isolation and structure of a brain constituent that binds to the cannabinoid receptor, *Science* **258**:1946 (1992).

3. L. Hanus, A. Gopher, S. Almog, and R. Mechoulam, Two new unsaturated fatty acid ethanolamides in brain that bind to the cannabinoid receptor, *J. Med. Chem.* **36**:3032 (1993).

4. R. Mechoulam, S. Ben-Shabat, L. Hanus, M. Ligumsky, N. E. Kaminski, A. R. Schatz, A. Gopher, S. Almog, B. R. Martin, D. R. Compton, R. G. Pertwee, G. Griffin, M. Bayewitch, J. Barg, and Z. Vogel, Identifation of an endogenous 2-monoglyceride, present in canine gut, that binds to cannabinoid receptors, *Biochem. Pharmacol.* **50**:83 (1995).

5. T. Sugiura, S. Kondo, A. Sukagawa, S. Nakane, A. Shinoda, K. Itoh, A. Yamashita, and K. Waku, 2-Arachidonoylglycerol: a possible endogenous cannabinoid receptor ligand in brain, *Biochem. Biophys. Commun.* **215**:89 (1995).

6. L. Hanus, S. Abu-Lafi, E. Fride, A. Breuer, Z. Vogel, D. E. Shalev, I. Kustanovich, R. Mechoulam R., 2-arachidonyl glyceryl ether, an endogenous agonist of the cannabinoid CB1 receptor. *Proc. Natl. Acad. Sci. U.S.A.* **98**:3662 (2001).

7. D. M. Lambert, and V. Di Marzo, The palmitoylethanolamide and oleamide enigmas : are these two fatty acid amides cannabimimetic? *Curr. Med. Chem.*; **6**:7571999.

8. V. Di Marzo, Biosynthesis and inactivation of endocannabinoids: relevance to their proposed role as neuromodulators. *Life Sci.* **65**:645 (1999).

9. V. Di Marzo, A. Fontana, H. Cadas, S. Schinelli, G. Cimino, J. C. Schwartz, and D. Piomelli D., Formation and inactivation of endogenous cannabinoid anandamide in central neurons. *Nature* **372**:686 (1994).

10. G. Petersen, and H. S. Hansen, N-acylphosphatidylethanolamine-hydrolysing phospholipase D lacks the ability to transphosphatidylate. *FEBS Lett.* **455**:41 (1999).

11. N. Ueda, Q. Liu, K Yamanaka K., Marked activation of the N-acyl-phosphatidyl-ethanolamine-hydrolyzing phosphodiesterase by divalent cations. *Biochim. Biophys. Acta* **1532**:121 (2001).

12. H. H. Schmid, P. C. Schmid, V. Natarajan, 1996 The N-acylation-phosphodiesterase pathway and cell signalling. *Chem. Phys. Lipids* **80**:133.

13. V. Di Marzo, L. De Petrocellis, T. Sugiura, and Waku, Potential biosynthetic connections between the two cannabimimetic eicosanoids, anandamide and 2-arachidonoyl-glycerol, in mouse neuroblastoma cells. *Biochem. Biophys. Res. Commun.* **227**:281 (1996).

14. N. Stella, P. Schweitzer P.D.. Piomelli, A second endogenous cannabinoid that modulates long-term potentiation. *Nature* **388**:773 (1997).

15. T. Bisogno, D. Melck, L. De Petrocellis, and V. Di Marzo, Phosphatidic acid as the biosynthetic precursor of the endocannabinoid 2-arachidonoylglycerol in intact mouse neuroblastoma cells stimulated with ionomycin, *J. Neurochem.* **72**:2113 (1999).

16. R. G. Pertwee, Pharmacology of cannabinoid CB1 and CB2 receptors, *Pharmacol. Ther.* **74**:129 (1997).

17. M. Herkenham, A. B. Lynn, M. D. Little, M. R. Johnson, L. S. Melvin, B. R. de Costa, and K. C. Rice, Cannabinoid receptor localization in brain, *Proc. Natl. Acad. Sci. U.S.A.* **87**:1932 (1990).

18. F. Maingret, A. J. Patel, M. Lazdunski, and E. Honore, The endocannabinoid anandamide is a direct and selective blocker of the background K(+) channel TASK-1, *EMBO J.* **20**:47 (2001).

19. J. Chemin, A. Monteil, E. Perez-Reyes, J. Nargeot, and P. Lory P, Direct inhibition of T-type calcium channels by the endogenous cannabinoid anandamide, *EMBO J.* **20**:7033 (2001).

20. P. M. Zygmunt, J. Petersson, D. A. Andersson, H. Chuang, M. Sorgard, V. Di Marzo, D. Julius, and E. D. Hogestatt , Vanilloid receptors on sensory nerves mediate the vasodilator action of anandamide, *Nature* **400**:452 (1999).

21. D. Smart, M. J. Gunthorpe, J. C. Jerman, S. Nasir, J. Gray, A. I. Muir, J. K. Chambers, A. D. Randall, and J. B. Davis, The endogenous lipid anandamide is a full agonist at the human vanilloid receptor (hVR1), *Br. J. Pharmacol.* **129**:227 (2000).

22. V. Di Marzo, T. Bisogno, and L. De Petrocellis L., Anandamide: some like it hot, *Trends Pharmacol. Sci.* **22**:346 (2001).

23. V. Di Marzo, L. De Petrocellis, F. Fezza, A. Ligresti, and T. Bisogno, Anandamide Receptors, *Prostagl. Leukotr. Essent. Fatty Acids.*, **66**:377-391 (2002).

24. L. De Petrocellis, T. Bisogno, M. Maccarone, J. D. Davis, A. Finazzi-Agrò, and V. Di Marzo, The activity of anandamide at vanilloid VR1 receptors requires facilitated transport across the cell membrane and is limited by intracellular metabolism, *J. Biol. Chem.* **276**:12856 (2001).

25. V. Di Marzo, T. Bisogno, T. Sugiura, D. Melck, and L. De Petrocellis, The novel endogenous cannabinoid 2-arachidonoylglycerol is inactivated by neuronal- and basophil-like cells: connections with anandamide, *Biochem. J.* **331**:15 (1998).

26. C. J. Hillard , and A. Jarrahian, The movement of N-arachidonoylethanolamine (anandamide) across cellular membranes, *Chem. Phys. Lipids* **108**:123 (2000).

27. F. Fezza, T. Bisogno, A. Minassi, G. Appendino, R. Mechoulam, and V. Di Marzo, Inactivation mechanisms and a sensitive method for the quantification of the putative novel endocannabinoid, noladin ether, in rat brain tissue and cells, *FEBS Letts.*, **513**:294-298 (2002).

28. C. J. Hillard, W. S. Edgemond, A. Jarrahian, and W. B. Campbell, Accumulation of N-arachidonoylethanolamine (anandamide) into cerebellar granule cells occurs via facilitated diffusion, *J. Neurochem.* **69**:631 (1997).

29. B. F. Cravatt, D. K. Giang, S. P. Mayfield, D. L. Boger, R. A. Lerner, and N. B. Gilula, Molecular characterization of an enzyme that degrades neuromodulatory fatty-acid amides, *Nature* **384**:83 (1996).

30. N. Ueda, R. A. Puffenbarger, S. Yamamoto, and D. G. Deutsch, The fatty acid amide hydrolase (FAAH), *Chem. Phys. Lipids* **108**:107 (2000).

31. B. F. Cravatt, K. Demarest, M. P. Patricelli, M. H. Bracey, D. K. Giang, R. R. Martin, and A. H. Lichtman, Supersensitivity to anandamide and enhanced endogenous cannabinoid signaling in mice lacking fatty acid amide hydrolase, *Proc. Natl. Acad. Sci. U.S.A.* **98**:9371 (2001).

32. V. Di Marzo, L. De Petrocellis, and T. Bisogno, Emerging Therapeutic Targets from the Endocannabinoid System. 1. Molecular bases of endocannabinoid formation, action and inactivation, and development of selective inhibitors, *Emerging Therapeutic Targets* **5**:241 (2001).

33. A. C. Howlett, and S. Mukhopadhyay, Cellular signal transduction by anandamide and 2-arachidonoylglycerol, *Chem. Phys. Lipids* **108**:53 (2000).

34. V. Di Marzo, D. Melck, T. Bisogno, L. De Petrocellis, Endocannabinoids: endogenous cannabinoid receptor ligands with neuromodulatory action, *Trends Neurosci.* **21**:521 (1998).

35. E. Schlicker, and M. Kathmann, Modulation of transmitter release via presynaptic cannabinoid receptors; *Trends Pharmacol. Sci.* **22**:565 (2001).

36. C. Levenes, H. Daniel, P. Soubrie, and F. Crepel, Cannabinoids decrease excitatory synaptic transmission and impair long-term depression in rat cerebellar Purkinje cells, *J. Physiol.* **510**:867 (1998).

37. B. Szabo, I. Wallmichrath, P. Mathonia, and C. Pfreundtner, Cannabinoids inhibit excitatory neurotransmission in the substantia nigra pars reticulata, *Neuroscience* **97**:89 (2000).

38. V. Morisset, and L. Urban, Cannabinoid-induced presynaptic inhibition of glutamatergic EPSCs in substantia gelatinosa neurons of the rat spinal cord, *J. Neurophysiol.* **86**:40 (2001).

39. D. Robbe, G. Alonso, F. Duchamp, J. Bockaert, and O. J. Manzoni, Localization and mechanisms of action of cannabinoid receptors at the glutamatergic synapses of the mouse nucleus accumbens, *J. Neurosci.* **21**:109 (2001).

40. C. W. Vaughan, M. Connor, E. E. Bagley, and M. J. Christie, Actions of cannabinoids on membrane properties and synaptic transmission in rat periaqueductal gray neurons in vitro, *Mol. Pharmacol.* **57**:288 (2000).

41. N. Auclair, S. Otani, P. Soubrie, and F. Crepel, Cannabinoids modulate synaptic strength and plasticity at glutamatergic synapses of rat prefrontal cortex pyramidal neurons, *J. Neurophysiol.* **83**:3287 (2000).

42. L. Ferraro, M. C. Tomasini, G. L. Gessa, B. W. Bebe, S. Tanganelli, and T. Antonelli, The cannabinoid receptor agonist WIN 55,212-2 regulates glutamate transmission in rat cerebral cortex: an in vivo and in vitro study, *Cereb Cortex*; **11**:728(2001).

43. N. Hajos, C. Ledent, and T. F. Freund, Novel cannabinoid-sensitive receptor mediates inhibition of glutamatergic synaptic transmission in the hippocampus, *Neuroscience* **106**:1(2001)..

44. P. K. Chan, S. C. Chan, and W. H. Yung, Presynaptic inhibition of GABAergic inputs to rat substantia nigra pars reticulata neurones by a cannabinoid agonist, *Neuroreport* **9**:671 (1998).

45. K. Tsou, K. Mackie, M. C. Sanudo-Pena, and J. M. Walker, Cannabinoid CB1 receptors are localized primarily on cholecystokinin-containing GABAergic interneurons in the rat hippocampal formation, *Neuroscience* **93**:969 (1999).

46. I. Katona, B. Sperlagh, Z. Magloczky, E. Santha, A. Kofalvi, S. Czirjak, K. Mackie, E. S. Vizi, and T. F. Freund T. F., GABAergic interneurons are the targets of cannabinoid actions in the human hippocampus, *Neuroscience* **100**:797 (2000).

47. C. W. Vaughan, I. S. McGregor, and M. J. Christie M, Cannabinoid receptor activation inhibits GABAergic neurotransmission in rostral ventromedial medulla neurons in vitro, *Br. J. Pharmacol.* **127**:935 (1999).

48. E. A. Jennings, C. W. Vaughan, and M. J. Christie M. J., Cannabinoid actions on rat superficial medullary dorsal horn neurons in vitro, *J. Physiol.* **534**:805 (2001).

49. J. Romero, R. de Miguel, J. A. Ramos, and J. J. Fernandez-Ruiz, The activation of cannabinoid receptors in striatonigral GABAergic neurons inhibited GABA uptake, *Life Sci.* **62**:351 (1998).

50. Y. P. Maneuf, J. E. Nash, A. R. Crossman, and J. M. Brotchie, Activation of the cannabinoid receptor by delta 9-tetrahydrocannabinol reduces gamma-aminobutyric acid uptake in the globus pallidus, *Eur. J. Pharmacol.* **308**:16 (1996).

51. R. I. Wilson, and R. A. Nicoll, Endogenous cannabinoids mediate retrograde signalling at hippocampal synapses, *Nature* **410**:588 (2001).

52. A. C. Kreitzer, and W. G. Regehr, Retrograde inhibition of presynaptic calcium influx by endogenous cannabinoids at excitatory synapses onto Purkinje cells, *Neuron* **29**:717 (2001).

53. M. A. Diana, C. Levenes, K. Mackie, and A. Marty, Short-Term Retrograde Inhibition of GABAergic Synaptic Currents in Rat Purkinje Cells Is Mediated by Endogenous Cannabinoids, *J. Neurosci.* **22**:200 (2002).

54. T. Maejima, K. Hashimoto, T. Yoshida, A. Aiba, and M. Kano, Presynaptic inhibition caused by retrograde signal from metabotropic glutamate to cannabinoid receptors, *Neuron* **31**:463 (2001).

55. R. I. Wilson, G. Kunos, and R. A. Nicoll, Presynaptic specificity of endocannabinoid signaling in the hippocampus, *Neuron* **31**:453 (2001).

56. N. Varma, G. C. Carlson, C. Ledent, and B. E. Alger, Metabotropic glutamate receptors drive the endocannabinoid system in hippocampus, *J. Neurosci.* **21**:RC188 (2001).

57. A. S. Rice, Cannabinoids and pain, *Curr. Opin. Investig. Drugs* **2**:399 (2001).

58. R. G. Pertwee, Cannabinoid receptors and pain, *Prog. Neurobiol.* **63**:569 (2001).

59. C. Ledent, O. Valverde, G. Cossu, F. Petitet, J. F. Aubert, F. Beslot, G. A. Bohme, A. Imperato, T. Pedrazzini, B. P. Roques, G. Vassart, W, Fratta, and M. Parmentier, Unresponsiveness to cannabinoids and reduced addictive effects of opiates in CB1 receptor knockout mice, *Science* **283**:401 (1999).

60. A. Zimmer, A. M. Zimmer, A. G. Hohmann, M. Herkenham, and T. I. Bonner, Increased mortality, hypoactivity, and hypoalgesia in cannabinoid CB1 receptor knockout mice, *Proc. Natl. Acad. Sci. U.S.A.* **96**:5780 (1999).

61. J. M. Walker, S. M. Huang, N. M. Strangman, K. Tsou, and M. C. Sanudo-Pena, Pain modulation by release of the endogenous cannabinoid anandamide, *Proc. Natl. Acad. Sci. U.S.A.* **96**:12198 (1999).

62. I. D. Meng, B. H. Manning, W. J. Martin, and H. L. Fields, An analgesia circuit activated by cannabinoids, *Nature* **395**:381 (1998).

63. J. D. Richardson, L. Aanonsen, and K. M. Hargreaves, Hypoactivity of the spinal cannabinoid system results in NMDA-dependent hyperalgesia, *J. Neurosci.* **18**:451 (1998).

64. J. D. Richardson, S. Kilo,and K. M. Hargreaves, Cannabinoids reduce hyperalgesia and inflammation via interaction with peripheral CB1 receptors, *Pain* **75**:111 (1998).

65. A. Calignano, G. La Rana, A. Giuffrida, and D. Piomelli, Control of pain initiation by endogenous cannabinoids, *Nature* **394**:277 (1998).

66. L. Hanus, A. Breuer, S. Tchilibon, S. Shiloah, D. Goldenberg, M. Horowitz, R. G. Pertwee, R. A. Ross, R. Mechoulam, and E. Fride, HU-308: a specific agonist for CB(2), a peripheral cannabinoid receptor, *Proc. Natl. Acad. Sci. U.S.A.* **96**:14228 (1999).

67. P. Beaulieu, T. Bisogno, S. Punwar, W. P. Farquhar-Smith, G. Ambrosino, V. Di Marzo, and A. S. Rice, Role of the endogenous cannabinoid system in the formalin test of persistent pain in the rat, *Eur. J. Pharmacol.* **396**:85 (2000).

68. W. P. Farquhar-Smith, and A. S. Rice, Administration of endocannabinoids prevents a referred hyperalgesia associated with inflammation of the urinary bladder, *Anesthesiology* **94**:507 (2001).

69. A. Calignano, G. La Rana, and D. Piomelli, Antinociceptive activity of the endogenous fatty acid amide, palmitylethanolamide, *Eur. J. Pharmacol.* **419**:191 (2001).

70. D. J. Mason, J. Lowe, and S. P. Welch, Cannabinoid modulation of dynorphin A: correlation to cannabinoid-induced antinociception, *Eur. J. Pharmacol.* **378**:237 (1999).

71. S. P. Welch , and M. Eads, Synergistic interactions of endogenous opioids and cannabinoid systems, *Brain Res.* **848**:183 (1999).

72. S. P. Welch, Characterization of anandamide-induced tolerance: comparison to delta 9-THC-induced interactions with dynorphinergic systems, *Drug Alcohol Depend.* **45**:39 (1997).

73. V. Di Marzo, C. Breivogel, T. Bisogno, D. Melck, G. Patrick, Q. Tao, A. Szallasi, R. K. Razdan, and B. R. Martin, Neurobehavioral activity in mice of N-vanillyl-arachidonyl-amide, *Eur. J. Pharmacol.* **406**:363 (2000).

74. J. W. Brooks, G, Pryce, T. Bisogno, S. I. Jaggar, D. J. R. Hankey, P. Brown, D. Bridges, C. Ledent, M. Bifulco, A. S. C. Rice, V. Di Marzo, and D. Baker, Arvanil-induced inhibition of spasticity and persistent pain: evidence for therapeutic non-VR1, non-CB$_1$, non-CB$_2$ sites of action, *Eur. J. Pharmacol.*, **439**:83-92 (2002).

75. M. Tognetto, S. Amadesi, S. Harrison, C. Creminon, M. Trevisani, M. Carreras, M. Matera, P. Geppetti, and A. Bianchi, Anandamide excites central terminals of dorsal root ganglion neurons via vanilloid receptor-1 activation, *J. Neurosci.* **21**:1104 (2001).

76. S. D. Gauldie, D. S. McQueen, R. Pertwee, and I. P. Chessell, Anandamide activates peripheral nociceptors in normal and arthritic rat knee joints, *Br. J. Pharmacol.* **132**:617 (2001).

77. J. Harris, L. J. Drew, V. Chapman, Spinal anandamide inhibits nociceptive transmission via cannabinoid receptor activation in vivo, *Neuroreport* **11**:2817 (2000).

78. V. Morisset, J. Ahluwalia, I. Nagy, and L. Urban, Possible mechanisms of cannabinoid-induced antinociception in the spinal cord, *Eur. J. Pharmacol.* **429**:93 (2001).
79. J. Ahluwalia, L. Urban, M. Capogna, S. Bevan, and I. Nagy I., Cannabinoid 1 receptors are expressed in nociceptive primary sensory neurons, *Neuroscience* **100**, 685 (2000).
80. B. F. Cravatt, O. Prospero-Garcia, G. Siuzdak, N. B. Gilula, S. J. Henriksen, D. L. Boger, R. A. Lerner, Chemical characterization of a family of brain lipids that induce sleep, *Science* **268**:1506 (1995).
81. I. Fedorova, A. Hashimoto, R. A. Fecik, M. P. Hedrick, L. O. Hanus, D. L. Boger, K. C. Rice, and A. S. Basile, Behavioral evidence for the interaction of oleamide with multiple neurotransmitter systems, *J. Pharmacol. Exp. Ther.* **299**:332 (2001).
82. D. L. Boger, S. J. Henriksen, and B. F. Cravatt, Oleamide: an endogenous sleep-inducing lipid and prototypical member of a new class of biological signaling molecule,. *Curr. Pharm. Des.* **4**:303 (1998).
83. W. B. Mendelson, and A. S. Basile, The hypnotic actions of the fatty acid amide, oleamide, *Neuropsychopharmacology* **25**:S36 (2001).
84. J. F. Cheer, A. K. Cadogan, C. A. Marsden, K. C. Fone, and D. A. Kendall, Modification of 5-HT2 receptor mediated behaviour in the rat by oleamide and the role of cannabinoid receptors, *Neuropharmacology* **38**:533 (1999).
85. W. B. Mendelson, and A. S. Basile, The hypnotic actions of oleamide are blocked by a cannabinoid receptor antagonist, *euroreport* **10**:3237 (1999).
86. R. Mechoulam, E. Fride, L. Hanus, T. Sheskin, T. Bisogno, V. Di Marzo, M. Bayewitch, and Z. Vogel, Anandamide may mediate sleep induction, *Nature* **389**:25 (1997).
87. V. Santucci, J. J. Storme, P. Soubrie, and G. Le Fur, Arousal-enhancing properties of the CB1 cannabinoid receptor antagonist SR 141716A in rats as assessed by electroencephalographic spectral and sleep-waking cycle analysis, *Life Sci.* **58**:PL103 (1996).
88. M. Martinez-Vargas, E. Murillo-Rodriguez, R. Gonzalez-Rivera, A. Landa, J. Velazquez-Moctezuma, O. Prospero-Garcia, and L. Navarro, Cannabinoid receptor 1 increases with sleep rebound, *Soc. Neurosci. Abstr.* **524**.22 (2001).
89. E. Murillo-Rodriguez, A. Giuffrida, F. Desarnaud, O. Prospero-Garcia, and D. Piomelli, Diurnal variations of endogenous cannabinoid compounds in csf and brain regions of the rat, *Soc. Neurosci. Abstr.* **805**.2 (2001)
90. G. Lees, M. D. Edwards, A. A. Hassoni, C. R. Ganellin, and D. Galanakis, Modulation of GABA(A) receptors and inhibitory synaptic currents by the endogenous CNS sleep regulator cis-9,10-octadecenoamide (cOA), *Br. J. Pharmacol.* **124**:873 (1998).
91. A. D. Laposky, G. E. Homanics, A. Basile, and W. B. Mendelson, Deletion of the GABA(A) receptor beta 3 subunit eliminates the hypnotic actions of oleamide in mice, *Neuroreport* **12**:4143 (2001).
92. M. D. Aceto, S. M. Scates, R. K. Razdan, B. R. Martin, Anandamide, an endogenous cannabinoid, has a very low physical dependence potential, *J. Pharmacol. Exp. Ther.* **287**:598 (1998).
93. T. W. Klein, B. Lane, C. A. Newton, and H. Friedman, The cannabinoid system and cytokine network, *Proc. Soc. Exp. Biol. Med.* **225**:1 (2000).
94. G. Kunos, Z. Jarai, S. Batkai, S. K. Goparaju, E. J. Ishac, J. Liu, L. Wang, and J. A. Wagner, Endocannabinoids as cardiovascular modulators, *Chem. Phys. Lipids* **108**:159 (2000).

EFFECT SITES OF NEUROMUSCULAR BLOCKING AGENTS AND THE MONITORING OF CLINICAL MUSCLE RELAXATION

Claude Meistelman[*]

1. INTRODUCTION

The main goals of muscular relaxation during induction of anaesthesia are the paralysis of the vocal cords and jaw muscles to facilitate tracheal intubation and the relaxation of the respiratory muscles. Paralysis of the abdominal muscles and the diaphragm is often required intraoperatively, particularly during abdominal surgery. During recovery of neuromuscular blockade, restoration of complete skeletal muscular strength is essential to ensure adequate spontaneous ventilation and the permeability of the upper airway. For practical reasons, it is almost impossible to monitor the response of the respiratory or abdominal muscles during anaesthesia. Paton and Zaimis demonstrated in 1951 that respiratory muscles were more resistant to curare than other muscles.[1] In humans, several studies have reported some discrepancies between the level of peripheral paralysis and respiratory depression or the intubating conditions.[2,3] Therefore, both understanding and knowledge of the relationship between neuromuscular function at the monitored muscle and the other muscles are important in the interpretation of monitoring.

2. RESPIRATORY MUSCLES

2.1 Diaphragm

In awake volunteers, minute volume and end-tidal pCO_2 are little affected, if at all, by doses of d-tubocurarine which abolish grip strength almost completely.[4,5] For example, after injection of d-tubocurarine, 0.2 mg/kg, grip strength is only 3% of control,

[*] Claude Meistelman, Department of Anaesthesiology, Nancy, France

Advances in Modelling and Clinical Application of Intravenous Anaesthesia
Edited by Vuyk and Schraag, Kluwer Academic/Plenum Publishers, 2003

but tidal volume is normal.[6] It is tempting to suggest that patients need only partial peripheral muscle recovery to have an adequate respiratory function, because normal gas exchange can be maintained. In fact, it is necessary to ensure return of full respiratory reserve because a decrease in vital capacity impairs the ability to cough.

The cumulative dose-response curve for the diaphragm is shifted to the right compared with that of the adductor pollicis for pancuronium,[7] atracurium, vecuronium or rocuronium.[8] The ED_{50} ratios are 1.56 for atracurium and 1.47 for vecuronium, suggesting that both atracurium and vecuronium exhibit a similar degree of sparing at the diaphragm. Thus, complete paralysis of the diaphragm is not expected with a dose of relaxant that barely blocks the adductor pollicis. Smith et al. have demonstrated that the diaphragm sparing effect of succinylcholine was comparable to that previously reported for non depolarising muscle relaxants.[9]

Waud and Waud in cats, found that, following d-tubocurarine administration, neuromuscular transmission occurs when approximately 18 % of the receptors are free at the diaphragm, whereas 29% free receptors are required at the tibialis muscle. This indicates that the diaphragm does not necessarily have a different acetylcholine receptor, but may have a higher receptor density, higher acetylcholine release, or smaller acetylcholinesterase activity.[10] Sterz et al demonstrated that differences in the density of ionic channels could exist between muscles. This lower density of acetylcholine receptors in slow muscle could explain, at least in part, the lower margin of safety for neuromuscular transmission compared with fast muscle.[11]

Surprisingly, the onset of neuromuscular blockade is significantly more rapid at the diaphragm than at the adductor pollicis despite the resistance of the diaphragm to muscle relaxants in human. The diaphragm receives a larger blood flow than limb skeletal muscles, because of its main role for breathing and its proximity from the aorta. It follows that the diaphragmatic muscle tends to be paralysed more rapidly than more peripheral less perfused muscles, such as the adductor pollicis. When subparalyzing doses of relaxants are given, time to maximum blockade is shorter at the diaphragm than at the adductor pollicis. This seems to contradict the concept that the diaphragm is resistant to the effects of relaxants. The apparent paradox is resolved if one considers that plasma concentrations decrease rapidly after a bolus dose. Thus, they are greater when the diaphragm is blocked maximally than when the adductor pollicis is.[12]

Because the diaphragm recovers at higher plasma concentrations, recovery from diaphragmatic blockade occurs sooner than does adductor pollicis recovery (Figure 1). With vecuronium 0.1 mg/kg, the twitch height (TH) at the diaphragm returned to 25% of control value after 27 min compared to 41 min at the adductor pollicis.[13] It is likely that the concentrations of muscle relaxant are the same at both muscles. Thus, blood flow plays a minor role in recovery from blockade.

2.2 Accessory respiratory muscles

No data have been obtained using single twitch or train-of-four stimulation of a nerve supplying intercostal, or accessory muscles of respiration. However, indirect data in awake subjects suggest that these muscles are less resistant to non depolarising drugs than the diaphragm is. Spontaneous EMG during partial paralysis is greater for the diaphragm than for other muscles of respiration. The abdominal muscles of the lateral wall are less resistant to non depolarising muscle relaxants than the diaphragm.[14] However, the lateral abdominal muscles and the rectus abdominis are resistant as compared with peripheral muscles such as the adductor pollicis.[15,16] These results confirm the concept of a relative sparing effect of non-depolarising muscle relaxants among expiratory respiratory muscles.

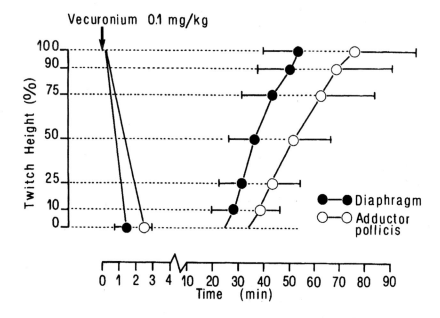

Figure 1. Simultaneous evolution of the neuromuscular blocking effects of 0.1 mg/kg vecuronium at the diaphragm and the adductor pollicis (with permission).[13]

2.3 Laryngeal muscles

Laryngeal adductor muscles are more resistant to non depolarising muscle relaxants than is the adductor pollicis. The ED_{90} of vecuronium is 46 µg/kg at the adductor pollicis and 80 µg/kg at the vocal cords.[17] The same sparing effect on the laryngeal muscles has been also described with rocuronium[18] and mivacurium[19] in man. Therefore complete paralysis of vocal cords requires greater doses, greater than those that block the adductor pollicis. No information is available on the margin of safety of the laryngeal muscles. However, the reasons for this resistance might be explained by histological and physiological differences between laryngeal and peripheral muscles as the adductor pollicis. These differences in sensitivity of different muscles might be due to the larger number of acetylcholine receptors in fast-twitch fibres. Recovery from neuromuscular blockade at the vocal cords occurs sooner than adductor pollicis. Following administration of twice the ED_{95}, recovery of the vocal cords to 90 % of control value occurred in approximately in 23 minutes whereas similar recovery at the adductor pollicis took 40 minutes for both vecuronium[17] or rocuronium. This was probably due to the sparing effects of non-depolarising muscle relaxants on fast-contracting muscles, an effect previously observed at the diaphragm. Onset of neuromuscular blockade is faster at the vocal cords than at the adductor pollicis. Following approximately twice the ED_{95}, maximum blockade of the laryngeal adductor muscles occurred 3.3 min and 1.3 min after vecuronium or rocuronium administration respectively, whereas the adductor pollicis was blocked in 5.7 min and 2.4 min respectively.[17] These findings, already reported for the diaphragm, are probably due to the greater visualization and the proximity to the central circulation of the laryngeal muscles, compared to peripheral muscles.

Unlike non-depolarising muscle relaxants, suxamethonium produces a more profound blockade at the vocal cords than at the adductor pollicis. After 0.25 mg/kg, blockade of first twitch is 66 % of control at the vocal cords and 45 % at the adductor pollicis. With 0.5 mg/kg maximum blockade is slightly greater at the vocal cords (93 %) than at the adductor pollicis (84 %). These sparing effects on the adductor pollicis might also be related to the different sensitivities of different fibre types and muscle relaxants. Experimental data in cats and pigs suggest that contrary to non-depolarising blockers, suxamethonium was more effective in blocking the fast contracting tibialis than the slow contracting soleus. Suxamethonium produces more rapid vocal cord neuromuscular blockade when compared with the adductor pollicis. With 0.5 mg/kg time to maximum neuromuscular blockade was 0.9 min at the vocal cords and 1.7 min at the adductor pollicis, with the onset at the laryngeal muscles occurring during fasciculations of peripheral muscles.[20] Therefore rapid onset of action and some selectivity for laryngeal adductor muscles make this drug particularly suitable for tracheal intubation.

2.4 Compared pharmacokinetic/pharmacodynamic relationship

Although the respiratory muscles studied are more resistant to muscle relaxants, paralysis of the respiratory muscles may occur before complete paralysis of the adductor pollicis. This apparent discrepancy can be explained by considering the factors, which influence peak neuromuscular effect, particularly the rate of equilibration between plasma and the effect site. After a bolus dose, equilibrium between plasma and the neuromuscular junction will be reached sooner at the muscle group with the more rapid equilibration. Peak concentration at the muscle group with more rapid equilibration will be greater than at the muscle group with the slower equilibration.[12] Even if the muscle group with the more rapid equilibration is resistant, the greater peak concentration will offset this to produce a more intense peak effect. Thus, more rapid equilibration of the respiratory muscles results in higher peak concentrations producing paralysis earlier and possibly of greater magnitude compared to the adductor pollicis.

This hypothesis has been confirmed by Plaud et al. who have shown, following rocuronium administration, that the rate constant of transport between plasma and the effect compartment (k_{eo}) was significantly greater at the laryngeal muscles (0.260 minutes) than at the adductor pollicis (0.168 minutes)[21] (Figure 2). Fisher et al. have found that vecuronium also equilibrated more rapidly with the laryngeal adductor muscles than with the adductor pollicis.[22] Even if the laryngeal muscles require a 30% greater concentration than the adductor pollicis for 50% effect, the markedly greater concentration of vecuronium at the laryngeal adductor muscles, following injection, results in earlier onset and a greater magnitude of paralysis.

The k_{eo} is dependant mainly on circulatory factors (muscle blood flow) and the partitioning of the relaxant between blood and muscle. It is likely that the more rapid equilibration of the laryngeal adductor muscles or the diaphragm when compared with the adductor pollicis is the result of the greater perfusion of the respiratory muscles.

The greater EC_{50} (concentration in the effect compartment producing 50% block) at the respiratory muscles [12, 21] explains why they recover from neuromuscular block before the adductor pollicis does. Recovery is a very slow phenomenon compared with onset of paralysis, and it occurs during the elimination phase. During recovery a pseudoequilibrium is reached between plasma and the neuromuscular junction at both muscles. Recovery occurs more rapidly at the respiratory muscles than the adductor pollicis because lower blood concentrations must be achieved at the adductor pollicis, compared with the respiratory muscles, before recovery begins.

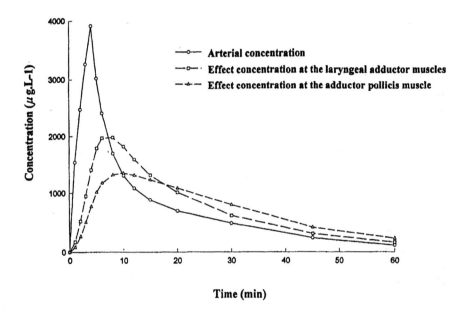

Figure 2. Rocuronium plasma concentration and calculated concentration in the effect compartment at the laryngeal adductor muscles and the adductor pollicis versus time (with permission).[21]

3. UPPER AIRWAY MUSCLES

Unlike the laryngeal adductor muscles or the diaphragm, the muscles of the upper airway are particularly sensitive to the effects of relaxants. Pavlin et al. reported that total airway obstruction was achieved with a dose of d-tubocurarine, that produced an inspiratory pressure of 45 cm H2O, i.e. as much as 50% of control.[5] Small doses of pancuronium (0.02 mg/kg) depress the swallowing reflex to a greater extent than the strength of peripheral muscles.[23] This indicates that muscles involved with maintenance of airway patency are more sensitive to relaxants than other respiratory muscles and possibly peripheral muscles. Thus, following administration of small doses of non depolarising muscle relaxants such as used during the priming technique, there is a risk of aspirating gastric content by paralysis of upper airway muscles.[24]

The cumulative dose-response curve at the masseter is shifted to the left compared with the adductor pollicis, i.e., the masseter is approximately 15% more sensitive to the drug. Onset of action is more rapid at the masseter, for all drugs tested, and both in adults and children.[25] These data indicate that jaw relaxation, which is required for adequate intubating conditions, can be obtained rapidly with small doses of neuromuscular blocking drugs. However, recovery of the masseter and possibly other upper airway muscles is probably delayed with respect to other respiratory muscles such as the diaphragm. The masseter has an unusual response to suxamethonium. A significant reduction in mouth opening and an increase in jaw stiffness occurs at a time when full relaxation of the limb muscles is obtained.[26] This reduction in mouth opening is observed within 60 seconds after loss of twitch at hand muscles and cessation of fasciculations. The increase in masseter tone may be greater than 500 g, usually occurs within one minute, returns to normal within 1 to 2 minutes after suxamethonium administration and is usually overcome easily by the laryngoscopist. However it is now accepted that the normal response of the masseter to suxamethonium is an increase in jaw stiffness which is maximal at the time of muscle fasciculations, is transient and is not accompanied by other signs of hypermetabolism.[27] The adductor pollicis also shows an increase in tension after suxamethonium, but of much less magnitude. This phenomenon is not observed after non-depolarising agents. The mechanism of action for this effect remains speculative, the increase in tone might be present even in the presence of total NMB at the masseter. The ineffectiveness of sub-paralysing doses of d-tubocurarine in preventing tension increases suggests that this effect of succinylcholine is not presynaptic. However, a paralysing dose of atracurium abolished the effect entirely, suggesting that nicotinic acetylcholine receptors either junctional or extrajunctional are involved.[28] A direct action on muscle is unlikely as atracurium, that acts at the neuromuscular junction, blocks this increase in tone.

It has been recently shown by Eriksson et al. that the upper oesophageal sphincter resting tone was significantly reduced at TOF ratios of 0.6, 0.7 and 0.8 at the adductor pollicis. This was associated with reduced muscle coordination required between oesophageal sphincter relaxation and contraction of the pharyngeal constrictor muscles for deglutition. Bolus transit time was shortened at a TOF ratio of 0.6.[29] Several volunteers showed misdirected swallowing with episodes of aspiration at TOF ratios less than 0.9. These results obtained during vecuronium-induced neuromuscular block have been confirmed during atracurium-induced paralysis.[30] This study has highlighted that the initiation of the swallowing reflex and the pharyngeal coordination was impaired during partial paralysis (Figure 3). This impairment causes a four- to fivefold increase in the incidence of misdirected swallowing resulting in penetration of bolus to the larynx.

4. CENTRAL RESPIRATORY EFFECTS

The increase in ventilation during hypoxia is mainly governed by afferent neuronal input from peripheral chemoreceptors of the carotid bodies. Acetylcholine is involved in the transmission of afferent neuronal activity from the carotid bodies to the central nervous system. Eriksson et al. have demonstrated that partial neuromuscular block (TOF ratio of 0.7) specifically reduces the ventilatory response to isocapnic hypoxia without altering the response to hypercapnia. At a mechanical adductor pollicis TOF of 0.7, the hypoxic ventilatory response was reduced by approximately 30% in the awake volunteer after atracurium, vecuronium and pancuronium.[31, 32] The ventilatory response to hypoxia returns to control values after recovery to a TOF above 0.9. The mechanism behind this interaction seems to be a spontaneous reversible depression of carotid body chemoreceptor activity during hypoxia. Wyon et al. have confirmed in rabbits, that chemosenstivity and the hypoxic response were significantly reduced after both 0.1 and 0.5 mg/kg vécuronium.[33] The effect was dose-dependant and the chemosensitivity remained significantly depressed at 30 and 60 min but had recovered spontaneously at 90 min after 0.5 mg vecuronium.

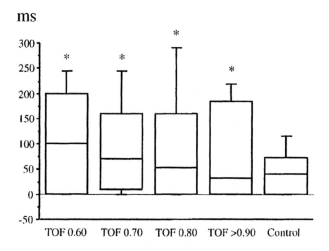

Figure 3. Duration of the swallowing reflex versus train-of-four ratio during partial relaxation (with permission).[30]

5. MONITORING OF CLINICAL MUSCULAR RELAXATION

Marked interindivdual variability in response to the effects of muscles relaxants is well known and for many years, stimulation of the ulnar nerve using train-of-four (TOF) in association with monitoring of the adductor pollicis has been used to determine the time course and intensity of neuromuscular blockade. It has become the gold standard for monitoring of neuromuscular transmission. However, new modes and sites of stimulation have been introduced to assess the time course and intensity of neuromuscular blockade from onset until complete recovery of neuromuscular transmission.

5.1 Onset of neuromuscular block

After induction of anaesthesia, the intensity of neuromuscular blockade must be assessed to determine the optimum time for tracheal intubation. Although intubating conditions can be affected by the depth of anaesthesia, good intubating conditions might not be obtained unless complete blockade of the respiratory muscles is obtained. Bencini and Newton have suggested that good intubating conditions could be obtained before complete paralysis at the adductor pollicis.[2] As previously discussed, paralysis of the adductor pollicis lags behind relaxation of the respiratory and the laryngeal adductor muscles. These findings could explain the discrepancies observed between the intubating conditions and the degree of peripheral neuromuscular blockade. If a dose sufficient to block the diaphragm or the laryngeal muscles is given, neuromuscular blockade at the adductor pollicis is not usually achieved when full relaxation of the respiratory muscles occurs. At the opposite, following administration of a subparalising dose of a NDMR at the respiratory muscles, their function may recover in the 3-6 minutes range, while adductor pollicis block becomes more intense.[34] Therefore monitoring of an other peripheral muscle during induction of anaesthesia could give more accurate information to determine the optimal time for intubation. Among the other peripheral muscles which can be easily monitored, the orbicularis oculi has been considered as an accurate monitoring of resistant muscles such as the diaphragm[34] or the laryngeal adductor muscles.[35] Le Corre et al. has demonstrated that when a NDMR was given at a dose sufficient to block respiratory muscles, complete blockade at the orbicularis oculi following train-of-four stimulation might predict good intubating conditions.[36] Following 0.5 mg/kg atracurium, intubation could be provided in all the patients approximately 1 minute before complete paralysis at the adductor pollicis.[35] However, the orbicularis oculi which is innervated by the temporal branch of the facial nerve is a thin muscle which covers the eyelid. In initial studies, movements recorded over the superciliary arch were attributed to the orbicularis oculi but close inspection of the response to facial nerve stimulation suggests that the movements observed over the superciliary arch corresponded to the contraction of the corrugator supercilii.[37] The corrugator supercilii receives, like the orbicularis oculi, facial innervation and pulls the eyebrow towards the nose. It may be a better choice than the adductor pollicis or the orbicularis oculi because its onset of paralysis approaches that of the laryngeal adductor muscles.[37] Since the sensitivity of the corrugator supercilii to NDMR is close to that of the laryngeal adductor muscles (Figure 4), its paralysis probably indicates complete blockade of almost all muscles whose relaxation is required for good intubating conditions. When a dose insufficient to block the respiratory muscles is given, monitoring of the adductor pollicis can be misleading because absence of a response at the adductor pollicis does not guarantee adequate intubating conditions.

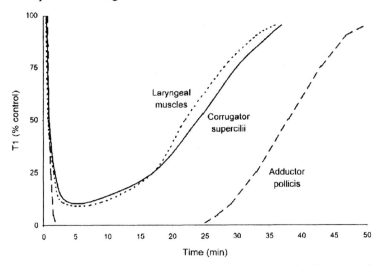

Figure 4. Time course of action of 0.5 mg/kg rocuronium at the laryngeal adductor muscles, corrugator supercilii and adductor pollicis (with permission).[37]

5.2 Maintenance of neuromuscular paralysis

The type of stimulation that one may elect to use intraoperatively will be influenced by the depth of block required for surgery. For practical reasons it is almost impossible to monitor the response of the diaphragm or the abdominal muscles during surgery. Disappearance of train-of-four (TOF) at the adductor pollicis does not necessarily indicates paralysis of the vocal cords or the diaphragm and does not eliminate the possibility of hiccups or extrusion of abdominal contents. During that phase of so called "period of no response", because no response to TOF occurs, two different techniques may allow the evaluation of very intense blockade when complete paralysis of the diaphragm is sought. Complete absence of post-tetanic count (PTC) suggests near 100% receptor occupancy with ablation of diaphragm response. The number of responses in the PTC is related inversely to the depth of neuromuscular block. PTC can also be used to predict the time that will be required for return of spontaneous twitch.[38] The major drawback of the technique is that it cannot be repeated more often than every 5 minutes as facilitation of subsequent responses may occur. Monitoring of the corrugator supercilii, using a TOF stimulus may also have a role during surgery because the response of the corrugator supercilii is a good reflection of the paralysis of the respiratory muscles.[37]

When profound blockade is not required, monitoring at the adductor pollicis using TOF is sufficient and allows easier assessment of antagonism of relaxation at the end of the case. When a twitch depression of approximately 90% is sought, usually one twitch at the adductor pollicis is visible. In this situation, neither PTC nor TOF at the corrugator supercilii provides more relevant information.

5.3 Recovery and detection of residual paralysis

The recovery phase begin with the reappearance of the fourth response to the TOF. The major goal of neuromuscular monitoring during recovery is to detect residual paralysis which can occur in at least 10% of the patients[39] and sometimes in more than 40% of the patients in the recovery room when there is no use of a nerve stimulator and no reversal.[40] It is recommended to monitor a muscle whom recovery will occur after recovery of respiratory muscles. Antagonism should never be attempted on the basis of information given by the TOF at the orbicularis oculi because its reappearance may be still associated with intense paralysis of muscles other than the diaphragm but which are also involved in respiration.

When the fourth response at the TOF at the adductor pollicis reappears, neuromuscular block is usually less than 75%. When the adductor pollicis has almost completely recovered, it can be assumed that no residual paralysis exist at both the diaphragm[41] and the laryngeal adductor muscles. However respiratory failure due to upper airway weakness,[24] impairment of the muscles of the pharynx[29,30] or of the ventilatory response to hypoxia[31] exists even in the presence of nearly complete recovery of the adductor pollicis. Therefore, monitoring needs to be used judiciously. Visual or tactile assessment of fade when the TOF ratio is above 40% is very difficult even for experienced anaesthesiologists and cannot exclude significant residual paralysis.[42] As the 50 Hz tetanus is not more accurate than TOF in detecting fade, its usefulness in monitoring recovery is doubtful.[42] Double-burst stimulation (DBS) can detect fade more easily than TOF, and improves manual assessment of neuromuscular block. However fade cannot be detected with DBS when the TOF ratio is above 60%[43] and does not eliminate the risk of remaining residual paralysis.[44] In cooperative patients a few clinical tests may reveal evidence of muscular weakness. The head lift test or the ability to lift the head for 5 s is passed for TOF ratio ranging from 45 to 75%. Kopman et al. have recently demonstrated that the most sensitive clinical tests were the ability to retain a tongue depressor clenched between the teeth or the lack of visual disturbance.[45] However, all clinical tests are imprecise and of limited use at the end of a case. In daily clinical practice the detection of residual paralysis could be improved by the use of objective measurements. Mechanomyography or electromyography are more research tools, and acceloromyography is more convenient in clinical practice. The objective measurement of the TOF ratio is the best way to detect and avoid residual paralysis in the recovery room. A TOF ratio above 0.9 at the adductor pollicis confirms the absence of residual block even at the upper airway muscles.[45]

6. CONCLUSION

The site and type of monitoring should be adapted to requirements during induction, maintenance and recovery from anaesthesia and neuromuscular block. A fast onset, resistant muscle, such as the corrugator supercilii, appears best suited for tracheal intubation and maintenance of deep neuromuscular block whereas the adductor pollicis is better adapted for monitoring of less intensive levels of paralysis and recovery. New methods of stimulation and recording of the evoked response have increased the sensitivity of neuromuscular monitoring during recovery from NMB.

7. REFERENCES

1. W. D. M. Paton and E. J. Zaimis, The action of d-tubocurarine and of decamethonium on respiratory and oher muscles in the cat. *J Physiol* **112**, 311-331 (1951).
2. A. F. Bencini and D. E. Newton, Rate of onset of good intubating conditions, respiratory depression and hand muscle paralysis after vecuronium. *Br J Anaesth* **56**, 959-965 (1984).
3. J. C. Carnie, M. K. Street and B. Kumar, Emergency intubation of the trachea facilitated by suxamethonium. *Br J Anaesth* **58**, 498-501 (1986).
4. T. J. Gal and T. C. Smith, Partial paralysis with d-tubocurarine and the ventilatory response to CO2: An example of respiratory sparing? *Anesthesiology* **45**, 22-28 (1976).
5. E. G. Pavlin, R. H. Holle and R. B. Schoene, Recovery of airway protection compared with ventilation in humans after paralysis with curare. *Anesthesiology* **70**, 381-385 (1989).
6. T. J. Gal and S. K. Goldberg, Diaphragmatic function in healthy subjects during partial curarization. *J Appl Physiol* **48**, 921-926 (1980).
7 F. Donati, C. Antzaka and D. R. Bevan, Potency of pancuronium at the diaphragm and the adductor pollicis muscle in humans. *Anesthesiology* **65**, 1-5 (1986).
8. J. P. Cantineau, F. Porte, G. D'Honneur and P. Duvaldestin, Neuromuscular effects of rocuronium on the diaphragm and adductor pollicis in anesthetized patients. *Anesthesiology* **81**, 585-590 (1994).
9. C. E. Smith, F. Donati and D. R. Bevan, Potency of succinylcholine at the diaphragm and at the adductor pollicis muscle. *Anesth Analg* **67**, 625-630 (1988).
10. B. E. Waud and D. R. Waud, The margin of safety of neuromuscular transmission in the muscle of the diaphragm. *Anesthesiology* **37**, 417-422 (1972).
11. R. Sterz, M. Pagala and K. Peper, Postjunctional characteristics of the endplates in mammalian fast and slow muscles. *Pflugers Arch* **398**, 48-54 (1983).
12. P. Bragg, D. M. Fisher, J. Shi, F. Donati, C. Meistelman, M. Lau and L. B. Sheiner, Comparison of twitch depression of the adductor pollicis and the respiratory muscles. Pharmacodynamic modeling without plasma concentrations. *Anesthesiology* **80**, 310-319 (1994).

13. M. Chauvin, C. Lebrault and P. Duvaldestin, The neuromuscular blocking effect of vecuronium on the human diaphragm. *Anesth Analg* **66**, 117-122 (1987).
14. K. Kirov, C. Motamed and G. Dhonneur, Differential sensitivity of abdominal muscles and the diaphragm to mivacurium: an electromyographic study. *Anesthesiology* **95**, 1323-1328 (2001).
15. J. M. Saddler, L. F. Marks and J. Norman, Comparison of atracurium-induced neuromuscular block in rectum abdominis and hand muscles of man. *Br J Anaesth* **69**, 26-28 (1992).
16. K. Kirov, C. Motamed, X. Combes, P. Duvaldestin and G. Dhonneur, [Sensitivity to atracurium in the lateral abdominal muscles]. *Ann Fr Anesth Reanim* **19**, 734-738 (2000).
17. F. Donati, C. Meistelman and B. Plaud, Vecuronium neuromuscular blockade at the adductor muscles of the larynx and adductor pollicis. *Anesthesiology* **74**, 833-837 (1991).
18. C. Meistelman, B. Plaud and F. Donati, Rocuronium (ORG 9426) neuromuscular blockade at the adductor muscles of the larynx and adductor pollicis in humans. *Can J Anaesth* **39**, 665-669 (1992).
19. B. Plaud, B. Debaene, F. Lequeau, C. Meistelman and F. Donati, Mivacurium neuromuscular block at the adductor muscles of the larynx and adductor pollicis in humans. *Anesthesiology* **85**, 77-81 (1996).
20. C. Meistelman, B. Plaud and F. Donati, Neuromuscular effects of succinylcholine on the vocal cords and adductor pollicis muscles. *Anesth Analg* **73**, 278-282 (1991).
21. B. Plaud, J. H. Proost, J. M. Wierda, J. Barre, B. Debaene and C. Meistelman, Pharmacokinetics and pharmacodynamics of rocuronium at the vocal cords and the adductor pollicis in humans. *Clin Pharmacol Ther* **58**, 185-191 (1995).
22. D. M. Fisher, J. Szenohradszky, P. M. Wright, M. Lau, R. Brown and M. Sharma, Pharmacodynamic modeling of vecuronium-induced twitch depression. Rapid plasma-effect site equilibration explains faster onset at resistant laryngeal muscles than at the adductor pollicis. *Anesthesiology* **86**, 558-566 (1997).
23. S. Isono, T. Ide, T. Kochi, T. Mizuguchi and T. Nishino, Effects of partial paralysis on the swallowing reflex in conscious humans. *Anesthesiology* **75**, 980-984 (1991).
24. G. D'Honneur, O. Gall, A. Gerard, J. M. Rimaniol, Y. Lambert and P. Duvaldestin, Priming doses of atracurium and vecuronium depress swallowing in humans. *Anesthesiology* **77**, 1070-1073 (1992).
25. C. E. Smith, F. Donati and D. R. Bevan, Differential effects of pancuronium on masseter and adductor pollicis muscles in humans. *Anesthesiology* **71**, 57-61 (1989).
26. A. F. L. Van Der Spek, W. B. Fang, J. A. Ashton-Miller, C. S. Stohler, D. S. Carlson and M. A. Schork, The effects of succinylcholine on mouth opening. *Anesthesiology* **67**, 459-463 (1987).
27. J. M. Saddler, Jaw stiffness-An ill understood condition. *Br J Anaesth* **67**, 515-516 (1991).
28. C. E. Smith, J. M. Saddler, J. C. Bevan, F. Donati and D. R. Bevan, Pretreatment with non-depolarizing neuromuscular blocking agents and suxamethonium-induced increases in resting jaw tension in children. *Br J Anaesth* **64**, 577-581 (1990).
29. L. I. Eriksson, E. Sundman, R. Olsson, L. Nilsson, H. Witt, O. Ekberg and R. Kuylenstierna, Functional assessment of the pharynx at rest and during swallowing in partially paralyzed humans: simultaneous videomanometry and mechanomyography of awake human volunteers. *Anesthesiology* **87**, 1035-1043 (1997).
30. E. Sundman, H. Witt, R. Olsson, O. Ekberg, R. Kuylenstierna and L. I. Eriksson, The incidence and mechanisms of pharyngeal and upper esophageal dysfunction in partially paralyzed humans: pharyngeal videoradiography and simultaneous manometry after atracurium. *Anesthesiology* **92**, 977-984 (2000).
31. L. I. Eriksson, M. Sato and J. W. Severinghaus, Effect of a vecuronium-induced partial neuromuscular block on hypoxic ventilatory response. *Anesthesiology* **78**, 693-699 (1993).
32. L. I. Eriksson, Reduced hypoxic chemosensitivity in partially paralysed man. A new property of muscle relaxants? *Acta Anaesthesiol Scand* **40**, 520-523 (1996).
33. N. Wyon, L. I. Eriksson, Y. Yamamoto and S. G. Lindahl, Vecuronium-induced depression of phrenic nerve activity during hypoxia in the rabbit. *Anesth Analg* **82**, 1252-1256 (1996).
34. F. Donati, C. Meistelman and B. Plaud, Vecuronium neuromuscular blockade at the diaphragm, the orbicularis oculi, and adductor pollicis muscles. *Anesthesiology* **73**, 870-875 (1990).
35. B. Debaene, M. Beaussier, C. Meistelman, F. Donati and A. Lienhart, Monitoring the onset of neuromuscular block at the orbicularis oculi can predict good intubating conditions during atracurium-induced neuromuscular block. *Anesth Analg* **80**, 360-363 (1995).
36. F. Le Corre, B. Plaud, E. Benhamou and B. Debaene, Visual estimation of onset time at the orbicularis oculi after five muscle relaxants: application to clinical monitoring of tracheal intubation. *Anesth Analg* **89**, 1305-1310 (1999).
37. B. Plaud, B. Debaene and F. Donati, The corrugator supercilii, not the orbicularis oculi, reflects rocuronium neuromuscular blockade at the laryngeal adductor muscles. *Anesthesiology* **95**, 96-101 (2001).
38. J. Viby-Mogensen, P. Howardy-Hensen, B. Chraemmer-Jorgensen, H. Ording, J. Engbaek and A. Nielsen, Posttetanic count (PTC): a new method of evaluating an intense non depolarizing neuromuscular blockade. *Anesthesiology* **55**, 458-461 (1981).

39. D. R. Bevan, C. E. Smith and F. Donati, Postoperative neuromuscular blockade: a comparison between atracurium, vecuronium, and pancuronium. *Anesthesiology* **69**, 272-276 (1988).
40. C. Baillard, G. Gehan, J. Reboul-Marty, P. Larmignat, C. M. Samama and M. Cupa, Residual curarization in the recovery room after vecuronium. *Br J Anaesth* **84**, 394-395 (2000).
41. G. D'Honneur, V. Slavov, J. C. Merle, K. Kirov, J. M. Rimaniol, L. Sperry and P. Duvaldestin, Comparison of the effects of mivacurium on the diaphragm and geniohyoid muscles. *Br J Anaesth* **77**, 716-719 (1996).
42. J. Y. Dupuis, R. Martin, J. M. Tessonnier and J. P. Tetrault, Clinical assessment of the muscular response to tetanic nerve stimulation. *Can J Anaesth* **37**, 397-400 (1990).
43. N. E. Drenck, N. Ueda, N. V. Olsen, J. Engbaek, E. Jensen, L. T. Skovgaard and J. Viby-Mogensen, Manual evaluation of residual curarization using double burst stimulation: a comparison with train-of-four. *Anesthesiology* **70**, 578-581 (1989).
44. K. Fruergaard, J. Viby-Mogensen, H. Berg and A. M. el Mahdy, Tactile evaluation of the response to double burst stimulation decreases, but does not eliminate, the problem of postoperative residual paralysis. *Acta Anaesthesiol Scand* **42**, 1168-1174 (1998).
45. A. F. Kopman, P. S. Yee and G. G. Neuman, Relationship of the train-of-four fade ratio to clinical signs and symptoms of residual paralysis in awake volunteers. *Anesthesiology* **86**, 765-771 (1997).

EFFECT SITE MODELLING AND ITS APPLICATION IN TCI

Eric Mortier and Michel Struys[*]

1. INTRODUCTION

Rational dosing of anaesthetic drugs derives from an understanding of both the pharmacokinetics and dynamics of the compound in use[1]. This knowledge can be applied to develop strategies to achieve a required therapeutic drug concentration. The pharmacokinetics of intravenous drugs can be described by a polyexponential function [2]:

$$Cp(t) = \sum_{i=1}^{n} c_i . e^{-\lambda_i t}$$

The polyexponential disposition function can be mathematically transformed to a more easily understood compartmental form[3]. In this mammillary model the drug is administered into a central compartment and transfer into peripheral compartments occurs by first-order processes. The classical ways of delivering an intravenous drug to achieve and maintain a specific therapeutic concentration are: single or repeated bolus administration, a zero-order continuous infusion without bolus administration, a bolus combined with a continuous infusion and a bolus combined with a profiled infusion. [4]

2. BOLUS ADMINISTRATION

The most simple technique is to give a single bolus. Obviously, with this approach it is impossible to maintain a constant concentration. If we want to maintain the concentration

---

[*] Eric P. Mortier and Michel M.R.F. Struys, Department of Anaesthesiology , Gent University Hospital, B-9000 Gent, Belgium

Advances in Modelling and Clinical Application of Intravenous Anaesthesia
Edited by Vuyk and Schraag, Kluwer Academic/Plenum Publishers, 2003

above the lowest therapeutic concentration for a prolonged time then we must choose the initial bolus extremely high. This may cause numerous side effects due to the initially high concentrations.[4] Another way to keep the drug concentration above the lowest therapeutic level is to administer smaller doses repeatedly. This repeated bolus technique produces a typical saw-tooth profile, which is hardly synonymous of a stable plasma concentration.[4]

3. BOLUS AND CONTINUOUS INFUSION

With a zero-order continuous infusion, it will take five times the elimination half-life to reach steady-state. For a propofol infusion, it will take more than one hour to equilibrate.[4] A more satisfactory strategy for reaching and maintaining adequate drug concentrations, is the use of a bolus followed by a continuous infusion. If the bolus is targeted to achieve a so-called steady state concentration in the central compartment, a decay occurs that takes some time to recover by the maintenance infusion. The decline in concentration between the initial concentration after the bolus and the concentration at equilibrium is due to the dilution of the bolus into a larger volume than the volume of the central compartment.[3] A compromise is Wagner's dual infusion regimen which uses a two-step infusion scheme with rates I_1 and I_2. With this technique it should be possible to reach the target concentration quickly, overshoot it only modestly and then maintain it at the desired level.[5] The duration of I_1 is chosen based on a compromise between time to reach steady-state and the degree of overshoot that is clinically accepted during the loading portion.[3]

4. BOLUS AND PROFILED INFUSION

Due to the work of Kruger-Thiemer, and later, Vaughan and Tucker and Schwilden and coworkers it became clear that the ideal profile can only be achieved at the price of a slightly more difficult regimen.[6,7,8] The resulting BET scheme (bolus, elimination, transfer) uses a loading dose, a final infusion rate which equates to the clearance and an interim infusion to match the distribution. The BET scheme can be accomplished only by using a computer controlled infusion device. The existing concept was expanded by Schwilden and incorporated into the first computer-controlled infusion system called CATIA.[8] The target concentration is achieved by the administration of a bolus of $C_T.V_1$. Concurrent with the bolus a maintenance infusion is started at the rate $I(t) = C_T.V_1 (k_{10}+ k_{12}e^{-k21t} + k_{13}e^{-k31t})$. Commercially available target-controlled infusion (TCI) devices for propofol incorporate an internal model of propofol pharmacokinetics to rapidly achieve and maintain a constant drug concentration in the plasma.[9] However, for anaesthetic agents, the site of drug-effect is not the plasma.[9] Unfortunately, the concentration of the drug at the site of action is not measurable.[10]

5. EFFECT SITE MODELLING OF PROPOFOL

The apparent rate of drug flow into and from the site of action can be characterised by the time course of drug effect.[3] Knowing this time course, the drug concentration in the biophase can be modelled with the introduction of an additional compartment, the "effect compartment"[2]. It is characterised by a first-order input rate constant (k_{1e}) and a first-order output rate constant (k_{eo}).[10] Assuming that the effect compartment is negligibly small, k_{1e} is an arbitrarily small fraction of k_{eo}.[3] As such, k_{1e} has no influence on the rate of plasma effect site equilibration. Knowing k_{eo}, the apparent concentration in the effect compartment can be calculated, since k_{eo} will precisely describe the temporal effects of equilibration between the plasma concentration and the corresponding drug effect.[11] In a linear, time-invariant, n-compartment model, the central compartment drug concentration resulting from a drug input can be predicted by convolving the drug input with the n-exponential unit disposition function.[12]

If the value of k_{eo} is defined, then there exists an n + 1 - exponential unit disposition function for the effect compartment and the drug concentration in the effect-site can be predicted by convolving the drug input with the n + 1 - exponential unit disposition function.[12] The convolution of the input from the central compartment with the first-order exponential function e^{-keot} (describing loss of drug from the effect site) predicts the amount of drug in the effect compartment. Mathematically [13] this can be expressed as:

$$A_e(t) = k_{1e} \int_0^t e^{-keo(t-\tau)} A_1(\tau) \, d\tau$$

Transforming this expression from the time to the Laplacian's domain (Laplace transformation) yields an expression relating output and input by a transfer function.[14] The time delay of the output profile of the effect site can then be characterised as a first-order process expressed as $1/1 + T_c s$ with $T_c = 1/k_{eo}$ and s being the Laplace operator.[14] Introducing the effect compartment concept into infusion rate control algorithms requires pharmacodynamic modelling. This can be either parametric or semiparametric. The first approach assumes a pharmacokinetic model with a k_{eo} and a pharmacodynamic model driven by the predicted effect site concentration. k_{eo} and the pharmacodynamic model allow us to attribute the effect data directly to the plasma concentration using non-linear regression data analysis.[10] In the semiparametric modelling k_{eo} is estimated without assuming a model.

The dose-plasma concentration relationship is linked with the appropriate k_{eo} to an effect-site concentration-effect relationship. The concentration at the effect site is calculated by means of numerical integration. k_{eo} is defined by a computer program in such a way that the area circumscribed by the hysteresis loop is minimised. By "collapsing the loop", k_{eo} resolves the equilibration delay between plasma concentration and effect-site concentration .[10] A model-independent descriptor of effect-site equilibration exists. It is the time to peak effect.

It can be established by giving a bolus and measuring the drug effect by means of an appropriately sensitive parameter.[15] The time to peak effect can be used to establish the appropriate value of k_{eo} for use with any pharmacokinetic model, provided that a submaximal effect is elicited and that the time of peak effect can be precisely observed. Although several pharmacokinetic sets have been defined for propofol, the Marsh kinetic set is the most popular since it is implemented in the Diprifusor® device developed by Astra Zeneca (Macclesfield, UK).[16] The numerical values of the Marsh set are shown in table 1.

Table 1: Numerical values of the Marsh kinetics of propofol.

Parameter	Value
V_1	0.228 Lkg^{-1}
k_{10}	0.119 min^{-1}
k_{12}	0.112 min^{-1}
k_{21}	0.055 min^{-1}
k_{13}	0.0419 min^{-1}
k_{31}	0.0033 min^{-1}

The accuracy of any parameter set can be described by Standard Performance Parameters, in pooled data as well as in intrasubject data when it is used in computer-assisted continuous infusion systems.[17] In the study of Coetzee and coworkers, the prediction errors and intrasubject performance indices of TCI performance for the Marsh parameter set were by all means acceptable.[18] Athough Wakeling and colleagues already pointed out that, compared with targeting plasma concentrations, targeting the effect site shortens the time to loss of consciousness without adverse cardiovascular effects, an optimal combined pharmacokinetic-pharmacodynamic model that best predicts the time course of propofol drug effect has not yet been validated.[19]

6. TCI CONTROL ALGORITHMS OF PROPOFOL

In a recently published report, Struys and colleagues tested the performance of three TCI control algorithms in one-hunderd twenty healthy female patients.[20] In all three groups the plasma concentrations were calculated by means of the Marsh pharmacokinetics.[16] In group I, the plasma concentration was controlled. In group II and III, the effect site was controlled. In group II, the effect site was computed using a k_{eo} of 0.20 min^{-1} as reported by Billard et al.[21] In group III, a k_{eo} of 1.21 min^{-1}, corresponding to a time to peak effect of 1.6 minutes was used (table 2).[15]

Table 2. Comparison of three different TCI algorithms.

Group I		Group II		Group III
Plasma Control	vs	Effect-site Control[21]	vs	Effect-site Control[15]
		k_{eo} = 0.20 min-1		k_{eo} = 1.21 min-1
		and		and
		time to peak		time to peak
		effect 4.5 min		effect 1.06 min

Each subject received a 12 minutes infusion of propofol to a target of 5.4 µg ml^{-1}. Propofol was administered by a Graseby syringe pump (SIMS Graseby Ltd, Herts,

England). The pump was controlled by RUGLOOP. The algorithms in RUGLOOP are adapted from STANPUMP (available at http: //pkpd.icon.palo-alto.med.va.gov). The PK/PD model was evaluated by six parameters: t_{peak} = the observed time required for reaching maximal drug effect (lowest BIS), within two minutes of loss of consciousness (LOC); t_{eq} = the calculated time required for equilibration between the calculated plasma concentration and the calculated effect-site concentration; $t_{error} = t_{eq}-t_{peak}$; Cp_{max} = the calculated maximum plasma propofol concentration; BIS_{peak} = the observed BIS at t_{peak}; t_{minMAP}: the observed time to lowest arterial blood pressure (defining the onset of cardiovascular side-effect).[20] Patients lost consciousness more slowly when the TCI device targeted the plasma [90 (44-601) seconds in group I, 68 (45-101) seconds in group II, 71 (43-110) seconds in group III]. In group II, the largest dose of propofol was administered (204±36 mg). In group III, the induction dose was similar to that in group I (group I = 114±39 mg; group III = 117±20 mg). Group II was associated with the largest overshoot in plasma propofol concentration (Cp_{max} 14.2 ± 0.4 µgml^{-1} vs. Cp_{max} 7.5 µgml^{-1} in group III) and the fastest onset of "side-effect", e.g. the shortest t_{minMAP}. Controlling the concentration in the effect compartment was more accurate in producing the desired time course of propofol drug effect than when the plasma compartment was controlled.[20]

7. CONCLUSIONS

Effect-site control produces a faster onset of drug effect, without adverse hemodynamic consequences with less variability in the time to loss of consciousness. Since k_{eo} is influenced by the pharmacokinetic model, it may be unwise to mix the k_{eo} from one study with the parmacokinetics of a different study.[22] A model-independent descriptor of equilibration such as time to peak effect is a better choice to define the k_{eo}. However, any value of k_{eo} will produce an overshoot when combined with the Marsh pharmacokinetics, since the Marsh kinetics are particularly poor at describing the rapid initial decrease in plasma concentration. Adjusting the k_{eo} for an incorrect input function can only provide a limited correction to a fundamental "wrong" PK model (Shafer SL, Schnider TW, personal communication). Nevertheless, although using the Marsh pharmacokinetics, combined with a k_{eo} to generate a time to peak effect of 1.6 minutes is not ideal, it is a lot better than targeting the plasma.[20]

8. REFERENCES

1. M. White, M. J. Schenkels, F. H. M. Engbers, A. Vletter, A. L. G. Burm, J.G. Bovill, G. N. C. Kenny, Effect-site modelling of propofol using auditory evoked potentials, *Br. J. Anaesth.* **82**, 333-9 (1999).
2. S. L. Shafer, K.M.Gregg, Algorithms to rapidly achieve and maintain stable drug concentrations at the site of drug effect with a computer-controlled infusion pump, *J. Pharmacokin. Biopharm.* **20**, 147-69 (1992).
3. S. L. Shafer, Principles of pharmacokinetics and pharmacodynamics. *Principles and Practice of Anesthesiology*, edited by: D. E. Longnecker, J. H. Tinker, E. C. Morgan, Mosby-Year Book, Inc., St-Louis, 1159-1210 (1998)
4. M. Struys, Study of the optimalization of anaesthetic-hypnotic drug administration during anaesthesia and sedation *PhD thesis, Ghent University* (1998)
5. J.G. Wagner, A safe method for rapidly achieving plasma concentration plateaus. *Clin. Pharmacol. Therap.* **16**, 691-700 (1974).
6. E. Kruger-Thiemer, Continuous intravenous infusion and multicompartment accumulation. *Eur. J. Pharmacol.* **4**, 317-24 (1968).

7. D. P. Vaughan, G. T. Tucker, General derivation of the ideal intravenous drug input required to achieve and maintain a constant drug concentration. Theoretical application to lignocaine therapy. *Eur. J. Clin. Pharmacol.* **10**, 433-40 (1976).
8. H. Schwilden, A general method for calculating the dosage scheme in linear pharmacokinetics. *Eur. J. Clin. Pharmacol.* **20**, 379-86 (1981).
9. S. L. Shafer, Towards optimal intravenous dosing strategies, *Sem. Anesth.* **12**, 222-34 (1993).
10. T. W. Schnider, C. F. Minto, D. R. Stanski, The effect compartment concept in pharmacodynamic modelling, *Anaesth. Pharmacol. Rev.* **2**, 204-13 (1994).
11. L. B. Sheiner, D. R. Stanski, S. Vozeh, R. D. Miller, J. Ham, Simultaneous modeling of pharmacokinetics and pharmacodynamics: application to d-turbocurarine. *Clin. Pharmacol. Therap.* **25**, 358-71 (1979).
12. R. J. Jacobs, Infusion rate control algorithms for pharmacokinetic model-driven drug infusion devices. *International Anesthesiology Clinics* **33**, 65-82 (1995).
13. J. G. Bovill, Targeting the effect site, in *On the Study and Practice of Intravenous Anaesthesia*, edited by J. Vuyk, F. Engbers, S. Groen-Mulder S, Kluwer Academic Publishers, Dordrecht, Boston, London (2000).
14. K. Morita, T. Kazama, S. Sato, K. Ikeda, Effect sites of intravenous anaesthetic agents, in *On the Study and Practice of Intravenous Anaesthesia*, edited by J. Vuyk, F. Engbers, S. Groen-Mulder S, Kluwer Academic Publishers, Dordrecht, Boston, London (2000).
15. T. W. Schnider, C. F. Minto, S. L. Shafer, P. L. Gambus, C. Andresen, D. B. Goodale, E. J. Youngs, The influence of age on propofol pharmacodynamics, *Anesthesiology* **90**, 1502-16 (1999).
16. B. Marsh, M. White, N. Morton, G. N. C. Kenny. Pharmacokinetic model driven infusion of propofol in children. *Br. J. Anaesth.* **67**, 41-8 (1991).
17. R. A. Veselis, P. Glass, A. Dnistrian, R. Reinsel, Performance of computer-assisted continuous infusion at low concentrations of intravenous sedatives. *Anesth. Analg.* **84**, 1049-57 (1997).
18. J. F. Coetzee, J. B. Glen, C. A. Wium, L. Boshoff, Pharmacokinetic model selection for target controlled infusions of propofol. *Anesthesiology* **82**, 1328-45 (1995).
19. H. G. Wakeling, J. B. Zimmerman, S. Howell, P. S. A. Glass, Targeting effect-compartment or central compartment concentration of propofol, *Anesthesiology* **90**, 92-7 (1999).
20. M. M. R. F. Struys, T. De Smet, B. Depoorter, L. F. M. Versichelen, E. P. Mortier, F. J. E. Dumortier, S. L. Shafer, G. Rolly, Comparison of plasma compartment versus two methods for effect compartment-controlled target-controlled infusion for propofol. *Anesthesiology* **92**, 399-406 (2000).
21. V. Billard, P. L. Gambus, N. Chamoun, D. R. Stanski, S. L. Shafer., A comparison of spectral edge, delta power and bispectral index as EEG measures of alfentanil, propofol and midazolam drug effect. *Clin. Pharmacol. Therap.* **61**, 45-58 (1997).
22. W. V. Gentry, T. C Krejcie, T. K Henthorn, C. A. Shanks, K. A. Howard, D. K. Gupta, M. J. Avram. Effect of infusion rate on thiopental dose-response relationships. Assessment of a pharmacokinetic-pharmacodynamic model. *Anesthesiology* **81**, 316-24 (1994).

REMIFENTANIL; FROM PHARMACOLOGICAL PROPERTIES TO CLINICAL PRACTICE

Frederique Servin[*]

1. INTRODUCTION

Remifentanil is a potent μ-agonist that retains all the pharmacodynamic characteristics of its class (analgesia, haemodynamic stability, respiratory depression, muscle rigidity, nausea and vomiting, pruritus) but with a unique pharmacokinetic profile due to a rapid metabolism by non-specific tissue esterases.[1] Its potency is in the same order of magnitude as that of fentanyl, and it is about 20 times more potent than alfentanil.[2] Its onset of action is similar to that of alfentanil, which reflects similar equilibration times between blood and effect site concentrations, but its duration of effect is much shorter,[3] and its measured context-sensitive half-time averages 3 minutes after an infusion of 3 hours.[4] All these characteristics needed to be integrated in clinical practice overcoming two major obstacles: remifentanil requires an important "cultural" change in the way opioids are dealt with intraoperatively, and in the way postoperative analgesia is planned and carried out. The scope of this review is to summarize remifentanil pharmacological properties and to analyse how these properties have influenced the clinical use of the drug.

2. REMIFENTANIL: BASIC PHARMACOLOGICAL PROPERTIES

2.1. Chemical and Physical Properties

Remifentanil is a μ-receptor agonist[5,6] of the 4-anilidopiperidine series, chemically related to fentanyl, alfentanil and sufentanil. It is the hydrochloride salt of the 3-(4-methoxycarbonyl-4-[(1-oxopropyl)-phenylamino]-1 piperidine) propanoic acid, methyl

[*] Frédérique S. Servin, Service d'Anesthésie-Réanimation, Hôpital Bichat, Paris, France

Advances in Modelling and Clinical Application of Intravenous Anaesthesia
Edited by Vuyk and Schraag, Kluwer Academic/Plenum Publishers, 2003

245

ester. Its molecular weight is 413 and it is a lipophylic drug with an octanol/water partition coefficient of 17.9 at a pH of 7.4. It does not have a chiral centre, and therefore exists in a single form. The modification of the basic anilidopiperidine structure by the introduction of a methylester group onto the N-acyl side chain of the piperidine ring confers to the molecule an increased susceptibility to hydrolytic metabolism by non-specific esterases, which leads to a rapid systemic elimination. It is not a substrate for butyrylcholinesterases and thus its clearance is not affected by cholinesterases deficiency or anticholinergic drugs.[7] It is presented as a water-soluble lyophilised powder containing the free base and glycine as a vehicle to buffer the solution (pH 3; pKa in water 7.07), to be reconstituted in water or 5% dextrose solution for injection. Glycine potentially produces reversible, naloxone insensitive motor dysfunction after continuous, but not after acute, bolus intrathecal administration in rodents.[8] Hence, the spinal or epidural administration of remifentanil in its current formulation is not recommended in humans.

2.2. Pharmacokinetics

Remifentanil was primarily designed to cover the need for a short acting opioid retaining the desirable pharmacodynamic features of fentanyl and its congeners. It was introduced at a time when the anaesthesiologists, through the works of S. Shafer et al.[9] and Hughes et al.[10] understood the importance of considering the decrease in concentration during the early phases after an infusion as opposed to terminal half-life. If a rapid decrease in concentration is desired after an infusion, simulation studies demonstrated that it was beneficial for a drug to exhibit a small central volume of distribution (V1) and a large elimination clearance (Cl_1).[11]

The concentration-time profile of remifentanil is best described by a triexponential function,[12,13] with a high elimination clearance (about 3 L/min) and a small volume of distribution at steady state (around 25 L). Remifentanil clearance is independent of the liver function, and thus is not modified by severe chronic liver disease,[14] or even by the anhepatic phase of liver transplant.[15] Similarly, remifentanil pharmacokinetics are unaffected by renal disease.[16] Nevertheless in this situation, the elimination of the active metabolite is markedly reduced.[16] Apart from the (expected) high clearance, another important feature of remifentanil pharmacokinetics is its quasi independency from body weight, with only the lean body mass appearing as a significant morphological covariate of the model. As a consequence, remifentanil pharmacokinetics are not appreciably different in obese versus lean subjects and in clinical practice, remifentanil dosing regimens should be based on lean body mass and not on total body weight.[17] Remifentanil crosses the placenta[18] but disappears rapidly from the neonate blood due to a high metabolic clearance,[19] and thus has no clinical consequences on the child. Remifentanil pharmacokinetics are very similar in children and in adult patients.[19] In the elderly, remifentanil clearance is reduced.[20] This observation, associated with the well-known increase of elderly patients susceptibility to the pharmacological action of opioids, should lead to markedly decreased dosing recommendations in this population.

2.3. Effect Site Concentration

Remifentanil has a brief half-time for equilibration between plasma and the effect compartment ($t_{1/2}k_{e0}$) of 1.0 – 1.5 min.[21] Its time to peak effect following a bolus dose is 1.5 min.[22] Thus, remifentanil has a short onset, similar to alfentanil, and much shorter than fentanyl or sufentanil.[2,9] After a bolus dose, and due to the rapid equilibration between plasma and the effect compartment, the peak effect site concentration of alfentanil represents a high percentage of the peak plasma concentration.[9] Nevertheless, as remifentanil plasma concentration decreases very quickly after a bolus dose, the peak effect site concentration of remifentanil is proportionally lower than that of alfentanil.

2.4. Context Sensitive Half Time

The time for the effect site concentration to decrease by 50% after the end of a remifentanil infusion (context sensitive half time, CSHT[10]) modelled from the early remifentanil pharmacokinetic analysis[1,12,21] was found to average 3 minutes and to be independent from the duration of infusion. This result was subsequently confirmed by an actual measurement in 30 volunteers receiving a 3 hours infusion of remifentanil or alfentanil.[4] Remifentanil CSHT was 3.2 ± 0.9 min, compared to 47.3 ± 12 min for alfentanil.[4]

2.5. Active Metabolite

Remifentanil is predominantly metabolised by non-specific esterases to an acid metabolite GI-90291 and to a lesser extend by N-dealkylation to a second metabolite GI-94219 [12]. GI-90291 is an analgesic, but its potency (about 0.1% of that of remifentanil) renders its clinical impact negligible. It is excreted through the kidney. Even when accumulation occurs in renal failure patients, the concentrations obtained after a few hours infusion are not sufficient to generate pharmacological effects.[16]

2.6. Pharmacodynamics

Remifentanil is a pure μ agonist analgesic drug which effects are antagonized by naloxone. The analgesic effect is mediated through coupling of a guanine nucleotide binding protein (G-protein), which concomitantly results presynaptically in an inhibition of excitatory neurotransmitter release and postsynaptically in an inhibition of cyclic adenosine monophosphatase, suppression of voltage-sensitive calcium channels and hyperpolarization of the postsynaptic membrane through increased potassium conductance.

2.6.1. Potency

Remifentanil is slightly more potent than fentanyl,[23] and about 20[2] to 40[3,24] times more potent than alfentanil. As a consequence, its range of clinically useful concentrations in anaesthesia is 1-20 ng/ml.

2.6.2. Respiratory Effects

Remifentanil induces a significant depression in the hypoxic drive, reversed by naloxone in a dose related fashion.[25] As might be expected from the pharmacokinetics of the drug, this depression disappears rapidly at the end of the administration.[26] After administration to healthy volunteers of a remifentanil bolus of 0.5 μg/kg, there was a decrease in slope and downward shift of the carbon dioxide ventilatory response curve which reached a nadir approximately 2.5 min after injection, and completely recovered within 15 minutes after injection.[27] This allowed the estimation of k_{e0} (0.34 min^{-1}) and EC_{50} (1.36 ng/ml) for respiratory effect. This ke0 value corresponds to a longer onset time than that observed by Egan for EEG effects.[2] This difference may be related in part to the fact that the EEG and ventilatory drive depend on different neural pathways, that local blood flows may also differ, as well as blood brain barrier characteristics and neural responsiveness to opioids.

2.6.3. Haemodynamic Effects

Remifentanil induces haemodynamic effects (dose-dependent decrease in heart rate, arterial blood pressure and cardiac output) consistent with μ-opioid agonism.[28] As fentanyl, remifentanil exerts a central vagotonic action, leading to bradycardia and hypotension, and associated with a marked increase in sympathetic nerve activity mediated by the arterial baroreflex.[29] These effects have a rapid onset and a short duration, but they may be marked if remifentanil potency is underestimated, specifically in elderly or β-adrenergic blockers treated patients.[30,31] In those patients, titration to effect and slow administration are advocated. When properly used, remifentanil conveys haemodynamic stability similar to that of sufentanil, with a more effective blunting of the increase in arterial pressure at intubation even in haemodynamically-compromised patients.[32] In isolated human right atrial fibers, remifentanil has no negative inotropic effect.[33] The haemodynamic effects of remifentanil are not related to histamine release.[34]

2.6.4. Central Nervous System

Like other μ-opioid agonists, remifentanil reduces cerebral blood flow in dogs.[35] This effect, which is independent from blood pressure control, is predominant in the forebrain and modest in lower brain regions. A positron emission tomography study in human volunteers further precised these topographic findings.[36] Remifentanil induces dose dependent changes in relative cerebral blood flow in areas involved in pain processing. At the highest infusion rate used (0.15 μg/kg/min), regional cerebral blood flow is also modified in structures known to participate in modulation of vigilance and alertness. Under remifentanil-N_2O anaesthesia the global cerebral blood flow is reduced.[37] As a consequence, intracranial pressure is reduced. Autoregulation is preserved.

Non-invasive assessment of cerebral capacity in awake volunteers showed no influence of low remifentanil infusion rates (0.1 μg/kg/min) on this parameter.[38] Remifentanil in rabbits did not influence cerebrospinal fluid formation nor resistance to reabsorption.[39] Under remifentanil /N2O anaesthesia, cerebrovascular reactivity to CO_2 remains intact.[37,40]

Remifentanil has a powerful spinal opioid action.[41] Nevertheless, supramaximal doses of intrathecal remifentanil sufficient to inhibit initial nociceptive behavioural response still permit sufficient glutamate release to allow spinal facilitation.[42] At high concentrations, remifentanil induces EEG changes similar to that of other μ-opioids.[22]

It also induces muscle rigidity with an incidence similar to that observed with equipotent doses of alfentanil.[43] This is probably related to the very rapid onset of effect of the drug.

2.7. Interactions With Hypnotics

Remifentanil acts synergistically with hypnotics, both volatile[23] and intravenous (propofol)[44] for control over intraoperative stimuli. At equipotent concentrations, the interaction is similar to that obtained with other potent μ-opioids,[45] but, due to its rapid offset of effect, the association which will allow a good intraoperative control over adrenergic stimuli and the quickest recovery is shifted towards high remifentanil-low hypnotic concentrations.[46] The synergistic interaction observed for the hypnotic effect in the absence of stimuli is of a lower magnitude.[47]

3. REMIFENTANIL: CLINICAL USE

Any dosage of remifentanil may be used during surgery without undue lengthening of emergence times.[48] In clinical practice, high doses of remifentanil may nevertheless have drawbacks: remifentanil reduces the MAC of isoflurane[23] and the EC_{50} of propofol. The hypnotics may be used at lower concentrations or infusion rates than when other opioids are considered,[49,50] but the reduction in the amount of hypnotics administered increases the risk of awareness during anaesthesia, specifically if the infusion of remifentanil is interrupted.[49] The incidence of postoperative nausea and vomiting is high in opioid-based anaesthetic techniques and remifentanil is no exception.[51] If spontaneous ventilation is planned, the suitable remifentanil concentrations will remain low, and the clinical difference with other potent μ-opioids difficult to demonstrate. The situations were remifentanil may represent a significant clinical improvement are therefore those were a potent analgesic effect is required with a short onset and a rapid offset, specifically if postoperative pain is easily controlled (i.e. with a regional technique).

3.1. Administration Modes

The pharmacokinetics of remifentanil renders its administration by continuous infusion quasi mandatory. Even though it is a forgiving drug, administration diluted through an infusion line by gravity[52] is not recommended if haemodynamics, drug interactions and even the recovery time are to be properly controlled. The 3 ways stopcock, which is usually used to bring remifentanil into the main infusion line, should be as close as possible to the patient to avoid dead space. If a one-way valve is not used, the infusion line should always be carefully purged before recovery and extubation, to avoid delayed boluses leading to apnea.[51,53] The risks of muscle rigidity at induction of anesthesia[54] and/or of haemodynamic instability in risk patients[30] preclude the use of important bolus doses. If a bolus is administered, it should be given over at least 30 seconds. Nevertheless, titration and experience will reduce the incidence of unwanted side effects.[55] A great help might also be the launching in clinical practice of a target controlled infusion (TCI) device for remifentanil, which might allow a direct application of the concentration-effect relationship[44] without risk of administration mistakes.[56] Such a device would be particularly helpful in obese, elderly or cardiac patients.[57] It might also represent a safer way to use remifentanil for postoperative pain control, either through doctor controlled or patient controlled administration.[58]

Closed loop control of hypnosis during anaesthesia and surgery is today feasible, provided any arousal reaction to intraoperative stimuli are blunted which in practice requires the use of remifentanil[59,60] or of epidural analgesia.

3.2. Remifentanil and Regional Anaesthesia

Due to the glycine contained in the current formulation, remifentanil should not be used in regional blocks, for fear of toxic motor impairment.[8]

It has been proposed, alone[61-63] or with propofol[64] for intraoperative sedation in patients undergoing surgery under regional anaesthesia. In this situation, remifentanil may offer some advantages in terms of sedation control, but respiratory depression should be monitored closely and antiemetic prophylaxis should be used in patients at risk. The adequate infusion rate in this situation is around 0.05 to 0.1 µg/kg/min, titrated to effect.

3.3. Tracheal Intubation Without the Use of a Muscle Relaxant

Neuromuscular blocking agents may cause serious side effects but remain in clinical use to facilitate tracheal intubation for lack of a suitable alternative. In the last few years, several anaesthetic protocols associating propofol for its depression of laryngeal reflexes[65] and various doses of opioids, usually alfentanil, have attempted to challenge the quality of intubation provided by muscle relaxants. Nevertheless, laryngoscopy and tracheal intubation are intensely stimulating but brief procedures, which therefore call for a very deep level of analgesia to be maintained only for a short time. The lingering effect of a bolus of fentanyl, sufentanil or alfentanil precludes the use of high opioid concentrations at the time of laryngoscopy for fear of subsequent haemodynamic effects and prolonged respiratory depression when the stimulation is reduced. The pharmacokinetic properties of remifentanil appear ideal for the purpose of blunting the haemodynamic and motor response to tracheal intubation without a needless prolonged effect.

Which is the proper concentration to reach this aim and which dosing regimen might provide it? Guignard et al.[66] have recorded the responses (haemodynamic, motor, EEG arousal) to tracheal intubation in patients receiving a propofol TCI (4 µg/ml) and randomly allocated remifentanil concentrations from 0 to 16 ng/ml. To adequately blunt the haemodynamic, motor and arousal responses to intubation, a concentration of 8 ng/ml remifentanil was required. To reach this concentration a bolus dose of at least 2 µg/kg is required (simulation from the Minto's model[20]). This pharmacokinetic estimation has been confirmed by clinical studies: intubating conditions, haemodynamic responses and duration of apnoea have been estimated in 60 ASA class1 adult patients after an induction of anaesthesia with propofol and either succinylcholine 1 mg/kg, remifentanil 2 µg/kg or remifentanil 4 µg/kg.[67] Intubation could be successfully performed in all patients but 2 in the remifentanil 2 µg/kg group, but only the remifentanil 4 µg/kg group reached the quality of intubating conditions provided by succinylcholine. The duration of apnoea, although acceptable, was longer in the remifentanil groups (2.6 and 2.9 min) than in the succinylcholine group (0.9 min) and the drop in arterial pressure greater (21 and 28% versus 8%). This drop in arterial pressure may reach dangerous levels in elderly or hypertensive patients [68,69], and this technique applies primarily to young healthy patients, including children.[70] The remifentanil dose required to insert a laryngeal mask is lower and was estimated as 0.25 µg/kg in association with propofol.[71,72]

3.4. Control over Intraoperative Stimuli

Clinically, titratability of remifentanil translates into a better control over adrenergic stimuli whatever the type of surgery or the patients.[32,54,73-78] Intraoperative high concentrations will not delay recovery.[4,75,79-88]

3.5. Absence of Residual Opioid Effect, an Advantage or a Drawback?

Microlaryngoscopy is a highly stimulating procedure, but its duration is short, and it is mandatory that the patients, often suffering from CPOD and with frequently some degree of airway obstruction, recover with as little respiratory impairment as possible. In this situation, the absence of residual remifentanil effect is clearly an advantage.[26] In upper intraabdominal surgery, a degree of postoperative respiratory impairment directly related to surgery is also present, and an effective postoperative analgesia is readily provided by central blockade. In this situation, remifentanil provides shorter time to extubation and fewer effects on postoperative SpO$_2$ than sufentanil in the first 7 hours after surgery.[80] On the contrary, remifentanil's lack of residual effect may be a major drawback if postoperative pain control is sub optimal.[89,90]

3.6. Remifentanil and Acute Tolerance

Opioids, as administered in animal studies, may rapidly induce acute tolerance to their effects.[91] In human studies remifentanil, administered for 4 hours to volunteers, induced an analgesic effect, which started to decrease after 60-90 min despite a constant rate infusion [92] After 3 hours of infusion; the effect was only one fourth of the peak value. This result was confirmed in the clinical setting, when Guignard et al. demonstrated an increase in morphine requirements associated with higher pain scores after high intraoperative doses of remifentanil.[93] This effect is not unheard of, and similar findings have already been published with fentanyl[94] and alfentanil.[95,96] Nevertheless, this acute tolerance to remifentanil is not always demonstrated in the clinical setting.[97,98] Schraag et al. administered remifentanil as a target controlled infusion for postoperative pain and could not demonstrate any change in the effectiveness of remifentanil over time.[98] This might nevertheless be compatible with tolerance associated to a reduction in the level of painful stimulus over the first postoperative hours. Cortinez et al. performed a study very similar to that of Guignard, using sevoflurane instead of desflurane.[97] The main difference was that they administered nitrous oxide which is an NMDA receptor antagonist[99] to their patients. Indeed acute tolerance to the effect of opioids seems, at least in part, mediated through the control of µ-opioid receptors by glutaminergic pathways in the central nervous system.[100] Several studies have attempted to demonstrate an improvement in postoperative pain control with infra analgesic doses of ketamine, an NMDA antagonist readily available to anesthesiologists.[101,102] These studies led to contradictory results which might be due to difficulties in defining the proper ketamine dose / concentration and to the wide interindividual variability.

Thus, remifentanil, like other potent opioids, induces acute tolerance, which, due to the rapid disappearance of its analgesic effect, may lead to difficult postoperative pain control after high doses. The co-administration of an NMDA receptor antagonist (ketamine, nitrous oxide) may be helpful.

3.7. Postoperative Analgesia

A major concern when using remifentanil during general anaesthesia is postoperative pain control, which must be planned and initiated before the end of the procedure. Local or regional analgesia, when available, is an obvious option, which brings satisfying results.[80] The absence of postoperative respiratory depression is an advantage in this situation.[80] In moderately painful surgery, adequate analgesia is usually obtained through multimodal analgesia associating various non-opioid analgesics. The major point is to administer the analgesics early enough to account for their onset time.[103]

In major surgery when regional techniques are not available, an elegant solution is to reduce the remifentanil infusion at the end of the procedure to allow spontaneous breathing and extubation while maintaining adequate analgesia.[104] After surgical procedures leading to significant postoperative pain, an infusion rate of remifentanil between 0.05 and 0.15 $\mu g.kg^{-1}.min^{-1}$ ensured adequate analgesia in 78% of the patients during the first hour after surgery, although some patients required doses well outside this range.[51] Even in the carefully controlled setting of a clinical investigation, 8% of the patients became apnoeic or required the administration of naloxone for severe respiratory depression. These events were usually triggered by the administration of a remifentanil bolus. Another risk is the rapid flush of an infusion line containing remifentanil. This risk can be avoided by reducing as much as possible the dead space between the remifentanil line and the patient's blood. The wide interindividual variability of the dosages required calls for patient's control over remifentanil infusion rates. This is best obtained with a patient controlled remifentanil TCI.[58] If postoperative remifentanil infusion is not considered, adequate analgesia can usually be obtained with morphine 0.15 to 0.20 mg/kg injected more than 30 minutes before the end of surgery, then titrated to effect in the PACU before the institution of a PCA.[105,106] An intraoperative dose of morphine 0.25 mg/kg would be excessive in some patients.[90] Adjuvant analgesics (paracetamol, ketamine) may reinforce morphine analgesia.

4. REMIFENTANIL FOR SPECIFIC CLINICAL SITUATIONS

Since it's marketing, remifentanil has been assessed in numerous clinical situations with rather predictable results when considering its pharmacology. Their description would unduly lengthen this review. Only specific fields, which have been an area for discussion, are therefore considered here.

4.1. Cardiac Anaesthesia

Administration of high doses of opioids is a very good way to blunt a stress response, which explains their wide use in cardiac compromised patients. Nevertheless, such administration may lead to delayed recovery and extubation if long acting opioids are used, and other possibly less optimal but cost saving anaesthetic regimen have therefore been advocated to shorten extubation and ICU stay in cardiac surgery.[107] Remifentanil might combine the requirement for intraoperative control of stress response and rapid recovery. A first step towards the use of remifentanil in cardiac surgery was to assess that remifentanil retained its unique pharmacokinetic profile during cardio pulmonary bypass and hypothermia. In fact, during hypothermic CPB, the volume of distribution of remifentanil increases with the institution of CPB and the elimination clearance decreases with hypothermia.[108] If the hypothermia remains mild (around 32°C), the effect of both CPB and hypothermia tend to maintain a fairly stable remifentanil concentration. Conversely a deeper hypothermia will lead to higher remifentanil concentrations, and the infusion rate should therefore be reduced during hypothermic CPB.

In open-heart clinical studies, haemodynamic stability in the remifentanil groups usually compares favourably with that in the fentanyl[74] or sufentanil[109,110] groups, with a better or an equivalent control over major stimuli (sternal spread) and an equivalent control during the rest of the procedure. Nevertheless, several reports of difficult haemodynamic control or of adverse events have been published.[30,111,112] An attentive examination of those reports brings out the difficulties in assessing the potency of the drug and its interactions with other anaesthetic agents, and in most cases a relative overdose in patients often taking β-blockers is likely. The initially recommended remifentanil infusion rate of 1 µg/kg/min generates a stable concentration around 27 ng/ml, whereas a bolus dose of 10 µg/kg fentanyl will allow the fentanyl concentration to peak at 11 ng/ml, when remifentanil is slightly more potent than fentanyl. Anaesthesia with high doses of remifentanil leads to alterations in myocardial perfusion not observed with lower remifentanil doses associated with propofol.[113] Only a careful titration of both the hypnotic and the analgesic component of the anaesthetic protocol may optimise intraoperative control. It might be helpful in that respect to titrate the hypnotic component through EEG monitoring and administer remifentanil through a TCI device. Apart from still sparse experiences of ultrafast track and minimally invasive surgery,[83,114] the time to extubation is usually not different whether remifentanil is used or not.[74,115-117] With the ability to readily obtain spontaneous ventilation, a new perspective is today planned extubation rather than fast-track.[57]

Of course another issue as to the use of remifentanil in cardiac surgery is postoperative pain control. Two analgesic protocol have demonstrated their efficiency: intrathecal administration of morphine[110,115] and i.v. morphine with patient controlled analgesia.[57,83] Please read the manuscript by Barvais et al. in this book for further details regarding remifentanil for cardiac anaesthesia.

4.2. Neuroanaesthesia

During craniotomy, the intensity of painful stimuli varies a lot, and a rapid and predictable emergence is warranted to assess early neurological status after surgery. Remifentanil therefore appears a useful drug in this situation. It allows a better intraoperative haemodynamic control than alfentanil[118] or fentanyl,[73] and less intraoperative isoflurane administration.[81] The recovery time is shorter with remifentanil [81,119] without naloxone administration.[73]

Remifentanil titrability, usually associated with propofol TCI, provides the necessary control over anaesthesia in minimally invasive neurosurgical procedures: awake craniotomies [120-122], stereotaxic neurosurgery,[123] epilepsy surgery,[124,125] magnetic resonance guided neurosurgery.[126]

4.3. Obstetrics

The gold standard for labour pain control is epidural analgesia. Nevertheless, this technique may be contraindicated in cases of sepsis or coagulation disorders for example. In this situation, remifentanil analgesia might be proposed considering the fact that newborns are able to metabolise remifentanil and are therefore not at risk of prolonged respiratory depression at birth.[18] Interest in this technique arose from several case reports describing successful remifentanil analgesia in labor.[127-130] Nevertheless, contradiction was brought by the results of a preliminary investigation of remifentanil as a labour analgesic, which was discontinued due to inadequate pain relief, and the presence of significant opioid-related side effects.[131] This issue was addressed by Saunders in an editorial outlining the fact that not only the pharmacological properties of the drug were important but also the administration mode.[132] The best way to administer remifentanil in labour is probably to provide basal analgesia through a small-dose continuous infusion to which small boluses are added by patient controlled administration. PCA without background infusions usually provides incomplete analgesia,[133] though superior to that provided by meperidine.[134] A patient-controlled remifentanil TCI[58] might be worth studying. Adequate continuous respiratory monitoring then is mandatory.

5. CONCLUSION

The pharmacodynamic profile of remifentanil in clinical practice corresponds to what was expected from this drug from the start: it is versatile, manageable, and when used adequately it increases the patient's safety, by suppressing the risk of delayed respiratory depression. Nevertheless, the current clinical studies have also confirmed that an adequate use of remifentanil could not be achieved without major changes in our management of analgesia, both intra and postoperatively, and in our prescribing habits. At a time when intravenous anaesthesia is maturing rapidly through the wide spread of TCI, remifentanil has taken an important part in this maturation process.

6. REFERENCES

1. T.D. Egan, Lemmens HJ, Fiset P, Hermann DJ, Muir KT, Stanski DR, Shafer SL, The pharmacokinetics of the new short-acting opioid remifentanil (GI87084B) in healthy adult male volunteers. *Anesthesiology* **79**, 881-92 (1993).
2. T.D. Egan, Minto CF, Hermann DJ, Barr J, Muir KT, Shafer SL: Remifentanil versus alfentanil: comparative pharmacokinetics and pharmacodynamics in healthy adult male volunteers. *Anesthesiology* **84**, 821-33 (1996).
3. P.S. Glass, Iselin-Chaves IA, Goodman D, Delong E, Hermann DJ: Determination of the potency of remifentanil compared with alfentanil using ventilatory depression as the measure of opioid effect. *Anesthesiology* **90**, 1556-63 (1999).
4. A. Kapila, Glass PS, Jacobs JR, Muir KT, Hermann DJ, Shiraishi M, Howell S, Smith RL: Measured context-sensitive half-times of remifentanil and alfentanil [see comments]. *Anesthesiology* **83**, 968-75 (1995).
5. T.D. Egan, Remifentanil pharmacokinetics and pharmacodynamics. A preliminary appraisal. *Clin Pharmacokinet* **29**, 80-94 (1995).
6. H. Burkle, Dunbar S, Van Aken H, Remifentanil: a novel, short-acting, mu-opioid, *Anesth Analg*, **83**: 646-51 (1996).
7. J. Manullang, Egan TD, Remifentanil's effect is not prolonged in a patient with pseudocholinesterase deficiency, *Anesth Analg*; **89**, 529-30 (1999).

8. H. Buerkle, Yaksh TL, Continuous intrathecal administration of shortlasting mu opioids remifentanil and alfentanil in the rat, *Anesthesiology*, **84**: 926-35 (1996).

9. S.L. Shafer, Varvel JR, Pharmacokinetics, pharmacodynamics, and rational opioid selection, *Anesthesiology*, **74**: 53-63 (1991).

10. M. Hughes, Glass P, Jacobs R, Context-sensitive half time in multicompartment pharmacokinetic models for intravenous anesthetic drugs, *Anesthesiology*, **76**: 334 - 341 (1992).

11. E.J. Youngs, Shafer SL, Pharmacokinetic parameters relevant to recovery from opioids. *Anesthesiology*, **81**: 833-42 (1994).

12. C.L. Westmoreland, Hoke JF, Sebel PS, Hug CC, Jr., Muir KT, Pharmacokinetics of remifentanil (GI87084B) and its major metabolite (GI90291) in patients undergoing elective inpatient surgery. *Anesthesiology*, **79**: 893-903 (1993).

13. C.F. Minto, Schnider TW, Egan TD, Young E, Lemmens HJM, Gambus PL, Billard V, Hoke JF, Moore KHP, Hermann DJ, Muir KT, Mandema JW, Shafer SL, Influence of age and gender on the pharmacokinetics and pharmacodynamics of remifentanil. I. Model development, *Anesthesiology*, **86**: 10-23 (1997).

14. M. Dershwitz, Hoke JF, Rosow CE, Michalowski P, Connors PM, Muir KT, Dienstag JL, Pharmacokinetics and pharmacodynamics of remifentanil in volunteer subjects with severe liver disease. *Anesthesiology*, **84**: 812-20 (1996).

15. V.U. Navapurkar, Archer S, Gupta SK, Muir KT, Frazer N, Park GR, Metabolism of remifentanil during liver transplantation, *Br J Anaesth*, **81**: 881-6 (1998).

16. J.F. Hoke, Shlugman D, Dershwitz M, Michalowski P, Malthouse-Dufore S, Connors PM, Martel D, Rosow CE, Muir KT, Rubin N, Glass PS, Pharmacokinetics and pharmacodynamics of remifentanil in persons with renal failure compared with healthy volunteers, *Anesthesiology*, **87**: 533-41 (1997).

17. T.D. Egan, Huizinga B, Gupta SK, Jaarsma RL, Sperry RJ, Yee JB, Muir KT, Remifentanil pharmacokinetics in obese versus lean patients, *Anesthesiology*, **89**: 562-73 (1998).

18. R.E. Kan, Hughes SC, Rosen MA, Kessin C, Preston PG, Lobo EP, Intravenous remifentanil: placental transfer, maternal and neonatal effects, *Anesthesiology*, **88**: 1467-74 (1998).

19. A.K. Ross, Davis PJ, Dear Gd GL, Ginsberg B, McGowan FX, Stiller RD, Henson LG, Huffman C, Muir KT, Pharmacokinetics of remifentanil in anesthetized pediatric patients undergoing elective surgery or diagnostic procedures, *Anesth Analg* **93**, 1393-401 (2001).

20. C.F. Minto, Schnider TW, Shafer SL, Pharmacokinetics and pharmacodynamics of remifentanil. II Model application, *Anesthesiology*, **86**: 24-33 (1997).

21. P.S. Glass, Hardman D, Kamiyama Y, Quill TJ, Marton G, Donn KH, Grosse CM, Hermann D, Preliminary pharmacokinetics and pharmacodynamics of an ultra-short-acting opioid: remifentanil (GI87084B), *Anesth Analg*, **77**: 1031-40 (1993).

22. P.L. Gambus, Gregg KM, Shafer SL, Validation of the alfentanil canonical univariate parameter as a measure of opioid effect on the electroencephalogram, *Anesthesiology*, **83**: 747-56 (1995).

23. E. Lang, Kapila A, Shlugman D, Hoke JF, Sebel PS, Glass PS, Reduction of isoflurane minimal alveolar concentration by remifentanil, *Anesthesiology*, **85**: 721-8 (1996).

24. M.L. Black, Hill JL, Zacny JP, Behavioral and physiological effects of remifentanil and alfentanil in healthy volunteers, *Anesthesiology*, **90**: 718-26 (1999).

25. H.M. Amin, Sopchak AM, Esposito BF, Henson LG, Batenhorst RL, Fox AW, Camporesi EM, Naloxone-induced and spontaneous reversal of depressed ventilatory responses to hypoxia during and after continuous infusion of remifentanil or alfentanil, *J Pharmacol Exp Ther*, **274**: 34-9 (1995).

26. R. Wuesten, Van Aken H, Glass PS, Buerkle H, Assessment of depth of anesthesia and postoperative respiratory recovery after remifentanil- versus alfentanil-based total intravenous anesthesia in patients undergoing ear-nose-throat surgery, *Anesthesiology*, **94**: 211-7 (2001).

27. H.D. Babenco, Conard PF, Gross JB, The pharmacodynamic effect of a remifentanil bolus on ventilatory control, *Anesthesiology*, **92**: 393-8 (2000).

28. M.K. James, Vuong A, Grizzle MK, Schuster SV, Shaffer JE, Hemodynamic effects of GI 87084B, an ultra-short acting mu-opioid analgesic, in anesthetized dogs, *J Pharmacol Exp Ther*, **263**: 84-91 (1992).

29. K. Shinohara, Aono H, Unruh GK, Kindscher JD, Goto H, Suppressive effects of remifentanil on hemodynamics in baro-denervated rabbits, *Can J Anaesth*, **47**: 361-6 (2000).

30. P. Elliott, O'Hare R, Bill KM, Phillips AS, Gibson FM, Mirakhur RK, Severe cardiovascular depression with remifentanil, *Anesth Analg*, **91**: 58-61 (2000).

31. J.E. Reid, Mirakhur RK, Bradycardia after administration of remifentanil, *Br J Anaesth*, **84**: 422-3 (2000).

32. S. Mouren, De Winter G, Guerrero SP, Baillard C, Bertrand M, Coriat P, The continuous recording of blood pressure in patients undergoing carotid surgery under remifentanil versus sufentanil analgesia, *Anesth Analg*, **93**: 1402-9, table of contents (2001).

33. J.L. Hanouz, Yvon A, Guesne G, Eustratiades C, Babatasi G, Rouet R, Ducouret P, Khayat A, Bricard H, Gerard JL, The in vitro effects of remifentanil, sufentanil, fentanyl, and alfentanil on isolated human right atria, *Anesth Analg*, **93**: 543-9 (2001).
34. P.S. Sebel PS, Hoke JF, Westmoreland C, Hug CC, Jr., Muir KT, Szlam F, Histamine concentrations and hemodynamic responses after remifentanil, *Anesth Analg*, **80**: 990-3 (1995).
35. W.E. Hoffman WE, Cunningham F, James MK, Baughman VL, Albrecht RF, Effects of remifentanil, a new short-acting opioid, on cerebral blood flow, brain electrical activity, and intracranial pressure in dogs anesthetized with isoflurane and nitrous oxide, *Anesthesiology*, **79**: 107-13, 26A (1993).
36. K.J. Wagner, Willoch F, Kochs EF, Siessmeier T, Tolle TR, Schwaiger M, Bartenstein P, Dose-dependent regional cerebral blood flow changes during remifentanil infusion in humans: a positron emission tomography study, *Anesthesiology*, **94**: 732-9 (2001).
37. N.D. Ostapkovich, Baker KZ, Fogarty-Mack P, Sisti MB, Young WL, Cerebral blood flow and CO_2 reactivity is similar during remifentanil/N2O and fentanyl/N2O anesthesia, *Anesthesiology*, **89**: 358-63 (1998).
38. I.H. Lorenz, Kolbitsch C, Hormann C, Schocke M, Zschiegner F, Felber S, Benzer A, The effects of remifentanil on cerebral capacity in awake volunteers, *Anesth Analg*, **90**: 609-13 (2000).
39. A.A. Artru, Momota T, Rate of CSF formation and resistance to reabsorption of CSF during sevoflurane or remifentanil in rabbits, *J Neurosurg Anesthesiol*, **12**: 37-43 (2000).
40. K.Z. Baker, Ostapkovich N, Sisti MB, Warner DS, Young WL, Intact cerebral blood flow reactivity during remifentanil/nitrous oxide anesthesia, *J Neurosurg Anesthesiol*, **9**: 134-40 (1997).
41. H. Buerkle, Yaksh TL, Comparison of the spinal actions of the mu-opioid remifentanil with alfentanil and morphine in the rat, *Anesthesiology*, **84**: 94-102 (1996).
42. H. Buerkle, Marsala M, Yaksh TL, Effect of continuous spinal remifentanil infusion on behaviour and spinal glutamate release evoked by subcutaneous formalin in the rat, *Br J Anaesth*, **80**: 348-53 (1998).
43. R. Jhaveri, Joshi P, Batenhorst R, Baughman V, Glass PS, Dose comparison of remifentanil and alfentanil for loss of consciousness, *Anesthesiology*, **87**: 253-9 (1997).
44. H. Ropcke, Konen-Bergmann M, Cuhls M, Bouillon T, Hoeft A, Propofol and remifentanil pharmacodynamic interaction during orthopedic surgical procedures as measured by effects on bispectral index, *J Clin Anesth*, **13**: 198-207 (2001).
45. J.E. Peacock, Luntley JB, O'Connor B, Reilly CS, Ogg TW, Watson BJ, Shaikh S: Remifentanil in combination with propofol for spontaneous ventilation anaesthesia, *Br J Anaesth*, **80**: 509-11 (1998).
46. J. Vuyk J, Pharmacokinetic and pharmacodynamic interactions between opioids and propofol, *J Clin Anesth* **9**: 23S-26S (1997).
47. C. Lysakowski, Dumont L, Pellegrini M, Clergue F, Tassonyi E, Effects of fentanyl, alfentanil, remifentanil and sufentanil on loss of consciousness and bispectral index during propofol induction of anaesthesia, *Br J Anaesth*, **86**: 523-7 (2001).
48. M. Dershwitz, Randel GI, Rosow CE, Fragen RJ, Connors PM, Librojo ES, Shaw DL, Peng AW, Jamerson BD, Initial clinical experience with remifentanil, a new opioid metabolized by esterases, *Anesth Analg*, **81**: 619-23 (1995).
49. C.W. Hogue, Jr., Bowdle TA, O'Leary C, Duncalf D, Miguel R, Pitts M, Streisand J, Kirvassilis G, Jamerson B, McNeal S, Batenhorst R, A multicenter evaluation of total intravenous anesthesia with remifentanil and propofol for elective inpatient surgery, *Anesth Analg*, **83**: 279-85 (1996).
50. J. Vuyk, Mertens MJ, Olofsen E, Burm AGL, Bovill JG, Propofol anesthesia and rational opioid selection. *Anesthesiology* **87**: 1549-1562 (1997).
51. T.A. Bowdle, Camporesi EM, Maysick L, Hogue CW, Miguel RV, Pitts M, Streisand JB, A multicenter evaluation of remifentanil for early postoperative analgesia, *Anesth Analg* **83**: 1292-97 (1996).
52. R.J. Fragen, Fitzgerald PC, Is an infusion pump necessary to safely administer remifentanil? *Anesth Analg* **90**: 713-6 (2000).
53. D. Fourel, Almanza L, Aubouin JP, Guiavarch M, Remifentanil, postoperative respiratory depression after purging of the infusion line, *Ann Fr Anesth Reanim* **18**: 358-9 (1999).
54. J. Schuttler, Albrecht S, Breivik H, Osnes S, Prys-Roberts C, Holder K, Chauvin M, Viby-Mogensen J, Mogensen T, Gustafson I, Lof L, Noronha D, Kirkham AJ, A comparison of remifentanil and alfentanil in patients undergoing major abdominal surgery, *Anaesthesia* **52**: 307-17 (1997).
55. G.P. Joshi Jamerson BD, Roizen MF, Fleisher L, Twersky RS, Warner DS, Colopy M, Is there a learning curve associated with the use of remifentanil? *Anesth Analg* **91**: 1049-55 (2000).
56. S.E. Milne SE, Kenny GN, Future applications for TCI systems, *Anaesthesia* **53** Suppl 1: 56-60 (1998).
57. P. Olivier, Sirieix D, Dassier P, D'Attellis N, Baron JF, Continuous infusion of remifentanil and target-controlled infusion of propofol for patients undergoing cardiac surgery: a new approach for scheduled early extubation, *J Cardiothorac Vasc Anesth*, **14**: 29-35 (2000).

58. S. Schraag, Kenny GN, Mohl U, Georgieff M, Patient-maintained remifentanil target-controlled infusion for the transition to early postoperative analgesia, *Br J Anaesth*, **81**: 365-8 (1998).

59. S.E. Milne, Horgan PG, Kenny GN, Target-controlled infusions of propofol and remifentanil with closed-loop anaesthesia for hepatic resection, *Anaesthesia* **57**: 93 (2002).

60. M.M. Struys, De Smet T, Versichelen LF, Van De Velde S, Van den Broecke R, Mortier EP, Comparison of closed-loop controlled administration of propofol using Bispectral Index as the controlled variable versus "standard practice" controlled administration, *Anesthesiology* **95**: 6-17 (2001).

61. M. Lauwers, Camu F, Breivik H, Hagelberg A, Rosen M, Sneyd R, Horn A, Noronha D, Shaikh S, The safety and effectiveness of remifentanil as an adjunct sedative for regional anesthesia, *Anesth Analg* **88**: 134-40, (1999).

62. M.L. Mingus, Monk TG, Gold MI, Jenkins W, Roland C, Remifentanil versus propofol as adjuncts to regional anesthesia. Remifentanil 3010 Study Group, *J Clin Anesth* **10**: 46-53 (1998).

63. F.S. Servin, Raeder JC, Merle JC, Wattwil M, Hanson AL, Lauwers MH, Aitkenhead A, Marty J, Reite K, Martisson S, Wostyn L, Remifentanil sedation compared with propofol during regional anaesthesia, *Acta Anaesthesiol Scand*, **46**: 309-15 (2002).

64. A. Holas, Krafft P, Marcovic M, Quehenberger F, Remifentanil, propofol or both for conscious sedation during eye surgery under regional anaesthesia, *Eur J Anaesthesiol* **16**: 741-8 (1999).

65. E. Sundman, Witt H, Sandin R, Kuylenstierna R, Boden K, Ekberg O, Eriksson LI, Pharyngeal function and airway protection during subhypnotic concentrations of propofol, isoflurane, and sevoflurane: volunteers examined by pharyngeal videoradiography and simultaneous manometry, *Anesthesiology* **95**: 1125-32 (2001).

66. B. Guignard, Menigaux C, Dupont X, Fletcher D, Chauvin M, The effect of remifentanil on the bispectral index change and hemodynamic responses after orotracheal intubation, *Anesth Analg* **90**: 161-7 (2000).

67. I.A. McNeil, Culbert B, Russell I, Comparison of intubating conditions following propofol and succinylcholine with propofol and remifentanil 2 micrograms kg-1 or 4 micrograms kg-1, *Br J Anaesth* **85**: 623-5 (2000).

68. A.S. Habib, Parker JL, Maguire AM, Rowbotham DJ, Thompson JP, Effects of remifentanil and alfentanil on the cardiovascular responses to induction of anaesthesia and tracheal intubation in the elderly, *Br J Anaesth* **88**: 430-3 (2002).

69. A.M. Maguire AM, Kumar N, Parker JL, Rowbotham DJ, Thompson JP, Comparison of effects of remifentanil and alfentanil on cardiovascular response to tracheal intubation in hypertensive patients, *Br J Anaesth* **86**: 90-3 (2001).

70. U.M. Klemola, Mennander S, Saarnivaara L, Tracheal intubation without the use of muscle relaxants: remifentanil or alfentanil in combination with propofol, *Acta Anaesthesiol Scand* **44**: 465-9 (2000).

71. M.P. Lee, Kua JS, Chiu WK, The use of remifentanil to facilitate the insertion of the laryngeal mask airway, *Anesth Analg* **93**: 359-62 (2001).

72. K. Grewal, Samsoon G, Facilitation of laryngeal mask airway insertion: effects of remifentanil administered before induction with target-controlled propofol infusion, *Anaesthesia* **56**: 897-901 (2001).

73. J. Guy, Hindman BJ, Baker KZ, Borel CO, Maktabi M, Ostapkovich N, Kirchner J, Todd MM, Fogarty-Mack P, Yancy V, Sokoll MD, McAllister A, Roland C, Young WL, Warner DS, Comparison of remifentanil and fentanyl in patients undergoing craniotomy for supratentorial space-occupying lesions, *Anesthesiology* **86**: 514-24 (1997).

74. M.B. Howie, Cheng D, Newman MF, Pierce ET, Hogue C, Hillel Z, Bowdle TA, Bukenya D, A randomized double-blinded multicenter comparison of remifentanil versus fentanyl when combined with isoflurane/propofol for early extubation in coronary artery bypass graft surgery, *Anesth Analg* **92**: 1084-93 (2001).

75. D.P. Cartwright, Kvalsvik O, Cassuto J, Jansen JP, Wall C, Remy B, Knape JT, Noronha D, Upadhyaya BK, A randomized, blind comparison of remifentanil and alfentanil during anesthesia for outpatient surgery, *Anesth Analg* **85**: 1014-9 (1997).

76. J.R. Sneyd, Camu F, Doenicke A, Mann C, Holgersen O, Helmers JH, Appelgren L, Noronha D, Upadhyaya BK, Remifentanil and fentanyl during anaesthesia for major abdominal and gynaecological surgery. An open, comparative study of safety and efficacy, *Eur J Anaesthesiol* **18**: 605-14 (2001).

77. R.R. McGregor, Allan LG, Sharpe RM, Thornton C, Newton DE, Effect of remifentanil on the auditory evoked response and haemodynamic changes after intubation and surgical incision, *Br J Anaesth* **81**: 785-6 (1998).

78. M. Gemma, Tommasino C, Cozzi S, Narcisi S, Mortini P, Losa M, Soldarini A, Remifentanil provides hemodynamic stability and faster awakening time in transsphenoidal surgery, *Anesth Analg* **94**: 163-8 (2002).

79. P.W. Doyle, Coles JP, Leary TM, Brazier P, Gupta AK, A comparison of remifentanil and fentanyl in patients undergoing carotid endarterectomy, *Eur J Anaesthesiol*, **18**: 13-9 (2001).

80. A. Casati, Albertin A, Fanelli G, Deni F, Berti M, Danelli G, Grifoni F, Torri G, A comparison of remifentanil and sufentanil as adjuvants during sevoflurane anesthesia with epidural analgesia for upper abdominal surgery: effects on postoperative recovery and respiratory function, *Anesth Analg* **91**: 1269-73 (2000).

81. G. Balakrishnan, Raudzens P, Samra SK, Song K, Boening JA, Bosek V, Jamerson BD, Warner DS, A comparison of remifentanil and fentanyl in patients undergoing surgery for intracranial mass lesions, *Anesth Analg* **91**: 163-9 (2000).

82. A.Y. Bekker, Berklayd P, Osborn I, Bloom M, Yarmush J, Turndorf H, The recovery of cognitive function after remifentanil-nitrous oxide anesthesia is faster than after an isoflurane-nitrous oxide-fentanyl combination in elderly patients, *Anesth Analg* **1**: 117-22 (000).

83. J. Ohanen, Olkkola KT, Verkkala K, Heikkinen L, Jarvinen A, Salmenpera M, A comparison of remifentanil and alfentanil for use with propofol in patients undergoing minimally invasive coronary artery bypass surgery, *Anesth Analg* **90**: 1269-74 (000).

84. G. Natalini, Fassini P, Seramondi V, Amicucci G, Toninelli C, Cavaliere S, Candiani A, Remifentanil vs. fentanyl during interventional rigid bronchoscopy under general anaesthesia and spontaneous assisted ventilation, *Eur J Anaesthesiol* **16**: 605-9 (1999).

85. L.H. Wee, Moriarty A, Cranston A, Bagshaw O, Remifentanil infusion for major abdominal surgery in small infants, *Paediatr Anaesth* **9**: 415-8 (1999).

86. R.S. Twersky, Jamerson B, Warner DS, Fleisher LA, Hogue S, Hemodynamics and emergence profile of remifentanil versus fentanyl prospectively compared in a large population of surgical patients, *J Clin Anesth* **13**: 407-16 (2001).

87. L.A. Fleisher, Hogue S, Colopy M, Twersky RS, Warner DS, Jamerson BD, Tuman KJ, Glass PS, Roizen MF, Does functional ability in the postoperative period differ between remifentanil- and fentanyl-based anesthesia? *J Clin Anesth* **13**: 401-6 (2001).

88. W. Wilhelm, Schlaich N, Harrer J, Kleinschmidt S, Muller M, Larsen R, Recovery and neurological examination after remifentanil-desflurane or fentanyl-desflurane anaesthesia for carotid artery surgery. *Br J Anaesth* **86**: 44-9 (001).

89. P.J. Davis, Finkel JC, Orr RJ, Fazi L, Mulroy JJ, Woelfel SK, Hannallah RS, Lynn AM, Kurth CD, Moro M, Henson LG, Goodman DK, Decker MD, A randomized, double-blinded study of remifentanil versus fentanyl for tonsillectomy and adenoidectomy surgery in pediatric ambulatory surgical patients, *Anesth Analg* **90**: 863-71 (2000).

90. D. Fletcher, Pinaud M, Scherpereel P, Clyti N, Chauvin M, The efficacy of intravenous 0.15 versus 0.25 mg/kg intraoperative morphine for immediate postoperative analgesia after remifentanil-based anesthesia for major surgery, *Anesth Analg* **90**: 666-71 (2000).

91. B.M. Cox, Ginsburg M, Osman OH: Acute tolerance to narcotic analgesic drugs in rats, *British Journal of Pharmacology* **33**: 245-56 (1968).

92. H.R. Vinik, Kissin I: Rapid development of tolerance to analgesia during remifentanil infusion in humans, *Anesth Analg* **86**: 1307-11 (1998).

93. B. Guignard, Bossard AE, Coste C, Sessler DI, Lebrault C, Alfonsi P, Fletcher D, Chauvin M, Acute opioid tolerance: intraoperative remifentanil increases postoperative pain and morphine requirement, *Anesthesiology* **93**: 409-17 (2000).

94. Y.Y. Chia, Liu K, Wang JJ, Kuo MC, Ho ST, Intraoperative high dose fentanyl induces postoperative fentanyl tolerance, *Can J Anaesth* **46**: 872-7 (1999).

95. I. Kissin, Lee SS, Arthur GR, Bradley EL, Jr., Time course characteristics of acute tolerance development to continuously infused alfentanil in rats, *Anesth Analg* **83**: 600-5 (1996).

96. J.W. Mandema, Wada DR, Pharmacodynamic model for acute tolerance development to the electroencephalographic effects of alfentanil in the rat, *J Pharmacol Exp Ther* **275**: 1185-94 (1995).

97. L.I. Cortinez, Brandes V, Munoz HR, Guerrero ME, Mur M, No clinical evidence of acute opioid tolerance after remifentanil-based anaesthesia, *Br J Anaesth* **87**: 866-9 (2001).

98. S. Schraag, Checketts MR, Kenny GN, Lack of rapid development of opioid tolerance during alfentanil and remifentanil infusions for postoperative pain, *Anesth Analg* **89**: 753-7 (1999).

99. V. Jevtovic-Todorovic, Todorovic SM, Mennerick S, Powell S, Dikranian K, Benshoff N, Zorumski CF, Olney JW, Nitrous oxide (laughing gas) is an NMDA antagonist, neuroprotectant and neurotoxin, *Nat Med* **4**: 460-3 (1998).

100. I. Kissin, Bright CA, Bradley EL, Jr., The effect of ketamine on opioid-induced acute tolerance: can it explain reduction of opioid consumption with ketamine-opioid analgesic combinations? *Anesth Analg*; **91**, 1483-8 (2000).

101. E.S. Fu, Miguel R, Scharf JE, Preemptive ketamine decreases postoperative narcotic requirements in patients undergoing abdominal surgery, *Anesth Analg* **84**: 1086-90 (1997).

102. W. Jaksch, Lang S, Reichhalter R, Raab G, Dann K, Fitzal S, Perioperative small-dose S(+)-ketamine has no incremental beneficial effects on postoperative pain when standard-practice opioid infusions are used, *Anesth Analg* **94**: 981-6 (2002).

103. P.E. Pendeville, Kabongo F, Veyckemans F: Use of remifentanil in combination with desflurane or propofol for ambulatory oral surgery, *Acta Anaesthesiol Belg* **52**: 181-6 (2001).

104. E. Calderon, Pernia A, De Antonio P, Calderon-Pla E, Torres LM. A comparison of two constant-dose continuous infusions of remifentanil for severe postoperative pain, *Anesth Analg* **92**: 715-9 (2001).

105. E. Kochs, Cote D, Deruyck L, Rauhala V, Puig M, Polati E, Verbist J, Upadhyaya B, Haigh C, Postoperative pain management and recovery after remifentanil-based anaesthesia with isoflurane or propofol for major abdominal surgery, *Br J Anaesth* **84**: 169-73 (2000).

106. H.S. Minkowitz, Postoperative pain management in patients undergoing major surgery after remifentanil vs. fentanyl anesthesia, *Can J Anaesth* **47**: 522-8 (2000).

107. D.C.H. Cheng, Karski J, Peniston C, Raveendran G, Asokumar B, Carroll J, David T, Sandler A, Early tracheal extubation after coronary artery bypass graft srugery reduces costs and improves resource use, *Anesthesiology* **85**: 1300-1310 (1996).

108. L.G. Michelsen LG, Holford NH, Lu W, Hoke JF, Hug CC, Bailey JM, The pharmacokinetics of remifentanil in patients undergoing coronary artery bypass grafting with cardiopulmonary bypass, *Anesth Analg* **93**: 1100-5 (2001).

109. A. Lehmann, Zeitler C, Thaler E, Isgro F, Boldt J, Comparison of two different anesthesia regimens in patients undergoing aortocoronary bypass grafting surgery: sufentanil-midazolam versus remifentanil-propofol, *J Cardiothorac Vasc Anesth* **14**: 416-20 (2000).

110. P. Latham, Zarate E, White PF, Bossard R, Shi C, Morse LS, Douning LK, Chi L, Fast-track cardiac anesthesia: a comparison of remifentanil plus intrathecal morphine with sufentanil in a desflurane-based anesthetic, *J Cardiothorac Vasc Anesth* **14**: 645-51 (2000).

111. T. Möllhoff T, Herregods L, Moerman A, Blake D, MacAdams C, Demeyere R, Kirnö K, Dybvik T, Shaikh S, Group TRS, Comparative efficacy and safety of remifentanil and fentanyl in "fast track"coronary artery bypass graft surgery: a randomized, double-blind study, *Br J Anaesth* **87**: 718-26 (2001).

112. J.Y. Wang JY, Winship SM, Thomas SD, Gin T, Russell GN, Induction of anaesthesia in patients with coronary artery disease: a comparison between sevoflurane-remifentanil and fentanyl-etomidate, *Anaesth Intensive Care* **27**: 363-8 (1999).

113. S. Kazmaier S, Hanekop GG, Buhre W, Weyland A, Busch T, Radke OC, Zoelffel R, Sonntag H, Myocardial consequences of remifentanil in patients with coronary artery disease, *Br J Anaesth* **84**: 578-83 (2000).

114. G.N. Djaiani GN, Ali M, Heinrich L, Bruce J, Carroll J, Karski J, Cusimano RJ, Cheng DC, Ultra-fast-track anesthetic technique facilitates operating room extubation in patients undergoing off-pump coronary revascularization surgery, *J Cardiothorac Vasc Anesth* **15**: 152-7 (2001).

115. E. Zarate, Latham P, White PF, Bossard R, Morse L, Douning LK, Shi C, Chi L, Fast-track cardiac anesthesia: use of remifentanil combined with intrathecal morphine as an alternative to sufentanil during desflurane anesthesia, *Anesth Analg* **91**: 283-7 (2000).

116. M. Engoren, Luther G, Fenn-Buderer N, A comparison of fentanyl, sufentanil, and remifentanil for fast-track cardiac anesthesia, *Anesth Analg* **93**: 859-64 (2001).

117. D.C. Cheng, Newman MF, Duke P, Wong DT, Finegan B, Howie M, Fitch J, Bowdle TA, Hogue C, Hillel Z, Pierce E, Bukenya D, The efficacy and resource utilization of remifentanil and fentanyl in fast-track coronary artery bypass graft surgery: a prospective randomized, double-blinded controlled, multi-center trial, *Anesth Analg* **92**: 1094-102 (2001).

118. J.R. Sneyd, Whaley A, Dimpel HL, Andrews CJ, An open, randomized comparison of alfentanil, remifentanil and alfentanil followed by remifentanil in anaesthesia for craniotomy, *Br J Anaesth* **81**: 361-4 (1998).

119. J.P. Coles, Leary TS, Monteiro JN, Brazier P, Summors A, Doyle P, Matta BF, Gupta AK, Propofol anesthesia for craniotomy: a double-blind comparison of remifentanil, alfentanil, and fentanyl, *J Neurosurg Anesthesiol* **12**: 15-20 (2000).

120. H. Berkenstadt H, Perel A, Hadani M, Unofrievich I, Ram Z, Monitored anesthesia care using remifentanil and propofol for awake craniotomy, *J Neurosurg Anesthesiol* **13**: 246-9 (2001).

121. K.B. Johnson KB, Egan TD, Remifentanil and propofol combination for awake craniotomy: case report with pharmacokinetic simulations, *J Neurosurg Anesthesiol* **10**: 25-9 (1998).

122. T. Tijero, Ingelmo I, Garcia-Trapero J, Puig A: Usefulness of Monitoring Brain Tissue Oxygen Pressure During Awake Craniotomy for Tumor Resection: A Case Report, *J Neurosurg Anesthesiol* **14**: 149-152 (2002).

123. A.M. Debailleul, Bortlein ML, Touzet G, Krivosic-Horber R, Particularités anesthésiques de la neurochirurgie stéréotaxique, *Ann Fr Anesth Reanim* **21**: 170-8 (2002).

124. I.A. Herrick IA, Craen RA, Blume WT, Novick T, Gelb AW, Sedative doses of remifentanil have minimal effect on ECoG spike activity during awake epilepsy surgery, *J Neurosurg Anesthesiol* **14**: 55-8 (2002).

125. C.T. Wass, Grady RE, Fessler AJ, Cascino GD, Lozada L, Bechtle PS, Marsh WR, Sharbrough FW, Schroeder DR, The effects of remifentanil on epileptiform discharges during intraoperative electrocorticography in patients undergoing epilepsy surgery, *Epilepsia* **42**: 1340-4 (2001).

126. H. Berkenstadt, Perel A, Ram Z, Feldman Z, Nahtomi-Shick O, Hadani M, Anesthesia for magnetic resonance guided neurosurgery: initial experience with a new open magnetic resonance imaging system. *J Neurosurg Anesthesiol* **13**: 158-62 (2001).

127. R. Jones, Pegrum A, Stacey RG, Patient-controlled analgesia using remifentanil in the parturient with thrombocytopaenia. *Anaesthesia* **54**: 461-5 (1999).

128. F. Roelants, De Franceschi E, Veyckemans F, Lavand'homme P, Patient-controlled intravenous analgesia using remifentanil in the parturient, *Can J Anaesth* **48**: 175-8 (2001).

129. J.A. Thurlow, Waterhouse P, Patient-controlled analgesia in labour using remifentanil in two parturients with platelet abnormalities, *Br J Anaesth* **84**: 411-3 (2000).

130. M.D. Owen, Poss MJ, Dean LS, Harper MA, Prolonged intravenous remifentanil infusion for labor analgesia, *Anesth Analg* **94**: 918-9 (2002).

131. A.J. Olufolabi, Booth JV, Wakeling HG, Glass PS, Penning DH, Reynolds JD, A preliminary investigation of remifentanil as a labor analgesic. *Anesth Analg* **91**: 606-8 (2000).

132. T.A. Saunders, Glass PS, A trial of labor for remifentanil. *Anesth Analg* **94**: 771-3 (2002).

133. J.M. Blair, Hill DA, Fee JP, Patient-controlled analgesia for labour using remifentanil: a feasibility study. *Br J Anaesth* **87**: 415-20 (2001).

134. J.A. Thurlow, Laxton CH, Dick A, Waterhouse P, Sherman L, Goodman NW, Remifentanil by patient-controlled analgesia compared with intramuscular meperidine for pain relief in labour, *Br J Anaesth* **88**: 374-8 (2002).

135. P.O. Maitre, Vozeh S, Heykants J, Thomson JA, Stanski DR, Population pharmacokinetics of alfentanil: average dose-plasma concentraiton relationship and interindividual variability, *Anesthesiology* **66**: 3-12 (1987).

ADVANCES IN REGIONAL ANAESTHESIA AND ANALGESIA

Alain Borgeat, Georgios Ekatodramis[*]

1. INTRODUCTION: PAIN AS A REALITY

Despite intense research in the last three decades and exciting new revelations in the physiology and pharmacology of nociception, it remains a common misconception among anaesthesiologists that acute postoperative pain is a transient condition involving physiological nociceptive stimulation, with a variable effective component, that differs markedly in its pathophysiological basis from chronic pain syndromes. However, it is known that clinical pain differs from physiological pain and that acute and chronic pain share common mechanisms. Acute postoperative pain still remains a major problem after surgery. The significant improvements that have been observed over the last years have resulted mostly from better organization and management and more intensive application of long-established drugs and techniques rather than, to date, the synthesis of new "magic drugs". The introduction of acute pain teams with the use of patient-controlled analgesia and epidural infusions of either local anaesthetic or a mixture of local anaesthetic and opioid on surgical wards represent major advances in improving patient well being compared to previous decades.

Preoperative and post-traumatic pain therapy in clinical practice still has major deficits. The problem persists despite the fact that efficient drugs and adequate techniques (central or peripheral blocks) are available for the management of acute pain. Reasons that can explain this situation are insufficient education,[1] lack of interest especially of surgeons,[2] fear of side effects and a lack of the standards and organization of backgrounds necessary to improve acute pain therapy.[3] The beneficial impact of recent developments is illustrated by two surveys conducted among surgical patients in a university hospital.[4] In 1989, when asked about the severity of their pain on the second postoperative day, 71% of those patients not managed by an acute pain service (APS) had moder-

[*] Alain Borgeat and Georgios Ekatodramis, Department of Anesthesiology, Orthopedic University Clinic Zurich/Balgrist, CH-8008 Zurich, Switzerland

Advances in Modelling and Clinical Application of Intravenous Anaesthesia
Edited by Vuyk and Schraag, Kluwer Academic/Plenum Publishers, 2003

261

ate pain and 19% severe. Six years later after implementation of pain treatment guidelines in the same department, 73% of the patients rated their pain intensity as "low" and only 6% of patients rated their pain as severe. Although great progress has been made, a considerable scope remains for further improvement in postoperative care. Among the targets the surgeons have to be taken into account. Indeed, a recent survey showed the need for better education of the surgeons.[5] The survey demonstrated that

- 81% of the surgeons felt uncomfortable with pain management
- 50% of the surgical departments had no guidelines for the management
- 62% of the surgeons believed that an interdisciplinary pain service was needed.

One of the most recent discoveries is the implication of insufficient postoperative pain control in the process of pain chronification. Indeed, Hyes and Molloy found in patients with chronic pain problems that 14% believed that previous surgery was the initiating factor and many of these patients were thought to have neuropathic pain in the postoperative phase.[6] The foregoing suggests that there is a continuum of pain after surgery ranging from acute to chronic and, moreover, that effective treatment of the acute variety, particularly when accompanied by a neuropathic element, will prevent the development of chronic pain syndromes. These concepts emphasize on the need to apply the best drugs and techniques available. In this context recent studies have demonstrated the great efficacy of regional techniques to control postoperative pain.[7, 8] Anaesthesiologists have a place of choice to deal with pain. Brian Ready wrote ten years ago "Anaesthetists are a logical choice to provide pain relief in the immediate postoperative period, since they are familiar with the pharmacology of analgesics, ... are knowledgeable about pain pathways and their interruption and are skilled in the techniques needed to offer multiple forms of pain control ..."

2. ADVANTAGES OF REGIONAL ANAESTHESIA

There has been undoubtedly renewed interest in regional anaesthesia and analgesia. Apart from a renewed emphasis on perioperative analgesia, improved techniques, equipment and drugs, this increase can be attributed to a perceived improvement in outcome. With current improvements in both intraoperative general and regional anaesthesia, it is unlikely that for unselected patients, differences in outcome will be found for the intraoperative interval. Nevertheless, if advances in regional anaesthesia are to continue to add value to surgical patients, and if regional methods are to become more widely accepted by anaesthesiologists, surgeons and patients, more work is needed to prove that such techniques really offer measurable advantages over other methods that are perceived to be „easier", faster, and less dependent on specific technical skills, such as general anaesthesia or postoperative patient-controlled analgesia.

Furthermore, despite our major concerns about minimizing pain in all of our patients, the demonstrated advantages probably need to go beyond simply showing that pain assessment scores are improved or that less morphine is needed by patients. Without such concrete information on benefits, it becomes more difficult to introduce effectively the analgesic methods, particularly in the face of concerns about rare but severe complications such neuraxial hematoma.[9]

Traditionally, studies have focused on „major" outcomes like death, blood loss, cardiac and pulmonary complications. Davis and colleagues demonstrated that spinal anaesthesia reduced blood loss during hip replacement surgery.[10] Christopherson et al.[11] showed an improved surgical outcome among patients undergoing peripheral vascular surgery with epidural anaesthesia and analgesia, and Liu et al.[12] showed that for relatively healthy patients undergoing colon surgery, epidural anaesthesia and analgesia provided the best balance of analgesia and side-effect profile along with improved gastrointestinal function and time-to-reach-discharge criteria. Unfortunately, as noted, many of these studies have focused on big outcomes: transfusion requirements, death, and surgical revision rates. Such outcomes are critically important to the population studied but are not easily transferable to the great majority of healthy young patients in whom regional anaesthesia might be applicable.

There is no question that the field of regional anaesthesia and perioperative pain medicine needs studies to show that choosing general anaesthesia over regional produces outcome improvement. In this context, peripheral nerve blocks, using single-shot and continuous techniques have taken a front seat in recent years by their ability to improve home readiness, rehabilitation scores and patient satisfaction compared with i.v. narcotic therapy after orthopaedic surgery for both upper and lower extremity procedures.

A variety of factors influence discharge times after ambulatory surgery, but the most common reasons for delay in discharge are persistent pain, nausea, and drowsiness. Peripheral nerve blocks reduce the incidence of these factors by reducing the use of narcotics and eliminating the need of general anaesthesia. In a study of factors influencing home readiness, peripheral nerve blockade for upper extremity surgery improved home readiness time by more than 70 minutes compared with „fast track" general anaesthesia techniques.[13] D' Alessio and co-workers documented a 30 minute improvement in street readiness after shoulder arthroscopy with interscalene block compared with general anaesthesia.[14] For lower extremity surgery, peripheral nerve blockade techniques are less well established but likely to be at least as effective as upper extremity peripheral nerve blockade. Ankle block has long been recognized as a safe and effective technique with a very high patient satisfaction rating.[15] Vloka and colleagues recently compared popliteal block to spinal anaesthesia for short-vein stripping.[16] The patients who received peripheral nerve blockade were discharged 70 minutes faster than those who received spinal anaesthesia. Borgeat and colleagues improved pain scores and satisfaction for patients receiving continuous interscalene blockade for analgesia after major shoulder surgery compared with patients receiving i.v. narcotics.[17] These authors particularly noted the improvement in analgesia during physical therapy. In a more recent study the same researchers could show that the performance of interscalene block with a standardized technique and drug application is associated with a low rate of long term neurological complications (0.4%), which are not related to the use of an interscalene catheter.[18]

Rehabilitation is particularly important after total knee arthroplasty. Two studies have recently shown improvement in rehabilitation outcome after this procedure when continuous peripheral nerve blockade was compared with IV narcotics analgesia.[7, 19] Both studies confirmed lumbar plexus blockade to be as efficacious as epidural analgesia after total knee arthroplasty. However, continuous lumbar plexus blockade has several distinct advantages compared with epidural analgesia, including unilateral block, reduced urinary retention, and reduction of the low but real risk of spinal haematoma in the anticoagulated patient receiving epidural analgesia.

These results support clearly the concept that postoperative analgesia is moving toward peripheral nerve techniques. More studies, especially on the upper extremities, are needed to further show the positive effect of continuous peripheral nerve blockade on the surgical outcome in orthopaedic patients.

3.   WHY ARE LOCAL ANAESTHETICS BENEFICIAL?

How can we understand the clinical advantages associated with the use of local anaesthetics? By looking at the different pain pathways that follow surgical trauma, we may notice that two of them can be efficiently blocked only by local anaesthetics. These two are firstly the segmental reflex responses, responsible for the pain associated with muscular reflex spasms, decreased thoracic compliance, bronchoconstriction, ileus and urinary retention and secondly the supra-segmental reflex responses (associated with the activity of the sympathetic systems), responsible for an increased blood pressure and cardiac output. Their involvement is demonstrated by a generalized increase of body oxygen consumption. Opioids are ineffective to block either the segmental or supra-segmental responses.

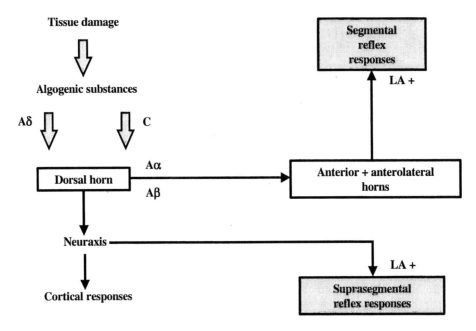

Figure 1. The implications of the operative surgical trauma on pain pathways. Only local anaesthetics (LA) are effective to block the segmental and supra-segmental reflex responses.

If we look closely at the interaction between drugs and nerves, we notice that opioids on the contrary to local anaesthetics are not very effective to block A delta nerve fibres, ineffective against A alpha, A beta and the sympathetic nerves. Opioids block the C nerves and have a strong modulation of pain within the central nervous system. The relative inefficacy of opioids on the group of A nerves is explained by the fact that opioids may act presynaptically to inhibit C, but not A delta, neurotransmission, and postsynaptically on dorsal horn cells that receive input from A delta and or C fibre-nociceptors.[20] Consistent with this is the fact that tonic postsurgical pain is generally well controlled by opioids, [21, 22] whereas wound movement pain requires much higher doses, [23] necessitating other drugs to attenuate A delta mediated pain.

Table 1. Interaction between drugs and nerves.

	Local Anaesthetics	Morphine
C	+++	+++
Aδ	+++	(+)
Aα	+++	-
Aβ	+++	-
Sympathetic	+++	-
CNS	?	+++

4. ADVANCES IN THE APPLICATION OF REGIONAL TECHNIQUES

Post-operative pain is a major problem, particularly after orthopaedic limb surgery. It not only causes the patient discomfort, but also compromises early physical therapy, which is the most influential factor for post-operative rehabilitation and ambulation.[24] Severe reflex muscular spasms may hinder mobilization particularly after major shoulder, hip or knee surgery.[25] A prolonged pain free period is today a requisite in orthopaedic surgery requiring the placement of perineural catheter since Salter[26] was able to demonstrate that continuous passive motion has a significant stimulating effect on the healing of articular tissues, including cartilage, tendons and ligaments, prevents adhesions and joint stiffness, does not interfere with the healing of incisions over the moving joint and, indeed, enhances such healing, and finally makes the regeneration of articular cartilage possible through neochondrogenesis, both with and without periostal grafts. The results of the study of Capdevila et al. are in accordance with this concept.[7] Indeed, the authors were able to show a significant better knee flexion and shorter rehabilitation in patients receiving regional analgesia as compared to those having a patient-controlled iv analgesia with morphine. Shoulder surgery is also associated with severe postoperative pain making early rehabilitation very difficult. Major progress has been made possible with the use of perineural catheter. The interscalene catheter has brought great progress to the management of postoperative pain therapy after major open shoulder surgery. Indeed, studies have shown that a continuous infusion of local anaesthetics through an interscalene catheter as compared to traditional PCA with opioids, provides significantly better control of pain, with statistically lower incidence of side-effects and greater patient's satisfaction.[17, 27, 28] The interscalene catheter is indicated in almost all open shoulder surgeries, the rotator cuff repair being the "gold indication". According to the type of surgery performed, the catheter may be used for 3 to 5 days.

Due to the great amount of periarticular structures rich with nociceptors in the shoulder, postoperative pain is not only severe during movement, but also at rest, making a bolus technique alone inadequate in this context, as shown by Singelyn et al.[28] The use of a continuous infusion of 0.125% bupivacaine at a rate of 0.125 ml kg^{-1} h^{-1} was shown to provide efficient pain relief, but at the cost of administrating a large volume of local anesthetics.[28] Moreover, a continuous infusion may not be the best way of administration for this purpose, since it does not comply with the dynamic nature of pain, which is moderate to severe at rest and severe to very severe during movement. The use of a continuous infusion with supplemental boli seems to be more appropriate.

When compared to the continuous technique,[29] a lower basal infusion of 5 ml h^{-1} of bupivacaine 0.125% associated with small PCA boli of 2.5 ml within 30 minutes provides similar pain control, but reduces the consumption of local anaesthetics by 37% and lowers the incidence of side-effects, such as Horner's syndrome or clinically apparent phrenic paresis.[28] Borgeat et al.[17, 27] have shown that both bupivacaine 0.15% or ropivacaine 0.2% at a rate of 5 ml h^{-1} with supplemental boli of 4 ml within 20 minutes were associated with better pain control, lower incidence of nausea, vomiting and pruritus and better patient's satisfaction, as compared to the classical PCA with opioids. In the PCIA (patient controlled interscalene analgesia), all patients were extremely satisfied with the possibility to rapidly reinforce the block shortly before and after a physical therapy session. In our department we have switched from bupivacaine to ropivacaine, since we demonstrated that PCIA with ropivacaine 0.2% compared to PCIA with bupivacaine 0.15% was associated with better preservation of hand strength 24 h and 48 h after the beginning of the infusion as well as 6 h after the infusion was stopped.[30] The incidence of paraesthesias in the fingers 48 h after the start and 6 h after the end of the infusion was also significantly higher in the bupivacaine group. Actually the application of the PCIA technique with a basal infusion and supplemental boli is the most appropriate technique for analgesia after major open shoulder surgery. The use of ropivacaine as compared to bupivacaine seems to have some advantages in terms of better sensorimotor dissociation.[31, 32] The concentration of ropivacaine 0.2% is adequate for most patients, but has to be increased up to 0.3 or 0.4% in some others, particularly young, athletic patients (unpublished data).

5. CONCLUSIONS

There is no doubt that the application of perineural catheters allowing prolonged continuance of local anaesthetics represents the most recent and most promising progress in regional anaesthesia. These techniques not only improve patient well being, but also have a positive impact on the surgical outcome. This is the new challenge for anaesthesiologists.

6. REFERENCES

1. T. H. Gould, P. M. Upton, and P. Collins, A survey of the intended management of acute postoperative pain by newely qualified doctors in the South West region of England in August 1992, *Anesthesia* **49**, 807-810 (1994).
2. E. Neugebauer and H. Trodl, Meeting report - Meran consensus conference on pain after surgery and trauma, *Thor. Surg.* **3**, 220-224 (1989).
3. C. Maier, J. Wawersik, and H. Wulf, Results of a survey on postoperative epidural analgesia in Western Germany, *Anästhesist* **40**, 61-70 (1991).
4. C. Maier, M. Raetzel, and H. Wulf, Audit in 1989 and 1994 of the Department of Anaesthesiology and Intensive Care, Hospital of Christian-Albrechts-University, Schwanenweg 21, D24105, Kiel, Germany.
5. E. Neugebauer, K. Hepel, S. Sauerland, M. Lempa, G. Koch, The status of perioperative pain therapy in Germany. Results of a representative, anonymous survery of 1,000 surgical clinics, *Chirurg.* **69**, 461-466 (1998).
6. C. Hayes and A. R. Molloy, Neuropathic pain in the perioperative period, *Int. Anaesth. Clin.* **35**, 67-81 (1997).
7. X. Capdevila, Y. Barthelet, P. Biboulet, Y. Ryckwaert, J. Rubenovitch, and F. d'Athis, Effects of perioperative analgesic technique on the surgical outcome and duration of rehabilitation after major knee surgery, *Anesthesiology* **91**, 8-15 (1999).
8. A. Rodgers, N. Walter, S. Schug, A. McKee, H. Kehlet, A. van Zundert, D. Sage, M. Futter, G. Saville, T. Clark, and S. MacMahon, Reduction of postoperative mortality and morbidity with epidural or spinal anaesthesia: results from overview of randomised trials, *Br. Med. J.* **321**, 1-12 (2000).
9. T. T. Horlocker and D. J. Wedel, Neuraxial block and low-molecular-weight heparin: Balancing perioperative analgesia and thromboprophylaxis, *Reg. Anesth. Pain Med.* **23**, 164-77 (1998).
10. F.M. Davis, E. McDermott, C. Hickton, E. Wells, D. C. Heaton, V. G. Laurenson, W. J. Gillespie, and J. Foate, Influence of spinal and general anaesthesia on haemostasis during total hip arthroplasty, *Br. J. Anaesth.* **59**, 561-571 (1987).
11. R. Christopherson, C. Beattie, S. M. Frank, E. J. Norris, C. L. Meinert, S. O. Gottlieb, H. Yates, P. Rock, S. D. Parker, B. A. Perler, and G. M. Williams, Perioperative morbidity in patiens randomized to epidural or general anesthesia for lower extremity vascular surgery, *Anesthesiology* **79**, 422-434 (1993).
12. S. S. Liu, R. L. Carpenter, D. C. Mackey, R. C. Thirlby, S. M. Rupp, T. S. J. Shine, N. G. Feinglass, P. P. Metzger, J. T. Fulmer, and S. L. Smith, Effects of perioperative analgesic technique on rate of recovery after colon surgery, *Anesthesiology* **83**, 757-767 (1995).
13. D. J. Pavlin, S. E. Rapp, N. L. Polissar, J. A. Malmgren, M. Koerschgen, and H. Keyes, Factors affecting discharge time in adult outpatients, *Anesth. Analg.* **87**, 816-826 (1998).
14. J. G. D'Alessio, M. Rosenblum, K. P. Shea, and D. G. Freitas, A retrospective comparison of interscalene block and general anesthesia for ambulatory surgery shoulder arthroscopy, *Reg. Anesth.* **20**, 62-68 (1995).
15. T. H. Lee, K. L. Wapner, P. J. Hecht, and P. J. Hunt, Regional anesthesia in foot and ankle surgery. *Orthopedics* **19**, 577-580 (1996).
16. J. D. Vloka, A. Hadzic, R. Mulcare, J. B. Lesser, R. Koorn, and D. M. Thys, Combined popliteal and posterior cutaneous nerve of the thigh for short saphenous vein strippin gin outpatients: an alternative to spinal anesthesia. *J. Clin. Anesth.* **9**, 618-622 (1997).
17. A. Borgeat, B. Schäppi, N. Biasca, and C. Gerber, Patient-controlled analgesia after major shoulder surgery, *Anesthesiology* **87**, 1343-1347 (1997).
18. A. Borgeat, G. Ekatodramis, F. Kalberer, and C. Benz, Acute and nonacute complications associated with interscalene block and shoulder surgery, *Anesthesiology* **95**, 875-880 (2001).
19. F. J. Singelyn, M. Deyaert, D. Joris, E. Pendeville, and J. M. Gouverneur, Effects of intravenous patient-controlled analgesia with morphine, continuous epidural analgesia, and continuous three-in-one block on postoperative pain and knee rehabilitation after unilateral total knee arthroplasty, *Anesth. Analg.* **87**, 88-82 (1998).
20. V. Pirec, C. E. Laurito, Y. Lu, and D. C. Yeomans, The combined effects of N-type calcium challen blockers and morphine on Aβ versus C fiber mediated nociception, *Anesth. Analg.* **92**, 239-243 (2001).
21. H. E. Torebjörk and R. G. Hallin, Perceptual changes accompanying controlled preferential blockings of A and C fibre responses in intact human skin nerves, *Exp. Brain Res.* **16**, 321-321 (1973).
22. D. Le Bars, G. Guilbaud, and J. M. Besson, Differential effects of morphine on responses of dorsal horn lamina V type cells elicited by A and C fibre stimulation in the spinal cat, *Brain Res.* **115**, 518-524 (1976).
23. A. S. Keats, Postoperative pain: research and treatment, *J. Chronic Diseases* **4**, 72-83 (1956).
24. J. Ryu, S. Saito, K., and S. Sano, Factors influencing the postoperative range of motion in total knee arthroplasty. *B. Hosp. Joint Diseases* **53**, 35-40 (1993)

25. J. J. Bonica, Postoperative pain, in: *The Management of Pain*, edited by J. J. Bonica, Lea & Febiger, Philadelphia, 1990, pp. 461-480.

26. R. B. Salter, History of rest and motion and the scientific basis for early continuous passive motion, *Hand Clin.* **12**, 1- 11 (1996).

27. A. Borgeat, E. Tewes, N. Biasca, and C. Gerber, Patient-controlled interscalene analgesia with ropivacaine after major shoulder surgery: PCIA vs PCA, *Br. J. Anaesth.* **81**, 603-605 (1998).

28. F. Singelyn, S. Seguy S, and J. M. Gouverneur, Interscalene brachial plexus analgesia after open shoulder surgery: continuous versus patient-controlled infusion, *Anesth. Analg.* **89**, 1216-1220 (1999).

29. P. Pere, The effect of continuous interscalene brachial plexus block with 0.125% bupivacaine plus fentanyl on diaphragmatic motility and ventilatory function, *Reg. Anesth.* **18**, 93-97 (1993).

30. A. Borgeat, F. Kalberer, H. Jacob, Y. A. Ruetsch, and C. Gerber, Patient-controlled interscalene analgesia with ropivacaine 0.2% versus bupivacaine 0.15% after major open shoulder surgery: the effects on hand motor function, *Anesth. Analg.* **92**, 218-223 (2001).

31. P. H. Rosenberg and E. Heinonen, Differential sensitivity of A and C nerve fibres to long-acting amide local anaesthetics, *Br. J. Anaesth.* **55**, 163-167 (1983).

32. J. A. Wildsmith, D. T. Brown, D. Paul, and S. Johnson, Structure-activity relationships in differential nerve block at high and low frequency stimulation, *Br. J.Anaesth.* **63**, 444-452 (1989).

KETAMINE, REVIVAL OF A VERSATILE INTRAVENOUS ANAESTHETIC

Johan Raeder[*]

1. INTRODUCTION

Ketamine has been in clinical use for more than 35 years for emergency cases and field surgery. However, there still remains much to discover about this compound and the clinical applications of ketamine have expanded considerably from its initial use as a dissociative anaesthetic. Presently the analgesic and immunologic properties are continuously been explored, as well as its use for total intravenous anaesthesia.

2. BASIC PHARMACOLOGY

The main molecular target of ketamine is the NMDA glutamate receptor, where it acts as a non-competitive antagonist. In addition to binding to the NMDA receptor ketamine also reduces the pre-synaptic release of glutamate. Antagonism of muscarinic and nicotinic acetylcholine receptors also appear to be clinically relevant.[1] It has been suggested that actions at the nicotinic receptor may be responsible for the behavioural side effects of ketamine.[2] Potentiation of GABA inhibition [3] has also been reported with high doses of ketamine, although a study by Flood and colleagues using clinically relevant concentrations did not show any GABA effect.[4] A weak affinity for the opioid receptors has also been proposed. However, a recent study with sedative doses in volunteers showed that neither the effects of ketamine or ketamine-induced side effects were influenced by the opioid antagonist, naloxone.[5]

Durieux and colleagues have shown that ketamine inhibits the formation of nerve growth factor in a preparation of human smooth muscle cells. This may be a possible

---

[*] J. Raeder, Department of Anaesthesiology, Ullevaal University Hospital, N-0407 Oslo, Norway

Advances in Modelling and Clinical Application of Intravenous Anaesthesia
Edited by Vuyk and Schraag, Kluwer Academic/Plenum Publishers, 2003

mechanism for the proposed pre-emptive analgesic effect of ketamine and local anaesthetics in the periphery.[6] A pre-emptive effect of epidural ketamine has recently been reported in a clinical setting.[7] However, in a study of mechanisms of secondary hyperalgesia, Koppert et al. were not able to find any peripheral effect from intradermal injection of ketamine into an experimentally traumatised area.[8] High concentrations of ketamine did, have a weak local anaesthetic effect.

Ketamine is a racemic mixture of the isomers R(-)-ketamine and S(+)-ketamine. The latter is 3-4 times as potent as an analgesic and has a 35% higher clearance and similar distribution volumes compared with R(-)-ketamine.[9] Interestingly, both isomers have the same potency for interaction with cholinergic receptors, which may explain the higher incidence of pscomimetic side effects with R(-)-ketamine when given in equianalgesic doses of S(+)-ketamine.[2, 10] The main metabolite is norketamine, which has an analgesic potency close to that of R(-)-ketamine and may contribute significantly to analgesia when ketamine is given by the oral route and thus subjected to a high degree of first-pass metabolism.[1]

3. CEREBRAL AND ANAESTHETIC EFFECTS

Sakai et al. studied different doses of ketamine during concomitant propofol infusion (30 mg kg^{-1} h^{-1}) looking for effects of the combination on sleep, reaction to noxious stimuli and EEG bispectral analysis (BIS).[11] They found the interaction between propofol and ketamine to be additive, apart from the EEG response, where ketamine reversed the decrement in BIS value observed when sleep was induced with propofol alone. Whereas patients usually have a BIS value of 50-60 or lower during anaesthesia, Mok found that BIS increased above 90 when patients sedated with midazolam were put to sleep by adding ketamine.[12] In a study of patients with a BIS score of 44 (mean value) during unstimulated propofol sleep, the BIS score increased to 59 when ketamine was given.[13] Friedberg, however, showed that ketamine may block the increase in BIS otherwise observed when a patient is exposed to noxious stimuli during propofol hypnosis.[14] The positive effect of ketamine on noxious stimulation during anaesthetic induction was also studied by Hans and colleagues who compared thiopentone 5 mg with ketamine 2.5 mg kg^{-1} for intubation conditions one minute after rocuronium 0.6 mg kg^{-1} was given.[15] Although the degree of neuromuscular block was similar in the two groups, the vocal cord relaxation and the diaphragmatic response to intubation were significantly more favourable after ketamine. This could be due to the analgesic effect of ketamine contributing to better intubating conditions.

Whereas ketamine may increase intracranial pressure [1], recent studies suggest many aspects of ketamine's actions to indeed be of advantage for the patient with cerebral damage or otherwise in need of intracranial surgery. During propofol anaesthesia with normocapnoea, Sakai demonstrated that adding ketamine did not alter the middle cerebral artery blood flow or cerebrovascular CO_2 response.[16] Denz found increased arterial pressure and cerebral perfusion pressure with S(+)-ketamine in pigs after asystole, with no increase in brain edema which was favourable compared to saline controls during barbiturate and opioid anaesthesia.[17] Nagase found a reduced cerebrovascular vasodilatatory response to increased PCO_2 in patients given ketamine.[18] The response returned to normal values after administration of nitroglycerine, suggesting that ketamine inhibition of nitric oxide (NO) formation may be responsible for the blunted vasodilatation. However, during ketamine anaesthesia, cerebrovascular autoregulation seems to be preserved, whereas inhalational anaesthesia may impair and slow down the vasoregulatory response.[19] In a rat experimental model of cerebral glucose metabolism, S(+)-ketamine reduced or maintained cerebral metabolism in most regions of the brain, whereas R(-)-ketamine resulted in increased metabolism in one third of the regions and decreased metabolism in most of the remainder.[20]

4. CARDIOVASCULAR EFFECTS

It is commonly stated that ketamine acts as a myocardial depressant on isolated heart muscle preparations, but in vivo this is counteracted by the sympathomimetic effect that results in positive inotropy and chronotropy.[1] Research into this area is difficult. Animal experiments can be confounded by species differences and studies on human heart is limited, most often confined to atrial muscle obtained from patients with cardiovascular disease undergoing cardiac surgery. However, recent research has elucidated some of these aspects. Kienbaum and co-workers studied sympathetic activity in peroneal nerves and muscles in healthy volunteers receiving ketamine anaesthesia.[21] They found a decreased sympathetic output when systemic blood pressure increased during ketamine anaesthesia. The sympathetic nerve outflow normalised when the blood pressure was kept stable with nitroprusside, indicating that normal baroreflex control in response to increased blood pressure was maintained during ketamine anaesthesia. However, the plasma concentrations of both adrenaline and noradrenaline increased and they concluded that ketamine has a predominant effect of decreasing cathecholamine re-uptake, causing an increased sympatomimetic tone locally in the tissues. This is supported by the study of Kunst and co-workers who found that clinical doses of racemic ketamine increased the contractile force in isolated human myocardium.[22] This effect was more pronounced with S-ketamine, and was not seen with R-ketamine. The effect was blocked by the β-adrenoceptor antagonist esmolol and augmented by dopamine. At higher concentrations both isomers had negative effects on contractility.[22] In a study looking at propofol induction, the concomitant use of ketamine ressulted in significantly less drop in blood pressure than propofol induction alone.[23] In a study on renal blood flow in rats, ketamine produced better maintenance of renal blood flow compared with propofol anaesthesia, which again was better than barbiturates.[24]

5. RESPIRATORY EFFECTS

Whereas the respiratory effects of ketamine has been described as minor, with some reduction in airway reflexes with increasing dose[1], a study by Persson and co-workers has elucidated the effects of ketamine on alfentanil-induced hypoventilation in volunteers.[25] The alfentanil-induced reduction of ventilation rate was antagonised by ketamine in a dose dependant manner, whereas there was no effect on the response to increased carbon dioxide. In a study at high altitudes, Bishop found respiration and oxygenation to be surprisingly well preserved in spontaneously breathing patients during ketamine anaesthesia.[26]

6. EFFECTS ON IMMUNOFUNCTION

During sepsis and post-ischaemic reperfusion of brain or heart-muscle tissue, activation of neutrophil granulocytes with subsequent endothelial adhesion and tissue migration may worsen the outcome by production of cytokines and other reactive proteins. Whereas ketamine has little effect on the vascular endothelium, studies by both Zahler and Weigand demonstrated a significant reduction by ketamine in leucocyte activation during hypoxia or sepsis.[27, 28] Ketamine suppressed pro-inflammatory cytokine production in human whole blood in vitro.[29] In a study of the different isomer effects on isolated guinea pig hearts, S-ketamine was more effective in reducing neutrophil adhesion whereas R-ketamine had a negative effect by worsening the coronary vascular fluid leakage into surrounding tissue.[30] A reduction in cellular adhesion by ketamine has been demonstrated both on leucocytes and platelets.[31]

7. USE FOR SEDATION

Frey and colleagues compared the combination of propofol and ketamine with propofol alone for sedation of elderly patients during retrobulbar block.[32] They found a faster onset and better quality of sedation in the ketamine plus propofol group, without side effects such as hallucinations or any need for assistance of ventilation. In a study of children during MRI, Haeseler and coworkers used midazolam and ketamine combination rectally for induction and intravenously for maintenance with excellent clinical characteristics.[33]

Administration of ketamine with the Stanpump target control system [34] at plasma concentrations of 100 –200 ng ml^{-1}, in combination with alfentanil 50 ng ml^{-1} in volunteers, produced subjective effects of abnormal perception in almost all subjects, whereas a ketamine concentration of 50 ng ml^{-1} did not result in such effects.[25] One volunteer (out of eight) developed reversible anxiety and agitation with the 200 ng/ml concentration. Ketamine is also been increasingly used as a narcotic drug in addicts, with reports of hallucinations containing both pleasant and very frightening elements.[35, 36] In a study of ketamine titrated for intravenous sedation Gruber and colleagues found amnesia in 133 out of 134 patients, 14 patients developed transient oxygen desaturation, but there was only one case of hallucinations or bad dreams.[37] Friedberg reported on 2059 office-based plastic surgery procedures performed successfully with 2 mg midazolam, adding a propofol infusion until sleep, then adding 50 mg ketamine before application of local anaesthesia and further continuation with propofol.[38] Ninety nine percent of the patients had SpO2 > 90% breathing room air, and only 2% of the patients needed anti-emetic medication. The high degree of safety and beneficial clinical characteristics of ketamine sedation and analgesia have also resulted in the use of ketamine for emergency patients by non-anaesthesiologists. A practice recently discussed and recommended, provided appropriate guidelines are adhered to [39].

8. USE IN GENERAL ANAESTHESIA

Recent reviews by Bergman and by Granry have elucidated the use of ketamine for sedation, general anaesthesia and pain control in children.[3, 40] In a case report of severe status asthmaticus in an 8-month-old infant, Nehama reported excellent results with an infusion of ketamine.[41] He also provided a comprehensive review of the use of ketamine in children. In a study of etomidate induction and low dose rocuronium (0.6 mg kg^{-1}) the addition of ketamine 0.5 mg kg^{-1} resulted in better intubating conditions than the addition of fentanyl 1.5 µg kg^{-1}.[42] When used for general anaesthesia in adults, premedication and co-administration of anticholinergics and benzodiazepines are recommended. Combinations of ketamine with opioids, propofol or midazolam provide a safe and stable total intravenous technique for maintenance of anaesthesia.[43] Depending on the choice and dose of concomitant drug(s), a typical induction dose of 1-2.5 mg kg^{-1} may be used, followed by an infusion of 2-6 mg kg^{-1}h^{-1}.

9. USE AS AN ANALGESIC

The use of low-dose ketamine in the management of acute postoperative pain has been reviewed by Schmid and colleagues in a survey covering the literature from 1966 – 1998.[44] They concluded that low-dose ketamine (i.e. less than 1mg kg^{-1} i.v. or epidural bolus, less than 20 µg kg^{-1} min^{-1} infusion or less than 2 mg kg^{-1} i.m.) is a valuable adjunct to other drugs for post-operative pain control. Some nausea or psychomimetic effects have been reported , but the overall incidence of side effects may also be reduced when an opioid sparing effect is accomplished by the use of ketamine. In a study of ketamine supplementation for pain control after outpatient surgery, a reduction in opioid requirements of 40% was demonstrated with ketamine 75 µg.kg^{-1} i.v., whereas 100 µg kg^{-1} resulted in increased drowsiness.[46] Infusing ketamine 150 µg kg^{-1} h^{-1} and Patient Controlled Analgesia (PCA) with morphine for 48 hours post-operatively reduced morphine requirements by almost 50% compared with placebo and also reduced the overall incidence of nausea.[47] In a study of epidural analgesia in terminal cancer patients, addition of ketamine 0.2 mg mg kg^{-1} to morphine increased the duration and quality of analgesia significantly.[48] A similar dose has also been used successfully i.v. in terminal cancer patients with severe pain despite high doses of opioids.[49]

The use of ketamine for chronic pain treatment is controversial. Whereas some authors report improved effects of morphine and possible less development of opioid tolerance with very low-dose infusion of ketamine, others are less enthusiastic.[50, 51] In patients with chronic neuropathic pain only 3 out of 21 patients experienced additional analgesia from adding oral ketamine to their analgesic regimen.[52] Many of these patients reported side effects, such as dizziness, somnolence, and strange feelings, but only one had bad dreams. In a recent review Sang discussed the role of ketamine and other NMDA-receptor antagonists in the treatment of neuropathic pain.[53] She concluded that although these drugs produce a definite effect, their use may be limited by dose restrictions due to occurrence of side effects.

10. PRE-EMPTIVE ANALGESIA AND SECONDARY HYPERALGESIA

Blocking pain mediators before pain is initiated may reduce the subsequent need for analgesics due to reduction of wind-up mechanisms in the spinal cord. The NMDA receptors in the spinal cord have been shown to be responsible for such wind-up, and NMDA receptor block with ketamine has been shown to induce pre-emptive analgesia in experimental models.[54] In a clinical study involving patients undergoing cholecystectomy an astonishing effect of giving a low dose of ketamine before surgery on postoperative pain was reported by Roytblat and colleagues.[55] A 10 mg dose of ketamine resulted in a 40% reduction in opioid consumption during the first five hours after cholecystectomy. However any pre-emptive analgesic effect of a low dose of ketamine pre-operatively compared with double-blind administration of the same dose post-operatively had not been confirmed in more recent studies. Mathisen and co-workers found no effect when R-ketamine 1 mg.kg^{-1} was given pre-operatively before laparoscopic cholecystectomy.[56] Adam et al. reported a similar negative result with racemic ketamine 0.15 mg.kg^{-1} for total mastectomy.[57] Dahl et al. found no pre-emptive effect of ketamine 0.4 mg.kg^{-1} in patients undergoing hysterectomy.[58] In these three studies ketamine given at the end of anaesthesia had a short-lasting hypnotic and analgesic effect compared with placebo, whereas the preoperative administration had no effects. In contrast Fu and colleagues found a significant analgesic effect lasting 48 hours after mastectomy with a preoperative dose of ketamine 0.5 mg kg^{-1} compared with postoperative administration.[59] The interpretation of this study is obscured by administration of a continuous perioperative ketamine infusion to the pre-emptive group but not to the control group. The administration of ketamine 0.15 mg kg^{-1} during arthroscopic knee anterior ligament repair was also without a pre-emptive effect, but interestingly this study demonstrated a reduction in analgesia and need of analgesic rescue for 48 hours in the two groups who received the low, single dose of ketamine.[60] Wu et al. found a significant pre-emptive effect of supplementing perioperative epidural lidocaine with a bolus epidural dose of ketamine 10 mg combined with morphine 1 mg in 10 ml of bupivacaine 0.085% in patients undergoing upper abdominal surgery.[7] In another study, Stubhaug and co-workers found significant reduction in post-operative hyperalgesia after 2 days by giving a continuous infusion of low-dose ketamine (1-2 μg kg^{-1} min^{-1}) peri-operatively and for two subsequent days.[61] Interestingly, the subjective pain and analgesic rescue consumption were not reduced in this meticulosly designed study, but the reduction in hyperalgesia strongly suggests an effect on wind-up phenomena with this regimen.

Thus, no studies have so far demonstrated a true pre-emptive clinical effect of a single dose of ketamine, and it still remains somewhat controversial as to whether ketamine may have analgesic effect outlasting the duration of adequate analgesic drug plasma concentrations. One problem with studies of the pre-emptive effect of ketamine is that an effect of a single drug may be concealed by possible pre-emptive effects of other drugs (e.g. opioids, local anaesthetics) used concomitantly. However, the use of continuous peri-operative low-dose ketamine in combination with other drugs in an i.v. or intrathecal multimodal mode seems promising for further studies.

11. CONCLUSION

Until recently the use of ketamine has mainly been restricted to induction of anaesthesia in hypovolaemic or cardiovascularly compromised patients, in paediatric anaesthesia or as a simple, almost complete general anaesthetic for anaesthesia under primitive or poorly equipped conditions. Recent research, however, seems to open the door for a wider use of this interesting and unique drug. The discovery of the role of the NMDA receptor in analgesia, wind-up phenomena and possible opioid tolerance is one major arena for ketamine. The immunomodulating property is another exciting area of research, which may yield results of importance during septicaemia and hypoxic injury of the brain, heart and other organs. The development of S-ketamine as a drug with better clinical properties and potency, less side effects and higher clearance compared with the currently used racemate ketamine is a third area of interest, which looks especially promising in neurosurgery and surgery of patients with cardiac disease.

The general picture of ketamine side effects such as increased intracranial pressure, increased cardiac risk, high rate of nausea and increased salivation needs to be greatly modified. Whereas concerns about dose-related psychomimetic effects and rare cases of hallucinations are still valid, the risks of these side effects may be greatly reduced by concomitant use of propofol, midazolam and other anaesthetic drugs. Ketamine anaesthesia has some unique characteristics and is not possible to monitor or titrate using EEG derived parameters, such as the bispectral index (BIS). However, ketamine is still, after more than 35 years, a safe and very useful anaesthetic, preserving haemodynamic and respiratory functions.

12. REFERENCES

1. R. Kohrs and M. E. Durieux, Ketamine: Teaching an Old Drug New Tricks, *Anesth. Analg.* **87**, 1186-1193 (1998).
2. P. Flood, Intravenous anesthetic inhibition of neuronal nAChRs, *Anesthesiology* **91**, A806(2000).
3. S. A. Bergman, Ketamine: review of its pharmacology and its use in pediatric anesthesia, *Anesth. Prog.* **46**, 10-20 (1999).
4. P. Flood and M. Krasowski, Ketamine: A general anesthetic that does not potentiate GABA-a receptors, *Anesth. Analg.* **90**, S408 (2000).
5. S. Mikkelsen, S. Ilkjaer, J. Brennum, F. M. Borgbjerg, and J. B. Dahl, The effect of naloxone on ketamine-induced effects on hyperalgesia and ketamine-induced side effects in humans, *Anesthesiology* **90**, 1539-1545 (1999).
6. M. E. Durieux, T. Sherer, W. Steers, and J. Tuttle, Local anesthetics and ketamine inhibit nerve growth factor secretion, *Anesthesiology* **91**, A856 (1999).
7. C. T. Wu, C. C. Yeh, J. C. Yu, M. N. Lee, P. L. Tao, S. T. Ho, and C. S. Wong, Pre-incisional epidural ketamine, morphine and bupivacaine combined with epidural and general anaesthesia provides pre-emptive analgesia for upper abdominal surgery, *Acta Anaesthesiol. Scand.* **44**, 63-68 (2000).
8. W. Koppert, S. Zeck, J. A. Blunk, M. Schmelz, R. Likar, and R. Sittl, The effects of intradermal fentanyl and ketamine on capsaicin-induced secondary hyperalgesia and flare reaction, *Anesth. Analg.* **89**, 1521-1527 (1999).
9. T. K. Henthorn, T. C. Krejcie, C. U. Niemann, C. Enders-Klein, and M. J. Avram, Ketamine distribution pharmacokinetics are not stereoselective, *Anesthesiology* **91**, A346 (1999).
10. T. Andoh, T. Sasaki, I. Watanabe, Y. Kamiya, and F. Okumura, Effects of ketamine stereoisomers on neuronal nicotinergic acetylcholine receptors, *Anesthesiology* **91**, A801 (1999).
11. T. Sakai, H. Singh, W. D. Mi, T. Kudo, and A. Matsuki, The effect of ketamine on clinical endpoints of hypnosis and EEG variables during propofol infusion, *Acta Anaesthesiol. Scand.* **43**, 212-216 (1999).
12. M. S. Mok, C. C. Wu, and S. R. Han, EEG-bispectral index monitoring of midazolam-ketamine anesthesia, *Anesth. Analg.* **90**, S224 (2000).
13. K. Hirota, T. Kubota, H. Ishihara, and A. Matsuki, The effects of nitrous oxide and ketamine on the bispectral index and 95% spectral edge frequency during propofol-fentanyl anaesthesia, *Eur. J. Anaesthesiol.* **16**, 779-783 (1999).
14. B. L. Friedberg, The effect of a dissociative dose of ketamine on the Bispectral Index (BIS) during propofol hypnosis, *J. Clin. Anesthesia* **11**, 4-7 (1999).
15. P. Hans, J. F. Brichant, B. Hubert, P. Y. Dewandre, and M. Lamy. Influence of induction of anaesthesia on intubating conditions one minute after rocuronium administration: comparison of ketamine and thiopentone, *Anaesthesia* **54**, 276-9 (1999).
16. K. Sakai, S. Cho, M. Fukusaki, O. Shibata, and K. Sumikawa. The effects of propofol with and without ketamine on human cerebral blood flow velocity and CO_2 response, *Anesth. Analg.* **90**, 377-382 (2000).

17. C. Denz, C. Janke, M. Weiss, P. Horn, K. Ellinger, and H. Krieter, Effects of (S)-ketamine on the brain in a porcine model of cardiopulmonary resuscitation, *Anesth. Analg.* **90**, S116 (2000).

18. K. Nagase, H. Iida, S. Dohi, and A. Oda, Nitroglycerin restored the reduction of carbon dioxide reactivity of ketamine in humans, *Anesth. Analg.* **90**, S264 (2000).

19. K. R. Engelhard, O. Möllenberg, C. P. Werner, and E. F. Kochs, Effects of S+ ketamine/propofol and sevoflurane on dynamic cerebrovascular autoregulation in humans, *Anesthesiology* **91**, A174 (1999).

20. C. Ori, U. Freo, A. Merico, F. Innocente, and M. Dam, Effects of ketamine-enatiomers anesthesia on local glucose utilization in the rat, *Anesthesiology* **91**, A772 (1999).

21. P. Kienbaum, T. Heuter, M. C. Michel, and J. Peters, Racemic ketamine decreases muscle sympathetic activity but maintains the neural response to hypotensive challenges in humans, *Anesthesiology* **92**, 94-101 (2000).

22. G. Kunst, E. Martin, B. M. Graf, S. Hagl, and C. F. Vahl, Actions of ketamine and its isomers on contractility and calcium transients in human myocardium, *Anesthesiology* **90**, 1363-1371 (1999)

23. A. Furuya, T. Matsukawa, M. Ozaki, T. Nishiyama, M. Kume, and T. Kumazawa, Intravenous ketamine attenuates arterial pressure changes during the induction of anaesthesia with propofol, *Eur. J. Anaesthesiol.* **18**, 88-92 (2001).

24. Y. Shiga, K. Minami, K. Segawa, K. Uryuu, and A. Shigematsu, The effects of propofol, ketamine and thiamylal on renal blood flow in rats, *Anesthesiology* **91**, A424 (1999).

25. J. Persson, H. Scheinin, G. Hellstrom, S. Bjorkman, E. Gotharson, and L. L. Gustafsson, Ketamine antagonises alfentanil-induced hypoventilation in healthy male volunteers, *Acta Anaesthesiol. Scand.* **43**, 744-752 (1999).

26. R. A. Bishop, J. A. Litch, and J. M. Stanton, Ketamine anesthesia at high altitude, *High Alt. Med. Biol.* **1**, 111-114 (2000).

27. S. Zahler, B. Heindl, and B. F. Becker, Ketamine does not inhibit inflammatory responses of cultured human endothelial cells but reduces chemotactic activation of neutrophils, *Acta Anaesthesiol. Scand.* **43**, 1011-1016 (1999).

28. M. A. Weigand, H. Schmidt, Q. Zhao, K. Plaschke, E. Martin, and H. J. Bardenheuer, Ketamine modulates the stimulated adhesion molecule expression on human neutrophils in vitro, *Anesth. Analg.* **90**, 206-212 (2000).

29. T. Kawasaki, M. Ogata, C. Kawasaki, J. Ogata, Y. Inoue, and A. Shigematsu, Ketamine suppresses proinflammatory cytokine production in human whole blood in vitro, *Anesth. Analg.* **89**, 665-669 (1999).

30. A. Szekely, B. Heindl, S. Zahler, P. F. Conzen, and B. F. Becker, S(+)-ketamine, but not R(-)-ketamine, reduces postischemic adherence of neutrophils in the coronary system of isolated guinea pig hearts, *Anesth. Analg.* **88**, 1017-1024 (1999).

31. H. Hirakata, T. Nakagawa, K. Nakamura, and K. Fukada, Ketamine inhibits platelet aggregation ny suppressed calcium mobilization, *Anesthesiology* **91**, A438 (1999).

32. K. Frey, R. Sukhani, J. Pawlowski, A. L. Pappas, M. Mikat-Stevens, and S. Slogoff , Propofol versus propofol-ketamine sedation for retrobulbar nerve block: comparison of sedation quality, intraocular pressure changes, and recovery profiles, *Anesth. Analg.* **89**, 317-321 (1999).

33. G. Haeseler, O. Zuzan, G. Kohn, S. Piepenbrock, and M. Leuwer, Anaesthesia with midazolam and S-(+)-ketamine in spontaneously breathing paediatric patients during magnetic resonance imaging, *Paediatr. Anaesth.* **10**, 513-519 (2000).

34. S. L. Shafer, L. C. Siegel, J. E. Cooke, J. C. Scott, Testing computer controlled infusion pumps by simulation, *Anesthesiology* **62**, 234-241 (1988).

35. I. Øye, Ketamine analgesia, NMDA receptors and the gates of perception, *Acta Anaesthesiol. Scand.* **42**, 747-748 (1998).

36. I. Øye, Ketamin - medienes nye motedop? *Tidsskr. Nor. Lægeforen* **120**, 1464-1466 (2000).

37. R. P. Gruber and B. Morley, Ketamine-assisted intravenous sedation with midazolam: benefits and potential problems, *Plast. Reconstr. Surg.* **104**, 1823-5 (1998).

38. B. L. Friedberg, Propofol-Ketamine technique. Dissociative Anaesthesia for Office Surgery (A 5-Year review of 1264 cases), *Aesth. Plast. Surg.* **23**, 70-75 (1999).

39. R. M. Sobel, B. W. Morgan, and M. Murphy, Ketamine in the ED: Medical Politics Versus Patient Care, *Am. J. Emerg. Med.* **17**, 722-725 (1999).

40. J. C. Granry JC, L. Dube, F. Turrouques, and F. Conreaux, Ketamine - New uses of an old drug, *Curr. Opin. Anaest.* **13**, 299-302 (2000).

41. J. Nehama, R. Pass, A. Bechtler-Karsch, C. Steinberg, and D. A. Notterman, Continuous ketamine infusion for the treatment of refractory asthma in a mechanically ventilated infant: Case report and review of the pediatric literature, *Pediat. Int. Care* **12**, 294-309 (1996).

42. T. Ledowski and H. Wulf , The influence of fentanyl vs. s-ketamine on intubating conditions during induction of anaesthesia with etomidate and rocuronium, *Eur. J. Anaesthesiol.* **18**, 519-523 (2001).

43. M. M. Atallah, H. A. el Mohayman, and R. E. el Metwally, Ketamine-midazolam total intravenous anaesthesia for prolonged abdominal surgery, *Eur. J. Anaesthesiol.* **18**, 29-35 (2001).

44. R. L. Schmid, A. N. Sandler, and J. Katz , Use and efficacy of low-dose ketamine in the management of acute postoperative pain: a review of current techniques and outcomes, *Pain* **82**, 111-125 (1999).

45. S. M. Green, N. Kuppermann, S. G. Rothrock, C. B. Hummel, and M. Ho. Predictors of adverse events with intramuscular ketamine sedation in children, *Ann. Emerg. Med.* **35**, 35-42 (2000).

46. M. Suzuki, K. Tsueda, P. S. Lansing, M. M. Tolan, T. M. Fuhrman, C. I. Ignacio, and R. A. Sheppard, Small-dose ketamine enhances morphine-induced analgesia after outpatient surgery, *Anesth. Analg.* **89**, 98-103 (1999).

47. G. Adriaenssens, K. M. Vermeyen, V. L. Hoffmann, E. Mertens, and H. F. Adriaensen, Postoperative analgesia with i.v. patient-controlled morphine: effect of adding ketamine, *Br. J. Anaesth.* **83**, 393-396 (1999).

48. G. R. Lauretti, J. M. A. Gomes, M. P. Reis, and N. L. Pereira, Low doses of epidural ketamine or neostigmine, but not midazolam, Improve morphine analgesia in epidural terminal cancer pain therapy, *J. Clin. Anesthesia* **11**, 663-668 (1999).

49. P. G. Fine, Low-Dose Ketamine in the Management of Opioid Nonresponsive Terminal Cancer Pain, *J. Pain Symptom Manage.* **17**, 296-300 (1999).

50. R. F. Bell, Low-dose subcutaneous ketamine infusion and morphine tolerance. *Pain* **83**, 101-103 (1999).

51. G. R. Lauretti, I. C. Lima, M. P. Reis, W. A. Prado, and N. L. Pereira, Oral ketamine and transdermal nitroglycerin as analgesic adjuvants to oral morphine therapy for cancer pain management, *Anesthesiology* **90**, 1528-1533 (1999).

52. D. R. Haines and S. P. Gaines, N of 1 randomised controlled trials of oral ketamine in patients with chronic pain, *Pain* **83**, 283-7 (1999).

53. C. N. Sang, NMDA-Receptor Antagonists in Neuropathic Pain: Experimental Methods to Clinical Trials, *J. Pain Symptom Manage.* **19**, S21-S25 (2000).

54. F. Guirimand, X. Dupont, L. Brasseur, M. Chauvin, and D. Bouhassira, The effects of ketamine on the temporal summation (wind-up) of the R(III) nociceptive flexion reflex and pain in humans, *Anesth. Analg.* **90**, 408-414 (2000).

55. L. Roytblat, A. Korotkoruchko, J. Katz, M. Glazer, L. Greemberg, and A. Fisher, Postoperative pain: The effect of low-dose ketamine in addition to general anesthesia, *Anesth. Analg.* **77**, 1161-1165 (1993).

56. L. C. Mathisen, V. Aasbo, and J. Raeder, Lack of pre-emptive analgesic effect of (R)-ketamine in laparoscopic cholecystectomy, *Acta Anaesthesiol. Scand.* **43**, 220-224 (1999).

57. F. Adam, M. Libier, T. Oszustowicz, D. Lefebvre, J. Beal, and J. Meynadier, Preoperative small-dose ketamine has no preemptive analgesic effect in patients undergoing total mastectomy, *Anesth. Analg.* **89**, 444-447 (1999).

58. V. Dahl, P. E. Ernoe, T. Steen, J. C. Raeder, and P. F. White, Does ketamine possess pre-emptive effects in women undergoing abdominal hysterectomy procedures, *Anesth. Analg.* **90**, 1419-1422 (2000).

59. E. S. Fu, R. Migue, and J. E. Scharf, Preemptive ketamine decreases postoperative narcotic requirements in patients undergoing abdominal surgery, *Anesth. Analg.* **84**, 1086-1090 (1997).

60. C. Menigaux, D. Fletcher, X. Dupont, B. Guignard, F. Guirimand, and M. Chauvin. The benefits of intraoperative small-dose ketamine on postoperative pain after anterior cruciate ligament repair, *Anesth. Analg.* **90**, 129-135 (2000).

61. A. Stubhaug, H. Breivik, P. K. Eide, M. Kreunen, and K. Frey, Mapping of punctate hyperalgesia around a surgical incisison demonstrates that ketamine is a powerful suppressor of central sensitization to pain following surgery, *Acta Anaesthesiol. Scand.* **41**, 1124-1132 (1997).

INDEX